Advanced Health Assessment and Differential Diagnosis

Karen M. Myrick, DNP, APRN, FNP-BC, ANP-BC, is a professor of nursing and chair of interdisciplinary research and education in the School of Interdisciplinary Health and Science, Department of Nursing, University of Saint Joseph, West Hartford, Connecticut; and clinical associate professor of medical sciences, School of Medicine, Quinnipiac University, Hamden, Connecticut. Dr. Myrick also maintains a current clinical practice as a nurse practitioner. She has many years of experience in teaching health assessment and was nominated for an "Excellence in Teaching" award in 2015 and 2017 and was also the recipient of the National Organization of Nurse Practitioner Faculty's "Outstanding Researcher of the Year Award." Dr. Myrick's interdisciplinary research is focused on athletes and sports medicine. She has an extensive and ongoing program of research that has been widely published and presented globally. The recipient of multiple grants, she works to improve clinical health assessment, identify areas for injury prevention, and improve sports performance and fitness maintenance. This is evidenced by her development and testing of a newly designed physical examination technique for determining hip labral tears, "The Hip Internal Rotation with Distraction (THIRD) Test." In addition to publishing regularly in peer-reviewed journals, Dr. Myrick has authored books and book chapters, and is a senior editor for the interprofessional *Journal of Clinical Case Reports*.

Laima M. Karosas, PhD, APRN, FAANP, is clinical professor and chair of nursing programs at Quinnipiac University, Hamden, Connecticut. Dr. Karosas has been a nurse educator for more than 20 years and a practicing nurse practitioner for more than 25 years, with experience in settings such as direct patient care, urgent care, nursing homes and assisted living, and international healthcare clinics. Dr. Karosas has a keen interest in nontraditional roles for advanced practice nurses in addition to maintaining expertise and promoting creativity and entrepreneurship. She is a proponent of healthcare delivery by an interprofessional team as well as interprofessional research to improve the effectiveness and efficiency of the healthcare system. Dr. Karosas has collaborated with nurses internationally and has published multiple journal articles in the areas of nursing history, spiritual care, and mentorship. She has authored book chapters on the techniques of physical assessment and on cultural health assessment. Dr. Karosas has served as a member of the International Editorial Advisory and Review Board for *Nursing Education, Research & Practice* and is a fellow of the American Association of Nurse Practitioners.

Expert Consultant: Suzanne C. Smeltzer, EdD, RN, ANEF, FAAN, is director of nursing research and evaluation and The Richard and Marianne Kreider Endowed Professor in Nursing for Vulnerable Populations, College of Nursing, Villanova University, Villanova, Pennsylvania. Dr. Smeltzer is an internationally known scholar, researcher, educator, and author. Committed to making health promotion practices and services accessible and acceptable for those who are physically challenged, she has done extensive research on multiple sclerosis and other disabilities; how to improve the health and wellness of those who are disabled; and how to integrate disability content into the education and training of healthcare professionals. Dr. Smeltzer is a member of several national task forces devoted to improving the education of healthcare providers about healthcare of people with disabilities. She is a fellow in the American Academy of Nursing and has received numerous awards for her research and writing regarding health issues of women with disabilities, including the Villanova University Investigator Award of 2006.

Advanced Health Assessment and Differential Diagnosis

ESSENTIALS FOR CLINICAL PRACTICE

KAREN M. MYRICK, DNP, APRN, FNP-BC, ANP-BC

LAIMA M. KAROSAS, PhD, APRN, FAANP

EDITORS

EXPERT CONSULTANT: SUZANNE C. SMELTZER, EdD, RN, ANEF, FAAN

SPRINGER PUBLISHING COMPANY

Springer Publishing Company, LLC
11 West 42nd Street
New York, NY 10036
www.springerpub.com
http://connect.springerpub.com/home

Acquisitions Editor: Adrianne Brigido
Compositor: diacriTech

ISBN: 978-0-8261-6249-6
ebook ISBN: 978-0-8261-6255-7
Instructor's Manual ISBN: 978-0-8261-6265-6
Instructor's PowerPoints ISBN: 978-0-8261-6264-9
Instructor's Test Bank ISBN: 978-0-8261-6266-3
Image Bank ISBN: 978-0-8261-6256-4
DOI: 10.1891/9780826162557

Qualified instructors may request supplements by emailing textbook@springerpub.com

21 22 / 5 4 3

The author and the publisher of this Work have made every effort to use sources believed to be reliable to provide information that is accurate and compatible with the standards generally accepted at the time of publication. Because medical science is continually advancing, our knowledge base continues to expand. Therefore, as new information becomes available, changes in procedures become necessary. We recommend that the reader always consult current research and specific institutional policies before performing any clinical procedure. The author and publisher shall not be liable for any special, consequential, or exemplary damages resulting, in whole or in part, from the readers' use of, or reliance on, the information contained in this book. The publisher has no responsibility for the persistence or accuracy of URLs for external or third-party Internet websites referred to in this publication and does not guarantee that any content on such websites is, or will remain, accurate or appropriate.

Library of Congress Cataloging-in-Publication Data
Library of Congress Control Number: 2019917100

Contact us to receive discount rates on bulk purchases.
We can also customize our books to meet your needs.
For more information please contact: sales@springerpub.com

Publisher's Note: **New and used products purchased from third-party sellers are not guaranteed for quality, authenticity, or access to any included digital components.**

Printed in the United States of America.

This book is dedicated to my husband, Scott, and my daughter, Kayden. They keep me motivated and inspire me every day. Thank you for putting up with the many hours and hard work that went into this textbook. Many healthcare providers will now learn how to take the best care of their patients because of your patience and support for this important work.

—KAREN M. MYRICK

CONTENTS

5. ADVANCED HEALTH ASSESSMENT OF SKIN, HAIR, AND NAILS   111

Lindita Vinca

6. ADVANCED HEALTH ASSESSMENT OF THE CARDIOVASCULAR SYSTEM   159

Allison Rusgo

CONTRIBUTORS

Alexandra Armitage, MS, CNL, APRN
Nurse Practitioner
Baylor Scott and White Health
Department of Neurology
Temple, Texas

Erin Fusco, DNP, FNP-BC, RN
Assistant Professor
School of Nursing
Quinnipiac University
Hamden, Connecticut

Kristen Marie Guida, DNP, ANP-C, ACNP-BC, AGACNP-BC, FNP-C
Advanced Practice Registered Nurse
Hartford Healthcare
Hartford, Connecticut

Laima M. Karosas, PhD, APRN, FAANP
Clinical Professor of Nursing
Chair of Nursing Programs
School of Nursing
Quinnipiac University
Hamden, Connecticut

Jensen Lewis, PA-C
Assistant Professor
Physician Assistant Program
Case Western Reserve University
Cleveland, Ohio

Jacquelyn McMillian-Bohler, PhD, CNM, CNE
Assistant Professor
Duke University School of Nursing
Durham, North Carolina

Karen M. Myrick, DNP, APRN, FNP-BC, ANP-BC
Associate Professor
School of Interdisciplinary Health and Science
Department of Nursing
University of Saint Joseph
West Hartford, Connecticut
Clinical Associate Professor of Medical Sciences
School of Medicine
Quinnipiac University
Hamden, Connecticut

Susanne A. Quallich, PhD, ANP-BC, NP-C, CUNP, FAANP
Andrology Nurse Practitioner
Michigan Medicine
Department of Urology
University of Michigan
Ann Arbor, Michigan

Angela Richard-Eaglin, DNP, MSN, FNP-BC, CNE, FAANP
Assistant Clinical Professor
Co-director, VA Nursing Academic Partnership in Graduate Education and Adult Gerontology
Primary Care Residency Program
Duke University School of Nursing
Durham, North Carolina

Dale Robertson, PA-C, MCHS
Lecturer and Clinical Coordinator
Department of Family Medicine
University of Washington
MEDEX Northwest
Seattle, Washington

Allison Rusgo, MHS, MPH, PA-C
Assistant Clinical Professor
Physician Assistant Department
Drexel University College of Nursing and Health
  Professions
Philadelphia, Pennsylvania

Adrienne Small, DNP, FNP-C, CNE
Medical Instructor
Duke University School of Nursing
Durham, North Carolina

Suzanne C. Smeltzer, EdD, RN, ANEF, FAAN
The Richard and Marianne Kreider Endowed
  Professor in Nursing for Vulnerable Populations
Evaluation Coordinator
M. Louis Fitzpatrick College of Nursing
Villanova University
Villanova, Pennsylvania

Lindita Vinca, DNP, APRN
Nurse Practitioner
Dermatology Associates of Connecticut
Hamden, Connecticut

FOREWORD

Much of healthcare today depends on the expertise of nurse practitioners (NPs) and physician assistants (PAs). Well-honed skills in history-taking and physical examination are foundational to accurate diagnoses that result in efficient and cost-effective care. *Advanced Health Assessment and Differential Diagnosis: Essentials for Clinical Practice* is the first health assessment textbook designed specifically for and written solely by experienced NPs and PAs.

Drs. Myrick and Karosas have previously published books, chapters, and articles about advanced assessment techniques and bring more than 30 years of combined patient care experience to the writing of this text. In addition, both are nationally recognized educators who have taught advanced health assessment to graduate students for many years. The authors of each chapter are frontline clinicians carefully selected for their expertise in caring for diverse populations in varied settings. Many have also worked internationally.

In the cost-conscious healthcare environment of today, clinicians are increasingly faced with productivity goals. Each chapter therefore includes a comprehensive physical exam of a body system, as well as a more focused assessment. The authors ease the daunting challenge of synthesizing complex information into a correct diagnosis by providing a table of differential diagnoses for common disorders to assist novices in developing diagnostic and clinical-reasoning proficiency.

Economic, spiritual, cultural, and psychosocial aspects are key factors in determining realistic and holistic treatment options. Failing to recognize the impact of these social determinants on health can adversely influence patient outcomes. The authors draw attention to these and other issues pertaining to safety, distress, living situations, or other patient concerns that are critical yet often overlooked by providers. Considerations for transgender, geriatric, pregnant, and pediatric patients, as well as patients with disabilities, are highlighted throughout.

Unlike many classical textbooks on physical examination, this book further engages the learner in applying clinical reasoning skills by including chapter cases of varying complexity. These case studies offer sample documentation and appropriate ICD codes, the accuracy of which is essential to reimbursement.

These editors have succeeded in producing a reference that is well designed for the complexity of healthcare today. While this is the first health assessment book written solely for and by NPs and PAs, it is sure to be an excellent resource for all healthcare providers.

Jean W. Lange, PhD, RN, FAAN

PREFACE

Advanced Health Assessment and Differential Diagnosis: Essentials for Clinical Practice will offer a unique contribution to the existing market, filling a gap that has been identified by students, professors, and practitioners alike. Currently, there is a paucity of advanced health assessment books that are authored *by* nurse practitioners or physician assistants *for* nurse practitioners or physician assistants.

This book delivers accurate and in-depth primary care health assessment techniques, with a quick review of normal findings, followed by assessment techniques for abnormal findings, presented in a focused, clinically relevant approach that is designed to encourage sound clinical decision-making, and, in the end, develop proficient diagnosticians. Typically, special populations are discussed in a separate chapter or chapters; this health assessment book incorporates the special populations into each topical area. Special populations examined include pediatric, transgender, pregnant, and disabled patients. Suzanne C. Smeltzer, a world-leading disability advocate and expert, has provided insight and expertise on the disabled population in each chapter.

OBJECTIVES

The primary goal of the textbook is to provide up-to-date and clinically relevant health assessment techniques and normal findings; it then moves on to identify abnormal findings that require more in-depth assessment techniques. The scope of practice for nurse practitioners and physician assistants will be emphasized, including skills and procedures for students who are learning their professional role.

Integrating special populations (pediatric, transgender, pregnant, and disability patients) into each topical area, not as separate chapters, allows for the learner to compare and contrast the findings of the body system without separating out certain groups of individuals. Likewise, covering the examination of special populations (e.g., transgender) right within the topical area serves to illustrate the differences. This approach allows the textbook to be fully inclusive.

FEATURES

Each chapter includes the following sections:

- **Overview of Anatomy and Physiology**: Describes the relevant anatomy and physiology, with corresponding illustrations and images.

- **Screening Health Assessment and Normal Findings**: Describes health assessment techniques with rationale and expected normal findings in the healthy population.

- **Focused Health Assessment and Abnormal Findings**: Describes health assessment techniques with rationale and expected abnormal findings in the patient population with a focused problem in the respective body system. Sensitivity and specificity of examination techniques, including any special tests, are included.

- **Holistic Assessment**: Emphasizes the holistic components of the assessment of the body system. Holistic assessment includes any other factors that may be relevant, such as safety, distress, diet and exercise, living situation, or financial, spiritual, or other unique concerns of the patient.

- **Case Study**: Includes case studies of varying complexity with the body system as a main component of the patient's case, including documentation for the encounter and ICD-10-CM coding.

- **Assessment of Special Populations**: Includes key assessment variables for the transgender, geriatric, pregnant, and pediatric patient, as well as patients with disabilities. Special population assessments are included in the respective body system chapter, allowing the learner to compare and contrast findings with other groups of patients.

- **Diagnostic Reasoning Tables**: Common disorders and their differential diagnoses with rationales to promote clinical reasoning.

The textbook also includes robust instructor resources, including an instructor manual with chapter summaries, case studies, and discussion questions; test bank; image bank; and chapter PowerPoint slides.

It is our hope that this book proves to be a valuable resource for students, instructors, and all practicing healthcare practitioners.

Karen M. Myrick
Laima M. Karosas

ACKNOWLEDGMENTS

The editors would like to acknowledge RonZel Hendrix, who was pivotal to the quality photographs in Chapter 12. Thank you, RonZel, for your artistic ability and unwavering stamina in helping to obtain the best images possible for this important work.

Thank you to everyone at Plus One Defense Systems, including Darin Reisler, Elias Morales, Travis Johnson, John Peterson, Izzy Raviv, Chris Pasquini, Scott Myrick, Kayden Myrick, Emily and Alivia Pasquini, and RonZel Hendrix.

INSTRUCTOR RESOURCES

Advanced Health Assessment and Differential Diagnosis includes a robust ancillary package. Qualified instructors may obtain access to supplements by emailing textbook@springerpub.com.

Resources include:

- Instructor's Manual
  - Learning Objectives
  - Chapter Summaries
  - Case Studies and Discussion Questions
- Chapter-Based PowerPoint Presentations
- Test Bank
- Image Bank

1

HEALTH HISTORY, THE PATIENT INTERVIEW, AND MOTIVATIONAL INTERVIEWING

Laima M. Karosas

CHAPTER CONTENTS

Overview of the Health History

The health history is a crucial part of evaluating a patient's health status. It establishes a baseline for the patient and can reveal the patient's understanding about health and the factors that influence his or her health. Finally, it also provides a comprehensive, holistic picture of the patient, his or her support systems, habits, and daily life. Most experienced providers will confirm that a skillfully obtained health history points the provider to appropriate areas of examination and significantly assists in directing the provider to areas of concern. If this is a new patient to the practice, a full history and physical examination is warranted. For an established patient, a focused history and physical examination may be sufficient. Even during a focused visit, information in the established patient's chart should be routinely reviewed and updated.

Although there are no specific anatomical and physiological areas that correlate to eliciting the patient's health history, anatomy and physiology may change how a provider obtains the history. Therefore, a quick assessment of whether the patient is capable of providing accurate information is crucial to the entire process. The patient must be able to communicate, although not necessarily orally, in order to convey information. Mental status plays a role in history taking. Anyone whose mental status is altered may not provide accurate information. Memory and reasoning must be intact, again, to be able to relay past events and how they may have led to the patient's condition. A comatose patient cannot answer any questions. In order to obtain any information, the provider may need to speak to family, friends, or witnesses to the event that occurred.

During all provider–patient interactions, the provider's verbal and nonverbal communication may instill trust and confidence in the provider's skills or be detrimental to building rapport with the patient. The verbal and nonverbal communication is very important during the first meeting of patient and provider. If the provider conveys a judgmental attitude either by making derogatory statements to the patient or with nonverbal cues such as arms crossed in front of the body, the patient may not be honest in all communications. Every healthcare provider should remember that the goals of health history include not only obtaining an accurate health history, but also building rapport with the patient and understanding the patient's perception of health.

From the moment the provider first sees the patient, assessment is occurring. The provider is observing the patient's appearance including dress, hygiene, and behavior. Some patients will be slightly anxious in a provider's office due to potential or known health concerns, stressors, or distractors. This should not be ignored, but rather explored. The patient may not be able to focus on other aspects of the health assessment until his or her concerns are validated and explored. Therefore, beginning with the patient's concerns is not unusual at the start of the health history discussion.

THE PATIENT INTERVIEW

At the first visit with a new patient, a thorough review of all health issues and anything potentially impacting health should occur. This information serves as a baseline for future comparison and should be updated annually or as needed. Introductions set the tone of the interview. The provider introduces him- or herself and lets the patient know how to refer to him or her. The provider should then ask the patient's preferred name and not assume familiarity. The patient may or may not have a specific complaint. While gathering the history, specific areas of concern should be noted and explored.

In general, before starting the health history interview, the patient should be comfortable. If possible, the history should be taken before the patient prepares for the physical examination, that is, before changing into a gown. The patient may be interviewed with family or significant others present, but at some point the patient should be interviewed alone as well. The best approach is to usher accompanying family or friends to the waiting room as the patient prepares for the examination. There are cultures, however, in which the patient may not be alone with a provider. This cultural norm should be respected unless the provider has concerns about patient safety. In that case, involving a social worker or providing crisis intervention may be warranted.

The patient must be able to communicate although it may not be orally. Writing, typing, and drawing may be used to communicate information in addition to oral expression. Body language and how the patient conveys information are important. There should be congruence between the patient's words and mood. If the patient is recounting a sad event (such as the death of a loved one), the provider would expect the patient to be appropriately sad and not, for example, laughing. The time elapsed since the event is also important. If the death occurred 20 years ago, the provider would expect sadness, but not necessarily a severe grief reaction. Paying attention to these details adds information to the overall assessment of the patient.

It is not unusual to have a patient who does not speak English or not enough to express his or her health concerns. The patient may be hearing impaired and require a sign language interpreter to communicate concerns. Interpreters may be used either in person, via an app that gives you the translation for a phrase, or via phone. The provider still addresses the patient although the interpreter translates the language spoken. The provider should not be focused on the interpreter; rather, the patient remains the focus of the conversation. Family members can be used as interpreters although this may not be the best option. Patients may not answer questions honestly in front of family members. In addition, family members as interpreters may not translate information accurately. An interpreter needs to translate the questions without adding his or her own perspectives. The privacy and confidentiality of the health information make it essential that a nonfamily member be the interpreter with language issues as well as sensory (deafness) issues.

Finally, exploring a patient's health history involves asking different types of questions. For example, if you ask a patient if he or she smokes, the answer will be yes or no. The provider does not know if the patient ever smoked, when he or she quit, or how much he or she smoked. The better approach may be to introduce the topic of habits and ask about habits that the patient has currently or has had. There will be closed-ended questions requiring a "yes" or "no," but starting with open-ended questions will capture more detail and help the provider focus on areas to clarify. The patient's story is reviewed until the provider is certain that the documentation accurately reflects the patient's responses. There is no judgment placed on the information from the patient. As a provider, the goal is to create a foundation from which to help the patient lead a healthy life and/or manage illness.

The entire health history is subjective information as it is what the patient tells the provider. The physical examination is objective information gathered by the provider. It is important to distinguish between these two types of information in a history and physical examination. What the patient tells the provider may be confirmed or opposed to the findings of the provider. Incongruent findings may lead to more questions to determine the reason for the discrepancies. Often providers can uncover a misunderstanding about wellness or illness and educate the patient about physiology and disease process.

The sections of the health history are noted in Table 1.1. The list can be daunting to a novice provider, but efficiency increases along with the skill of the provider as more and more assessments are completed. During the first patient visit, allot enough time to collect the full history in addition to completing a comprehensive physical examination. The health history ends with the review of systems (ROS) at which point documentation of the physical examination begins.

CHIEF COMPLAINT

The interview begins with the patient stating the reason for coming to see the provider, the *chief complaint*. If it is for a routine or annual visit, the provider should not assume there are no other

TABLE 1.1 The Complete Health History	
Section	**Information Gathered**
ID	Age, gender, occupation
CC	The reason for the visit; may be a direct quote or brief summary of patient's comments
HPI	The onset, location, duration, frequency, intensity, and aggravating and relieving factors surrounding the patient's symptom(s)
PM/SH	Any health issues that the patient may have had during his or her lifetime, including mental illness and surgeries. For women, number of pregnancies, live births, abortions (spontaneous or therapeutic)
Allergies	Any reactions to medications, food, other materials; when the reactions occurred; and what the reactions were
FH	The illnesses in the patient's parents, grandparents, and children. Generally, this is in first-degree relatives only
Social	Support system, living situation, profession, exercise, dietary and other habits, safety at home and work
ROS	Review of each system from head to toe to ensure all issues are documented. The review includes skin; head, eyes, ears, nose, throat, neck; lymphatic; cardiovascular, respiratory, gastrointestinal, genitourinary, musculoskeletal, neurological (including mental status), and endocrine.

CC, chief complaint; FH, family history; HPI, history of the present illness; ID, identification; PM/SH, past medical/ surgical history; ROS, review of systems.

complaints. The provider must ask what has happened since the last visit, or in the case of an initial visit, if there are any issues of concern.

HISTORY OF THE PRESENT ILLNESS

If there is a specific complaint, the *history of the present illness (HPI)* must be fully explored. The onset, location, and duration of the symptom as well as any accompanying symptoms, aggravating or relieving activities, and what the patient has tried for treatment must be discussed. These areas are known as the seven attributes of a symptom, which may be recalled with the mnemonic OLD CART:

O: **O**nset

L: **L**ocation

D: **D**uration

C: **C**haracteristics

A: **A**ggravating factors

R: **R**elieving factors

T: **T**reatment

The patient's perception of the symptom may shed light on how the patient perceives illness. This may provide an opportunity to discuss possible cause and effect and explore the meaning of illness to the patient.

PAST MEDICAL AND SURGICAL HISTORY

The *past medical and surgical history* is a listing of any illnesses that the patient has had. The provider should note which illnesses are continuing or chronic and which have been resolved. If a patient reports a sinus infection every autumn for the last 3 years or pneumonia for three winters in a row, the provider should ask about surrounding factors. For example, does the patient work with a large group of people or travel often in the fall or winter, or have allergies. All of these factors may influence when the patient becomes ill and can direct the provider to discuss strategies for prevention. For women, the number of pregnancies, live births, and abortions (spontaneous or therapeutic) are also documented.

ALLERGIES

Allergies must be written in the patient chart including, if the patient recalls, when the allergy occurred and what the reaction was. At times, patients may list an allergy to a substance when the actual offending agent may be different.

FAMILY HISTORY

Family history may be documented in a narrative format or a genogram may be constructed. The family history should include relatives in a direct relationship to the patient such as the parents, grandparents, and children of the patient, and any illnesses they may have had, including cause of death. Patterns may indicate genetic predisposition to certain illnesses, but environmental influences should not be overlooked. Families generally share the same living environments, which can also lead to patterns of illness. The challenge for the provider is to identify these patterns and determine whether they are influenced by genetics or environment. The plan for the patient will differ depending on the findings.

SOCIAL HISTORY

The *social history* is extremely important and often overlooked or not explored in detail. This section fills in the gaps regarding the living situation and support system for the patient. The provider learns about the patient's family, significant others, friends, coworkers, and anyone else who the patient considers part of the support system. In addition, the provider must ask about habits including diet, exercise, smoking, use of other substances, sleeping habits, safety in and outside the home, and anything else the patient may reveal. Not enough attention is generally paid to safety from using seat belts and smoke detectors to feeling safe in the home or at work. Healthcare providers are uniquely positioned to uncover difficult situations that patients may find themselves in. For this reason, it is imperative to be able to interview patients individually, without others present, so that they can truthfully respond and know that anything they reveal is confidential. Keeping this in mind, providers also need to know what agencies or services patients can be referred to, from crisis teams to mental health specialists to caregiver support services and even to law enforcement officers.

REVIEW OF SYSTEMS

The *ROS* allows the provider to gather information about each body system. This may seem repetitive, but it is necessary to ensure all aspects of a patient's health have been documented. The patient may not consider shortness of breath after walking 50 steps as a problem. This may only be uncovered in the ROS. The provider asks about any symptoms in each body system: skin; head, eyes, ears, nose, and throat (HEENT); neck and lymphatics; respiratory; cardiovascular; gastrointestinal; genitourinary; musculoskeletal; neurological; and endocrine. The provider should ask questions using nonmedical terminology such as asking about double vision rather than diplopia. See Table 1.2 for the types of questions to ask for each body system.

An important technique while collecting information and when, in the provider's opinion, all information has been collected is summarizing. At the conclusion of a section and again at the conclusion of the health history, reviewing information and providing a summary back to the patient is essential. The patient has the opportunity to correct information or a misunderstanding on the part of the provider. Often, the patient may add to the information upon hearing the summary to clarify the complaint. Summarizing provides a way to verify that the provider's understanding truly reflects the patient's story.

TABLE 1.2
Review of Systems: Key Questions

Body system	Ask the patient if he or she has experienced:
Skin	Rashes, dry skin, itching, open areas, changes in freckles or moles, discolorations, easy bruising
Head	Hair loss or thinning, excessive dandruff, itching, trauma
Eyes	Blurry vision, double vision, redness, excessive tearing, pain, dryness, discharge, use of glasses
Ears	Loss of hearing, ringing in the ears, discharge, pain, itching, use of hearing aids, previous cochlear implants
Nose	Loss of smell perception, discharge, difficulty breathing, bleeding
Throat	Soreness, hoarseness, difficulty swallowing, discharge, enlarged tonsils
Neck	Pain, enlarged lymph nodes
Respiratory	Shortness of breath, wheezing, congestion, cough, inability to lay flat
Cardiovascular	Chest pain, swelling of the legs, shortness of breath when walking short distances or up a flight of stairs
Gastrointestinal	Nausea, vomiting, heartburn, pain, constipation, diarrhea
Genitourinary	Pain; difficulty urinating, including frequency or hesitation; discharge; bleeding; menstrual changes or difficulties for women
Musculoskeletal	Joint pain or stiffness, swelling of joints, difficulty walking or running, back or neck pain, decreased range of motion, use of assistive devices (cane, walker, crutches, wheelchair, motorized wheelchair or scooter) for mobility
Neurological	Headaches, dizziness, difficulty speaking or finding words, weakness, fatigue, insomnia, anxiety
Endocrine	Low or high sugars, sensitivity to heat or cold, changes in skin color

Screening Health Assessment and Normal Findings

Not all assessments need to be comprehensive. A patient with an identified problem will need an assessment that explores the symptom(s). Only areas that relate to the symptom are investigated in order to develop a plan for physical examination and assessment. For a patient whose chief complaint is a sore throat, the provider must do a thorough history in the area of head, eyes, ears, nose, throat, and respiratory as well as reviewing habits such as smoking that can worsen the symptoms. In addition, work and home environments are explored to ensure no contributing factors are present at home or work. The focused assessments help to direct the physical examination to the body systems which are affected.

There is no recipe for a focused examination. Each patient has a unique presentation and set of findings; therefore, the provider must question the patient about each symptom in detail. The findings may lead to one illness or multiple. The interview should not end prematurely with the provider assuming a diagnosis. All possible paths should be considered before closing in on a diagnosis. In addition, it is just as important to rule out diagnoses as well as ruling in a diagnosis. To come to a conclusion, the provider must follow the clues to eliminate possibilities as well as to determine the most likely diagnoses.

Holistic Assessment

During the health assessment, every finding requires exploration and clarification. Providers begin to build relationships with their patients as soon as they see their patients and, in fact, the entire encounter should be patient-focused and patient-driven. The provider needs to gather information, but also needs to answer questions that the patient may have. Holistic assessment requires the provider to understand the factors surrounding a patient's answers and the history leading to the findings.

The provider cannot shy away from asking important questions. If a patient has a bruised left eye, the circumstances of that injury must be explored. Questions about who the patient lives with, the support system, and whether the environment at home or outside the home is safe are paramount to ask. Violence in the home, school, workplace, and other locations has become more prevalent. The patient may be a victim of human trafficking, being bullied for his or her sexual orientation, or suffering from anxiety in the wake of a national or natural disaster. Without asking the questions, the provider cannot uncover the issues

that the patient is facing and therefore cannot offer any support or assistance.

Holistic assessment also involves paying attention to patient comfort and positioning during the interview and exam. Elderly clients may require different positioning or assistive hearing devices. Family members may need to be included in the interview to confirm and verify information. Much of this is true for younger patients as well. Every patient, however, also deserves time to express him- or herself freely, in confidence. The patient's perspective helps the provider understand the patient and illness more fully. The provider learns how the illness impacts the patient's daily life. A holistic approach requires more than just determining diagnosis, but also understanding its impact. The provider, then, is able to work with the patient to tailor interventions that are reasonable for the patient. Holistic assessment also involves paying attention to patient comfort and positioning during the interview and exam. Elderly clients or those with disabilities may require different positioning or assistive hearing devices.

Motivational interviewing is a skill that can help a provider move to a more patient-centered approach during the health history interview. Motivational interviewing helps the patient explore pros and cons of change and the implications of change. The health history interview becomes less provider-driven and more patient-centered. The patient considers the reasons for or against changes in health behaviors. The provider guides the patient in the process of thinking about a behavior. The provider should listen, ask open-ended questions, and offer information as needed. The behavioral change, then, comes from a desire within the patient rather than the provider telling the patient what to do. Often there are many priorities and eliciting what is most important for the patient provides a place to start. For providers interested in learning more about and using motivational interviewing, there are many in-depth courses, articles, and books written on the subject.

CASE STUDY

Mr. G., a retired accountant, is a new patient in the practice. He is 64 years old and comes to this practice because his previous provider retired. He states he will have his records sent to the practice, but in the meantime, he is getting supplemental life insurance and needs a complete physical examination. The provider begins with introducing himself or herself and then asks the patient for his or her preferred name. In this case, the patient prefers to be called by his childhood nickname, Mac. The provider begins by asking if there are any questions that Mac would first like to ask. Mac shrugs his shoulders and says not really. The provider reassures him that he can bring up any issues while he is there. The provider ensures Mac is comfortable and then explains that first they will discuss his health and then move onto the physical examination.

Mac states that he has no current problems although he says occasionally he has difficulty urinating. He has been relatively healthy his entire life. His previous provider suggested he take a baby aspirin daily and he has been doing so. His wife also insists that he take a multivitamin daily. His wife is the cook at home. He prefers meat and potatoes, but his wife also insists that he eat salad or vegetables with meat and either potatoes or pasta. He is of Italian descent. His wife is French and has always been a very good cook. He tries to stay healthy by taking a walk with his wife every morning and every afternoon. They walk around the neighborhood or through the town center. Mac states the walk is usually about an hour in the morning and afternoon.

Mac is active in the local chamber of commerce. He owned his own accounting business for 30 years. He enjoys working with others who want to establish businesses. In addition, he and his wife volunteer for the town soup kitchen, and look for other opportunities. Every Tuesday, a few of his childhood friends

(continued)

(continued)

and their wives come over for a round of cards and socializing. Mac has one to two glasses of wine on Tuesday nights only. He has never smoked cigarettes or anything else. He tried marijuana once in high school and didn't like it. He has lived in the same town for his entire life and went to college not far from home.

Mac and his wife have been married 34 years and raised two children. His wife is 60 years old and states she is healthy and active. Their eldest child is a daughter who is 30 years old, works as a nurse, and just got married last year. She lives in a neighboring state about 2 hours away. They have no children. His son is 27 years old and also works as an accountant. He lives about 6 hours away and is not married. Mac and his wife see their children during holidays and make a point to visit each one for about a week in the summer. Mac has two dogs, so they do not like to travel far or long from home. He and his wife own their own home. His wife was a secretary for a local business and when he retired, she did as well. She will occasionally help out when asked, but that occurs maybe once or twice a year. He states he feels safe at home and has a good relationship with his wife. Others may comment that she controls everything, but for many years, he worked and she was the "queen" of the house. He does not have any issues with his wife's management of the household and has no intention of changing anything. They are Catholic and attend Mass every Sunday morning. Mac and his wife take turns hosting the coffee hour after Mass as well. He stated that his religion is a source of strength for him. When his business was not profitable, his wife and the Church parishioners were the main sources of support for him. He doesn't think he was technically depressed, but it was a very difficult time for him. For this reason, he feels indebted and needs to give back to the Church and community.

As far as illnesses are concerned, Mac does not think he has any. He is allergic to penicillin and thinks his reaction is a rash. He thinks he took it for strep throat when he was a child and that's when the allergy was discovered. Mac takes antacids (Tums) sometimes after eating a full meal. He has never had chest pain. He stays active. He does take an aspirin daily and vitamin. He doesn't think he has ever been told that he has high cholesterol or hypertension. He had an inguinal hernia repair 20 years ago and an appendectomy and tonsillectomy as a child. He is not sure about his vaccines, but thinks he did have the pneumonia vaccine and the flu vaccine this year. He said his wife writes everything down, but, unfortunately, she could not come with him to his appointment today. His wife's mother is 93 years old and in a nursing home, so she likes to visit her often. His parents are deceased. His father died in a car accident when he was 45 years old. Mac does not know if he had any illnesses. His mother died at the age of 82 from a massive stroke.

(continued)

(continued)

He thinks that is why his previous provider told him to take aspirin. Mac has a younger sister who is 60 years old and still working as a university professor. She is married and has three boys and one daughter. To his knowledge, all of them are healthy.

Mac confides that he does worry about his son. He lives farther away, and he thinks he is working too much. Mac states that he worked too much in the beginning and the stress was overwhelming. He was lucky, he found a "good wife" who helped him see that work wasn't everything. He worries that his son is alone and does not have balance in his life. He also understands, though, that his son has to lead his own life and that commenting on his work patterns generally results in an argument. Nonetheless, he does worry.

He does wear seat belts while driving and tries to stick to the speed limit, but admits he generally drives faster. Mac has a smoke detector on each level of his house. He feels secure at home. In the future, he and his wife may move to a warmer climate or at least a smaller home, but for now they are happy where they are. They know the neighbors and many of the people in the town.

At this point, the provider moves into the ROS and asks the patient to answer a series of questions. Mac states the only rashes he has had are from penicillin. He has no itching, open areas, discolorations, or easy bruising. He does not have dandruff, any scalp itching, and has not had trauma to the head. Mac denied blurry vision, double vision, redness, excessive tearing, pain, dryness, and eye discharge. He gets a cold a few times per year. He does not have seasonal allergies. He has a pool in his backyard, so Mac does like to swim and sit in the sun. He has no moles or unusual freckles. Mac wears progressive lens glasses so he can see near and far. He has worn glasses since he was about 12 years old for distance. At about the age of 45, Mac also required reading glasses. He has not had double vision or conjunctivitis. He has no eye, ear, mouth, or nose pain. As far as he knows, he has not had a change in his ability to smell odors. He denied hearing loss, ringing in the ears, discharge, pain, and itching in the ears. Mac did have strep throat a few times in high school and infectious mononucleosis in his first year of college. He denied current throat soreness, hoarseness, difficulty swallowing, discharge, and enlarged tonsils. He has not noticed any lumps in his neck, throat, or underarms. He does not have neck pain. Mac denied shortness of breath, cough, congestion, wheezing, fevers, and weight loss. He sleeps on one pillow unless he is reading in bed. He uses two pillows in bed to read. He does not have insomnia and falls asleep quickly at night. He does not have palpitations, chest pain, swelling of the

(continued)

(continued)

legs, or shortness of breath when walking short distances or up a flight of stairs. His bowel movements are regular, generally every morning. He does not take any laxatives although his wife does give him prune juice every other morning. He has not had nausea, vomiting, constipation, or diarrhea. He has no abdominal pain. Mac repeated that he occasionally has to strain in order to urinate. He denied frequency, hesitancy, and pain. He drinks plenty of fluids during the day and urinates about four times a day. He wakes usually once per night to urinate as well. He has not had urinary tract infections and has never been told he has an enlarged prostate gland. Mac states he has difficulty urinating once or twice per week. He tries to drink less at dinner and after dinner to decrease the need to urinate at night. He is sexually active with his wife and believes it has been a monogamous relationship for their entire marriage of 36 years. Mac has never had a sexually transmitted disease (STD) or difficulty with an erection. He does not have any discharge or bleeding from his penis. Mac admits to joint aches and pains. He does enjoy the daily walks with his wife and says his joints feel better after the walks. He has not had any broken bones since high school when he played soccer. He fractured his collar bone in a soccer match when he was 17 years old. Mac says he knows when the weather is changing because his collar bone will start to ache. He has a slight bump where the fracture occurred. He has no difficulty walking. Mac has not experienced headaches, dizziness, difficulty speaking or finding words, weakness, fatigue, or anxiety. He has no numbness or tingling in any of his extremities. Mac denies any history of mental health difficulties. He does not have any issues with his blood glucose and has never been told he has diabetes. His hair has been thinning in the same pattern his grandfather's thinned. He does not remember if his father's hair had begun to thin. He has not noticed any unexplained bruising, changes in skin color, or increased sensitivity to heat or cold. Overall, Mac states he thinks he is in good health and plans to see his grandchildren, which he hopes he will have soon, grow up.

The provider thanks Mac for the information and asks him to remove his clothes down to his underwear and put on the examination gown. In the meantime, the provider will step out of the room and document the findings so far.

See Tables 1.3 and 1.4 for documentation of the Mac's full health history and ROS. The components of the history must be recorded to have a baseline for the patient and also for billing and reimbursement. A higher number of systems must be included in the history for a higher rate of reimbursement. For a focused history, anything pertinent to the patient problem must be explored and documented in the history.

TABLE 1.3
Mr. G.'s Health History

Section	Information Gathered
ID	64-year-old male, retired accountant, prefers to be called "Mac," Italian
CC	Needs insurance physical, c/o difficulty and straining with urination at times
HPI	Previous provider retired. Needs to establish care. Regarding urination, does not have a h/o UTIs. Has not been told he has an enlarged prostate gland. Denied dysuria and frequency. Wakes once/night to urinate and urinates three to four times daily. Has difficulty once or twice per week.
PM/SH	Tonsillectomy and appendectomy as a child; clavicular fracture in high school; inguinal hernia repair; takes prn Tums, multivitamin daily, and ASA 81 mg daily. Has had flu vaccine and pneumovax.
Allergies	PCN (rash), childhood
FH	Father deceased 45-year-old, car accident; mother deceased 82-year-old, CVA; son 27-year-old health; dtr 30-year-old healthy; sister 60-year-old healthy
Social	Church and wife are supportive, lives with wife, owns home, has two dogs. Retired accountant. Walks 1 hour 2× daily with wife. Wife cooks at home. Likes meat and potatoes, but wife also provides vegetables. Nonsmoker, no illicit drugs, drinks 1–2 glasses wine on Tues nights. Friends over every Tuesday for cards/socializing. Safe at home, has smoke detectors, wears seat belts. Dtr, married, lives 2 hour away and son single, lives 6 hour away.

ASA, acetylsalicylic acid (aspirin); CC, chief complaint; CVA, cerebrovascular accident; dtr, daughter; FH, family history; HPI, history of the present illness; ID, identification; PCN, penicillin; PM/SH, past medical/surgical history; prn, as needed; UTI, urinary tract infection.

TABLE 1.4
Mr. G.'s Review of Systems

System	Information Gathered
Skin	Rash only with PCN; denied dry skin, itching, open areas, changes in freckles or moles, discolorations, easy bruising
Head	+Hair thinning; denied dandruff, itching, trauma

(continued)

TABLE 1.4
Mr. G.'s Review of Systems (*continued*)

System	Information Gathered
Eyes	Wears glasses for near and far vision Denied blurry vision, double vision, redness, excessive tearing, pain, dryness, discharge
Ears	Denied hearing loss, ringing in the ears, discharge, pain, itching
Nose	Denied loss of smell perception, discharge, difficulty breathing, bleeding, seasonal allergies
Throat	Had strep throat in high school; denied current soreness, hoarseness, difficulty swallowing, discharge, enlarged tonsils
Neck	Denied pain, lymphadenopathy
Respiratory	Denied shortness of breath, wheezing, congestion, cough, inability to lay flat
Cardiovascular	Denied chest pain, palpitations, swelling of the legs, shortness of breath when walking short distances or up a flight of stairs
Gastrointestinal	Uses antacids (Tums) as needed for heartburn; daily BMs in the morning; denied nausea, vomiting, pain, constipation, diarrhea
Genitourinary	+Difficulty urinating, straining 1–2×/wk; denied frequency, hesitation, discharge, bleeding; sexually active with wife, no h/o STDs or ED
Musculoskeletal	+Mild joint pain/stiffness, improves with walking; +clavicular fracture in high school, aches with change in weather; denied swelling of joints, difficulty walking or running, back pain, decreased range of motion
Neurological	+Concern about son and his work schedule; denied headaches, dizziness, difficulty speaking or finding words, weakness, numbness, tingling, fatigue, insomnia, anxiety; denied mental health difficulties
Endocrine	Denied diabetes, sensitivity to heat or cold, changes in skin color

BM, bowel movement; ED, erectile dysfunction; h/o, history of; PCN, penicillin; STDs, sexually transmitted diseases.

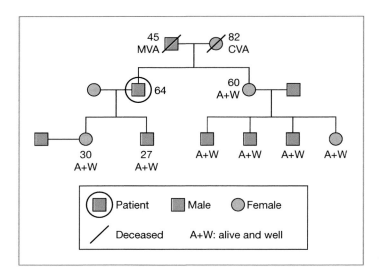

FIGURE 1.1 Mr. G.'s family history genogram. CVA, cerebrovascular accident; MVA, motor vehicle accident.

For family history, a genogram may be used. Mac's genogram is depicted in (Figure 1.1).

If Mac was an established patient and came to the office for difficult urinating, the information gathered would focus on the problem. The following case illustrates the information that would be gathered for this focused history.

FOCUSED HEALTH HISTORY

Mr. G., "Mac," a 64-year-old male and established patient, comes to the practice with a complaint of occasional difficulty urinating. Mac states he occasionally has to strain in order to urinate. He denies frequency, hesitancy, and pain. He drinks plenty of fluids during the day and urinates about four times a day. He wakes usually once per night to urinate as well. He has not had urinary tract infections and has never been told he has an enlarged prostate gland. Mac states he has difficulty urinating once or twice per week. He tries to drink less at dinner and after

dinner to decrease the need to urinate at night. He is sexually active with his wife and believes it has been a monogamous relationship for their entire marriage of 36 years. Mac has never had a STD or difficulty with an erection. He does not have any discharge or bleeding from his penis. His bowel movements are regular, generally every morning. He does not take any laxatives although he drinks prune juice every other morning. He has not had nausea, vomiting, constipation, or diarrhea. He has no abdominal pain.

The provider thanks Mac for the information and asks him to remove his clothes down to his underwear and put on the examination gown. In the meantime, the provider will step out of the room and document the focused history findings.

The documentation of the focused health history and ROS is found in Table 1.5. Just as with the full history, the components of the focused history must be recorded for documentation of the complaint as well as billing and reimbursement. For a focused history, anything pertinent to the patient problem must be explored and documented in the history.

TABLE 1.5
Mr. G.'s Focused Health History and Review of Systems

Section	Information Gathered
ID	64-year-old male, prefers to be called "Mac"
CC	Difficulty and straining with urination at times
HPI	Does not have a h/o UTIs Has not been told he has an enlarged prostate gland Denied dysuria and frequency Wakes once/night to urinate and urinates three to four times daily Has difficulty once or twice per week
ROS	
Gastrointestinal	Daily BMs in the morning Denied nausea, vomiting, pain, constipation, diarrhea
Genitourinary	+Difficulty urinating, straining 1–2×/wk Denied frequency, hesitation, discharge, bleeding Sexually active with wife, no STDs or ED

BM, bowel movement; CC, chief complaint; ED, erectile dysfunction; HPI, history of the present illness; ID, identification; ROS, review of systems; STDs, sexually transmitted diseases; UTI, urinary tract infection.

Assessment of Special Populations

The provider must be sensitive to patients and their abilities. Some may have physical or mental disabilities. Although the same type of information must be obtained, how questions are asked or what the expected answers are may differ. In a health history, the provider must remain nonjudgmental and supportive of the patient. For example, an overweight patient may not return to the provider's office if the patient knows that there will be another lecture about losing weight. The patient already knows that that is important. The difficulty for the patient may be determining how to approach losing weight and how to fit exercise into the schedule. Therefore, the provider's insistence that the patient lose weight is not helpful and, in fact, deters the patient from seeking assistance from the provider. An open patient–provider relationship serves to maintain communication and create an environment of wellness and healing for the patient. The provider may not scientifically agree with all the patient thinks and does, but at least the patient informs the provider and can have a dialogue with the provider.

The health history will take different forms depending upon the practice of the provider. In the case of a home care practice, the health history is conducted in the patient's home and may put the patient more at ease. The provider is able to observe the patient's living environment and obtain much information from observation. In the office setting, the patient may be more nervous and need more reassurance from the provider. The patient may have difficulty getting to the office or be unable to sit in a chair. Culture and language may also differ and the provider needs to ensure that the patient is understanding the provider's questions correctly and, conversely, that the provider is understanding the patient's questions and responses. Taking time to pause and rephrase is a good method to determine whether both parties are truly understanding each other.

For the person with a disability, the following are relevant issues: history of disability or disabling conditions (e.g., polio as a child), asking about obvious disability and its history; and making sure not to focus exclusively on the disability or disabling condition, but not ignoring it either. If a patient has a mobility-limiting disability, asking about how the disability affects the patient's ability to participate in physical activity, in health screening, and so on, seems warranted. If the patient has hearing loss, it is important to find out how the patient prefers to communicate (sign interpreter [who is not a family member]; lip reading; writing; communication board). Another important issue related to history is to be sure that all health issues are *not* attributed to an existing disability.

Diagnostic Reasoning

The health history is a necessary and important component in diagnostic reasoning and determining the differential diagnoses for a patient. The health history indicates problematic areas for the patient. The provider uses that information to conduct a full or focused physical examination as needed. Without the information in the health history, the provider does not have any direction in conducting the physical examination. When the patient is alert, oriented, and reliable, the information about symptoms is also reliable and the provider can tailor the examination to the areas in question.

When the patient is not reliable, the provider may need to reconcile findings with patient-reported information or information from a significant other, guardian, or family member. The examination may reveal misunderstandings regarding the disease process. In turn, this provides an opportunity for the provider to educate the patient.

A differential diagnosis cannot be determined until after both the history and the physical examination. However, the history provides direction and may help the provider determine which body systems to examine. However, a word of caution. The provider must not narrowly focus the examination in order to entertain all possibilities in the differential.

BIBLIOGRAPHY

Bickley, L. S. (2017). *Bates' guide to physical examination and history taking* (12th ed.). Philadelphia, PA: Wolters Kluwer.

Hickey, K. T., Katapodi, M. C., Coleman, B., Reuter-Rice, K., & Starkweather, A. R. (2017). Improving utilization of the family history in the electronic health record. *Journal of Nursing Scholarship, 49*(1), 80–86. doi:10.1111/jnu.12259

Lagu, T., Iezzoni, L. I., & Lindenauer, P. K. (2014). The axes of access–improving care for patients with disabilities. *New England Journal of Medicine, 370*(19), 1847–1851. doi:10.1056/NEJMsb1315940

Legg, C., Young, L., & Bryer, A. (2005). Training sixth-year medical students in obtaining case-history information from adults with aphasia. *Aphasiology, 19*(6), 559–575. doi:10.1080/02687030544000029

Maragh-Bass, A. C., Griffin, J. M., Phelan, S., Finney Rutten, L. J., & Morris, M. A. (2017). Healthcare provider perceptions of accessible exam tables in primary care: Implementation and benefits to patients with and without disabilities. *Disability and Health Journal, 11*(1), 155–160. doi:10.1016/j.dhjo.2017.04.005

Morrissey, J. (1994). Obtaining a "reasonably accurate" health history. *Plastic Surgical Nursing, 14*(1), 27–30.

Rolnick, S., Butler, C. C., Kinnersley, P., Gregory, J., & Mash, B. (2010). Motivational interviewing. *BMJ, 340*, c1900. doi:10.1136/bmj.c1900

2

ADVANCED HEALTH ASSESSMENT OF THE HEAD, NECK, AND LYMPHATIC SYSTEM

Erin Fusco

CHAPTER CONTENTS

(continued)

ASSESSMENT OF SPECIAL POPULATIONS
   Transgender Population
   Elderly Population
   Pregnant Population
   Pediatric Population
   Patients With Disabilities
   Veteran Population

DIAGNOSTIC REASONING
   Common Differential Diagnoses: Head and Neck Disorders

Overview of Anatomy and Physiology

HEAD AND NECK

The skull plays an important role in the function of the body (Figure 2.1). It is pivotal in protecting the brain, and the nerves and vessels that feed and control the brain, face, and scalp. In addition, the skull provides a site for attachment of muscles and tendons of the face and scalp. The skull is made of 22 bones: eight cranial bones and 14 facial bones. The eight cranial bones are the frontal bone, two temporal bones, two partial bones, a sphenoid bone, an ethmoid bone, and an occipital bone. The skull bones are separated by coronal, lambdoid, sagittal, and squamosal sutures. The 14 facial bones are two nasal conchae, two nasal bones, two maxilla bones, two palatine bones, two lacrimal bones, two zygomatic bones, the mandible, and the vomer. Each of these bones have structural and protective roles; they form the human face and lead to differences among human appearances.

The sternocleidomastoid muscle (SCM) plays a vital role in the posture of the neck and the body. The SCM is a large and easily recognizable and palpable muscle. The SCM is one of more than 20 pairs of muscles in the neck (Figure 2.2). The SCM divides the neck area into an anterior triangle and a posterior triangle. The posterior border of the SCM, the inferior border of the mandible, demarcates the anterior triangle inferiorly, and the medial line of the neck, medially. In the anterior triangle, the examiner can find the suprahyoid and infrahyoid muscles. The posterior triangle is demarcated by the SCM anteriorly, by the clavicle inferiorly, and by the trapezius muscle posteriorly. Scalene muscles reside in the posterior triangle. The hyoid bone borders the triangle inferiorly. The triangle's floor is shaped by the mylohyoid, behind the submandibular gland. The submandibular gland that helps produce salivary fluid secreted into the oral cavity takes up the majority of the space within the triangle. Additionally, the gland helps to facilitate lymphatic drainage from the lower gums, tongue, the floor of the mouth, and tonsils into the three to six lymph nodes within the triangle which lie next to the submandibular gland.

SCM has a dual-innervation and multiple functions. The vestibular area works with the SCM motoneurons to improve posture and neck movements; the

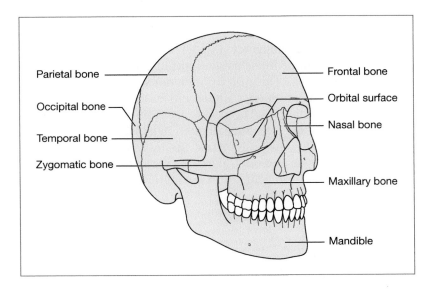

Parietal bone

Occipital bone

Temporal bone

Zygomatic bone

Frontal bone

Orbital surface

Nasal bone

Maxillary bone

Mandible

FIGURE 2.1 Anatomy of the skull.

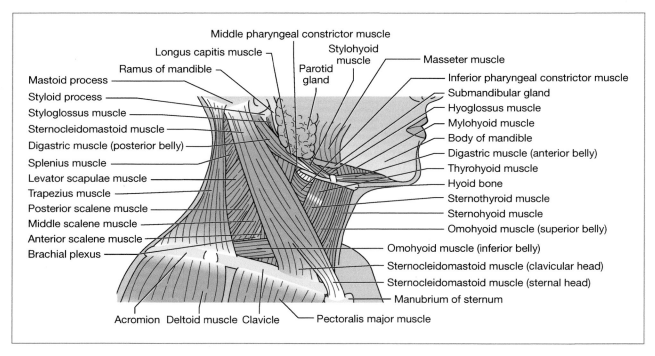

FIGURE 2.2 Muscles of the neck.

cervico-trigeminal reflexes put in direct contact the occlusive capacity of the temporomandibular joint and the electrical activity of the SCM, with a reciprocal influence, in particular with the masseter muscle. The inspiratory act is enabled by the contraction of the SCM muscle. The one-sided contraction of the SCM creates three movements: the rotation of the head on the side opposite to that of its contraction, the inclination from the side of its contraction, and extension.

LYMPH NODES

Lymph nodes are distinct structures (Figure 2.3). They are surrounded by a capsule composed of connective tissue and a few elastic fibrils. Lymph nodes usually occur in groups. Superficial nodes are located in subcutaneous connective tissues and can be palpated by the practitioner. They are the practitioner's access to assessing the health of the entire lymphatic system. Readily accessible to inspection and palpation, they provide some of the earliest clues to the presence of infection or malignancy. Deeper nodes lie beneath the fascia of muscles and within the various body cavities. The practitioner does not usually palpate these deeper nodes unless they are abnormally enlarged. The nodes are numerous and tiny, but some may have diameters as large as 0.5 to 1 cm. They defend against the invasion of microorganisms and other particles with filtration and phagocytosis, and aid in the maturation of lymphocytes and monocytes.

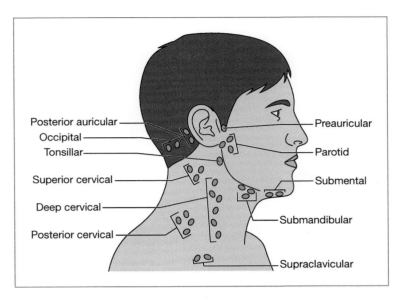

FIGURE 2.3 Lymph nodes of the head and neck.

Screening Health Assessment and Normal Findings

HEAD

The first step in assessing the head is to observe. What position is the head in? Note if the head is tilted. Are there any tremors? Then, inspect the skull and scalp for size, shape, symmetry, lesions, or trauma. Next, inspect facial features, including symmetry, shape, unusual features, tics, characteristic facial expressions, and pallor or pigmentation variations. At that point, palpate the head and scalp, noting symmetry, tenderness (particularly over areas of frontal and maxillary sinuses), scalp movement, sutures/fontanels, and hair texture, color, and distribution (Figure 2.4). Gloves may be worn if there is any suspicion for infestations such as lice. Finally, auscultate the temporal arteries and palpate, noting thickening, hardness, or tenderness. Inspect and palpate the salivary glands.

NECK

To start the exam of the neck, inspect for symmetry, alignment of the trachea, fullness, masses, webbing, and skinfolds. Palpate the neck, noting the tracheal

position and lymph nodes (Figure 2.5). Next, palpate the thyroid gland for size, shape, configuration, consistency, tenderness, and nodules (Figure 2.6). If the thyroid gland is enlarged, auscultate for bruits. Finally, evaluate the range of motion of the neck in three planes. First, ask the patient to look up and then down, placing the chin on the chest. Second, ask the patient to turn the head side to side. Finally, have the patient attempt to touch an ear to the shoulder on the same side.

LYMPH NODES

Inspect the visible nodes and surrounding area for edema, erythema, or red streaks. Next, palpate the superficial lymph nodes and compare side to side for size, consistency, mobility, discrete borders or matting, tenderness, or warmth. Using the pads of your index and middle fingers, press gently, moving the skin over the underlying tissues in each area. The patient should be relaxed, with the neck flexed slightly forward and, if needed, turned slightly toward the side being examined. You can usually examine

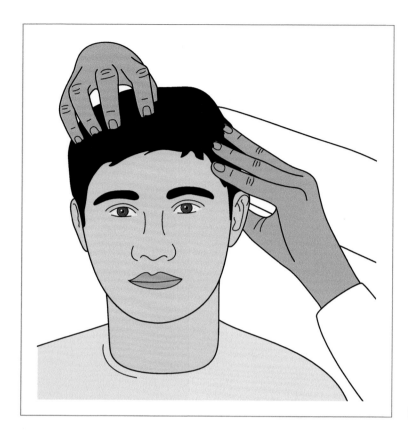

FIGURE 2.4 Inspection of the head.

both sides at once, noting both the presence of lymph nodes as well as asymmetry. For the submental node, however, it is helpful to feel with one hand while bracing the top of the head with the other. If you discover an enlarged node, consider the associated region drained by the node to suggest possible sources for a potential problem (Table 2.1).

SEQUENCE FOR EXAMINING LYMPH NODES

The location of lymph nodes can be seen in (Figure 2.7). The following list details the sequence for examining lymph nodes.

1. *Preauricular*—in front of the ear

2. *Posterior auricular*—superficial to the mastoid process

3. *Occipital*—at the base of the skull posteriorly

4. *Tonsillar*—at the angle of the mandible. A pulsating "tonsillar node" is really the carotid artery. A small hard tender "tonsillar node" high and deep between the mandible and the sternocleidomastoid is probably a styloid process.

5. *Submandibular*—midway between the angle and the tip of the mandible. These nodes are usually smaller and smoother than the lobulated submandibular gland against which they lie.

6. *Submental*—in the midline, a few centimeters behind the tip of the mandible

7. *Superficial cervical*—superficial to the sternocleidomastoid

8. *Posterior cervical*—along the anterior edge of the trapezius

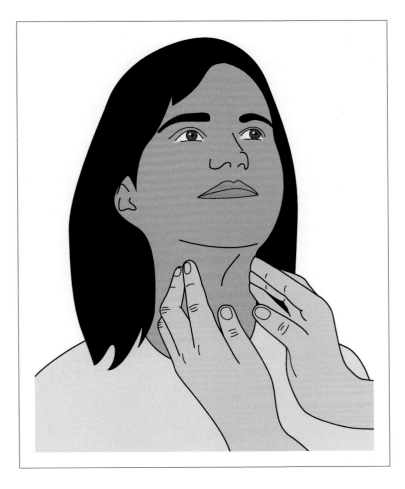

FIGURE 2.5 Palpation of the neck.

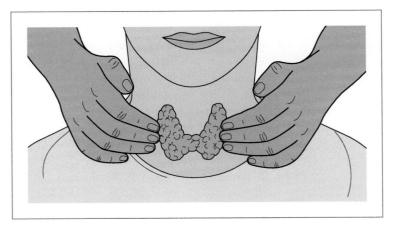

FIGURE 2.6 Palpation of the thyroid gland.

TABLE 2.1
Palpable Superficial Lymph Nodes and Associated Regions

Neck Region	Arms	Legs
Tonsillar	Axillary	Inguinal
Submandibular		Popliteal
Submental		
Superficial anterior cervical		
Superficial posterior cervical		
Preauricular		
Postauricular		
Sternocleidomastoid		
Occipital		

9. *Deep cervical chain*—deep to the sternocleidomastoid and often inaccessible to examination. Hook your thumb and fingers around either side of the SCM to find them.

10. *Supraclavicular*—deep in the angle formed by the clavicle and the sternocleidomastoid.

Palpate the preauricular nodes (Figure 2.8). Palpate the *anterior superficial* and *deep cervical chains*, located anterior and superficial to the sternocleidomastoid. Then palpate the *posterior cervical chain* along the trapezius (anterior edge) and along the sternocleidomastoid (posterior edge). Flex the patient's neck slightly forward toward the side being examined. Examine the supraclavicular nodes in the angle between the clavicle and the sternocleidomastoid.

Palpate the submandibular nodes (Figure 2.9) and then the supraclavicular nodes (Figure 2.10). Occasionally, you may mistake a band of muscle or an artery for a lymph node. Unlike a muscle or an artery, you should be able to roll a node in two directions: up and down, and side to side. Neither a muscle nor an artery will pass this test.

Focused Health Assessment and Abnormal Findings

Many symptoms of the head and neck represent common benign processes, but sometimes these symptoms reflect a serious underlying condition. Careful attention to the interview and physical examination, with a focus on features and findings that do not fit a typical benign pattern, can often distinguish a common condition of the head and neck from a serious underlying disease.

TRAUMATIC BRAIN INJURY

History should include an independent observer's description of event; the patient's state of consciousness after the injury: immediately and 5 minutes later; duration of unconsciousness; and if the patient is combative, confused, alert, or dazed. In addition, the history should include any

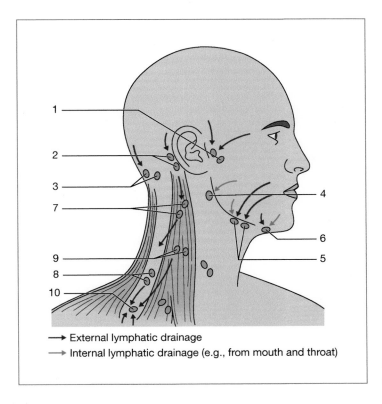

→ External lymphatic drainage

→ Internal lymphatic drainage (e.g., from mouth and throat)

FIGURE 2.7 Sequence for examining lymph nodes.

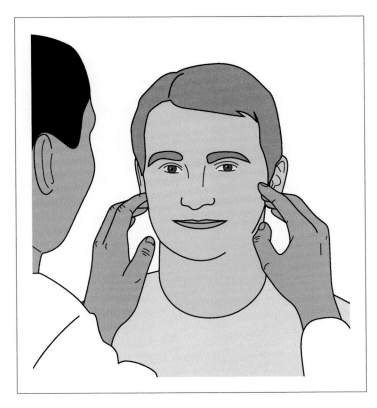

FIGURE 2.8 Palpation of the preauricular nodes.

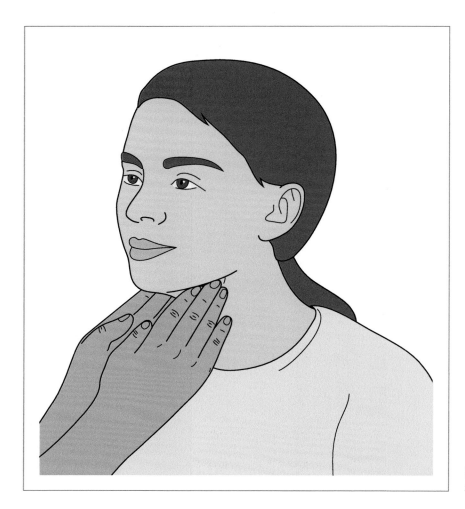

FIGURE 2.9 Palpation of the submandibular nodes.

predisposing factors: seizure disorder, hypoglycemia, poor vision, lightheadedness, syncope, and/or sports participation. Finally, the provider should review all associated symptoms: head or neck pain, laceration, local tenderness, change in breathing pattern, blurred or double vision, discharge from nose or ears, nausea or vomiting, urinary or fecal incontinence, and ability to move all extremities.

HEADACHE

History should include the following elements. See Tables 2.2 to 2.8 for characteristics of various headache types.

- Onset: Early morning, midday, nighttime; gradual versus abrupt.

- Location: Entire head, unilateral, specific site (neck, sinus region, behind eyes, hatband distribution)

- Duration: Minutes, hours, days, weeks; relieved by medication or sleep; resolves spontaneously; occurs in clusters; headache-free periods

- Character: Throbbing, pounding, boring, dull, nagging, constant pressure, aggravated with movement

- Severity: Grade each event severity on a scale from 1 (mild) to 10 (severe)

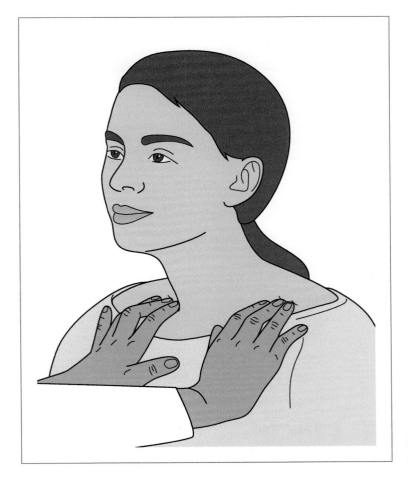

FIGURE 2.10 Palpation of the supraclavicular nodes.

- Visual prodrome: Scotoma; hemianopia (decreased vision or blindness takes place in half the visual field of one or both eyes); distortion of size, shape, or location

- Pattern: Worse in morning or evening, worse or better as day progresses, awakens patient from or occurs only during sleep episodes, closer together or worsening, lasting longer; change in level of consiousness as pain increases

- Associated symptoms: Nausea, vomiting, diarrhea, photophobia, visual disturbance, difficulty falling asleep, increased lacrimation, nasal discharge, tinnitus, paresthesias, mobility impairment, goiter

- Precipitating factors: Fever, fatigue, stress, food additives, prolonged fasting, alcohol, seasonal allergies, menstrual cycle, sexual intercourse, oral contraceptives, amount of caffeine intake

- Efforts to treat: Sleep, pain medication, need for daily medications, rebound if pain medications are not taken or if caffeine not consumed

- Medications: Antiepileptic drugs, antiarrhythmics, beta-blockers, calcium channel blockers, oral contraceptives, serotonin antagonists or agonists, selective serotonin reuptake inhibitors (SSRIs), antidepressants, nonsteroidal anti-inflammatory drugs (NSAIDs), narcotics, caffeine-containing medication

TABLE 2.2
Characteristics of Migraine Headaches

Age of onset	Childhood
Location	Unilateral or generalized
Duration	Hours to days
Time of onset	Morning or night
Quality of pain	Pulsating or throbbing
Prodromal event	Vague neurologic changes, personality change, fluid retention, appetite loss to well-defined neurologic event, scotoma, aphasia, hemianopsia, aura
Precipitating event	Menstrual period, missing meals, birth control pills, letdown after stress
Frequency	Twice a week
Gender predilection	Females
Other symptoms	Nausea, vomiting

TABLE 2.3
Characteristics of Muscular Tension Headaches

Age of onset	Adult
Location	Unilateral or bilateral
Duration	Hours to days
Time of onset	Anytime, commonly in afternoon or evening
Quality of pain	Band-like, constricting
Prodromal event	None
Precipitating event	Stress, anger, bruxism
Frequency	Daily
Gender predilection	Equal
Other symptoms	None

TABLE 2.4
Characteristics of Cluster Headaches

Age of onset	Adult
Location	Unilateral
Duration	0.5–2.0 hours
Time of onset	Night
Quality of pain	Intense burning, boring, searing, knifelike
Prodromal event	Personality changes, sleep disturbances
Precipitating event	Alcohol consumption
Frequency	Several times nightly for several nights, then none
Gender predilection	Male
Other symptoms	Increased lacrimation, nasal discharge

TABLE 2.5
Characteristics of Medication-Rebound Headaches

Age of onset	Any
Location	Generalized or diffuse
Duration	Hours to days
Time of onset	Predictably begins within hours to days of the last dose of the medication or caffeine
Quality of pain	Dull or throbbing
Prodromal event	Daily analgesics use and/or daily caffeine use
Precipitating event	Abrupt discontinuation of analgesics or caffeine
Frequency	Gradual increase in headache frequency to daily
Gender predilection	Female
Other symptoms	Alternate or preventive medications fail to control the headache

TABLE 2.6
Characteristics of Hypertensive Headaches

Age of onset	Adult
Location	Bilateral or occipital
Duration	Hours
Time of onset	Morning
Quality of pain	Throbbing
Prodromal event	None
Precipitating event	None
Frequency	Daily
Gender predilection	Equal
Other symptoms	Generally remits as day progresses

TABLE 2.7
Characteristics of Temporal Arteritis Headaches

Age of onset	Older adult
Location	Unilateral or bilateral
Duration	Hours to days
Time of onset	Anytime
Quality of pain	Throbbing
Prodromal event	None
Precipitating event	None
Frequency	Daily
Gender predilection	Equal
Other symptoms	None

TABLE 2.8
Characteristics of Space-Occupying Lesion Headaches

Age of onset	Any
Location	Localized
Duration	Rapidly increasing duration
Time of onset	Steady pain worse upon waking and better within a few hours
Quality of pain	Aching
Prodromal event	Aggravated by coughing or bending forward
Precipitating event	Develops in temporal relation to the neoplasm
Frequency	Progressive
Gender predilection	Equal

STIFF NECK

History should include neck injury or strain, traumatic brain injury, neck swelling, fever, associated headache, or other symptoms of meningitis (confusion, drowsiness/lethargy, photophobia, cranial nerve deficits, and seizure). Character of the stiffness: limitation of movement; pain with movement, pain relieved by movement; continuous or cramping pain; radiation patterns to arms, shoulders, hands, or down the back. Predisposing factors: unilateral vision or hearing loss, work position (e.g., long hours in front of a computer). Efforts to treat: heat, physical therapy, complementary medicine (e.g., chiropractor); medications: analgesics, muscle relaxants. Neck kyphosis may develop secondary to trauma.

Consider also symptoms of thyroid disease such as change in temperature preference with more or less clothing than worn by other members of the household, any history of neck swelling, difficulty swallowing, redness, pain with touch or swallowing, or hyperextension of the neck; change in texture of hair, skin, or nails; increased pigmentation of skin at pressure points; change in mood and energy, irritability, nervousness, lethargy, or disinterest; increased prominence of eyes (exophthalmos); periorbital swelling, blurred or double vision; cardiac symptoms of thyroid disease such as tachycardia or palpitations; change in menses; change in bowel habits. Medications: thyroid preparations.

LYMPHADENOPATHY

Tender nodes suggest inflammation; hard or fixed nodes (fixed to underlying structures and not movable on palpation) suggest malignancy. If you feel supraclavicular lymph nodes, a thorough work-up is warranted. Cancers of the head and neck account for about 3% of all cancer diagnoses in the United States.

Enlarged or tender nodes, if unexplained, call for reexamination of the regions they drain and careful assessment of lymph nodes elsewhere to distinguish between regional and generalized lymphadenopathy. Generalized lymphadenopathy is seen in multiple infectious, inflammatory, or malignant conditions such as HIV or AIDS, infectious mononucleosis, lymphoma, leukemia, and sarcoidosis.

Holistic Assessment

Distress with complaints of the head, neck, and lymph nodes is common. In one study of 113 patients, 49% of those with chronic headaches reported high psychological distress, which is significantly higher than in the general population. Mental health and a person's ability to work are hampered by physical complaints. In addition, patients who complained of headache and were extremely distressed evoked a negative response from healthcare professionals. Healthcare professionals should be more aware of their own response to patients in distress; this way, they will be more capable of managing this patient group.

Safety in caring for patients with head, neck, and lymph node disorders should be considered at all exams. When seeing patients with traumatic head and neck complaints, safe handling of the patient should be the provider's first consideration. Physical examination of patients with such complaints should be done carefully so as not to worsen any trauma that may already exist.

CASE STUDY

A man, aged 62 years, presents to the clinic with a neck mass. The patient has had a mass in the left side of the neck for approximately 1 year, and it had recently begun to grow. He had a long beard, which hid the growing mass. The patient reports the mass hurts when touched now, which brought him in. In addition, he reports some difficulty swallowing. The patient previously smoked for a long period, but no longer smokes. He reports a history of drinking four to five beers daily.

On Examination:

Head: Normocephalic

Neck: Fixed hard tender mass noted on the left tonsillar lymph node, measuring approximately 5 cm.

Throat: Left tonsil 3+, erythematous with lesion noted. Right tonsil pink, nonenlarged.

Plan: Referral to ear, nose, and throat (ENT) specialist made.

Diagnosis: Biopsy results indicated squamous cell carcinoma, and tested positive for human papillomavirus (HPV). The patient received a diagnosis of left tonsillar cancer that was considered stage IV because of the size of the obstructing tumor.

ICD-10-CM Diagnosis Code: C02.4 Malignant Neoplasm of Lingual Tonsil

Assessment of Special Populations

 ### TRANSGENDER POPULATION

Create an inclusive environment when providing care for the transgender patient. Screen transgender patients for cancer as this group has a higher rate of cancer than the general population. In addition, screen for sexually transmitted diseases as this patient population also has a higher rate than the general population. Lesions on the outside of the mouth should not be dismissed. Consider herpes and other causes such as viral zoster, other sexually transmitted diseases, or hand, foot, and mouth disease.

▪▫▫ ELDERLY POPULATION

Lymph nodes decrease with age in size and number. The teeth in the mouth may decrease in number, leading to a sunken appearance of the patient's mouth. The skin dries out with age, which may lead to more flaking of the scalp upon inspection.

▪▫▫ PREGNANT POPULATION

Hypertrophy during pregnancy is normal, causing some swelling of the gums. The "mask of pregnancy," or cholasma, is sometimes present. The thyroid can sometimes be palpable during pregnancy.

▪▫▫ PEDIATRIC POPULATION

Fontanels, or "soft spots," are present to allow for the growth of the head. The head is molded during the vaginal delivery of a baby but should reshape within days of delivery. Sinuses do not develop until 7 years of age. Tonsils are larger in childhood than in adolescence and lymph nodes are larger in children than adults.

▪▫▫ PATIENT WITH DISABILITIES

It is important for the provider to understand the patient's specific disability and tailor the assessment to that patient. Examples of assessing the head, neck, and lymph nodes in a patient with disabilities can include having a patient with quadriplegia who has no movement of the neck. This is the patient's baseline health status and should be treated as such. Another example could be dealing with trying to assess a patient with schizophrenia for problems with his or her head, neck, or lymph nodes. The patient may have a difficult time participating in the examination and the provider may need to use creative ways to engage the patient.

▪▫▫ VETERAN POPULATION

The provider should ask the patient if they served in the military. If so, the dates and capacity in which they served (e.g., pilot, ground forces, medical services) should be ascertained. Based upon this information, the provider will be aware of what potential hazards or chemicals of warfare the patient may have been exposed to.

Diagnostic Reasoning

Common Differential Diagnoses: Head and Neck Disorders

Body Part	Symptom/ Complaint	Diagnostics	Assessment (ICD-10-CM)
Head	Neuralgia pain of the face that is continuous or in spasms	History and physical exam	Trigeminal neuralgia (G50.0)
Head	Pain/Headache	MRI or CT scan	Migraine headache (G44.00) Cluster headache (G44.019) Tension headache (G44.201) Sinusitis (J01.90)

(continued)

Body Part	Symptom/ Complaint	Diagnostics	Assessment (ICD-10-CM)
Head	Temporomandibular joint pain	X-ray or MRI	Temporomandibular joint syndrome (M26.62)
Head	Trauma	X-ray	Trauma may lead to skull depression (S07.1XXA)
Lymph Nodes	Pain	CBC, CMP, X-ray, MRI, or CT	Lymphadenopathy secondary to infection (L04.9) or lymphoma (Non-Hodgkin's C85.9; Hodgkin's C81)
Lymph Nodes	Swelling	CBC, CMP, throat cultures, X-ray, MRI, or CT	Lymphadenopathy secondary to infection (L04.9) or lymphoma (Non-Hodgkin's C85.9; Hodgkin's C81)
Neck	Decreased ROM	X-ray, MRI, or CT	Unspecified injury of the neck (S19.9XXA)
Neck	Mass	Ultrasound, MRI, or CT scan, thyroid function tests	Thyroid nodule E04.1 Thyroid cancer C73 Goiter E04.9 Hashimoto's disease E06.3
Neck	Pain	X-ray, MRI, or CT	Trauma may lead to vertebral dysfunction, which may need surgical intervention (S13)

Common Differential Diagnoses: Head and Neck Disorders (*continued*)

CBC, complete blood count; CMP, comprehensive metabolic panel.
Source: Data from World Health Organization (1992). *International classification of diseases and related health problems* (10th rev., ICD-10). Geneva, Switzerland: Author.

BIBLIOGRAPHY

Anderson, B. W., & Al Kharazi, K. A. (2018, January). *Anatomy, head and neck, skull.* Treasure Island, FL: StatPearls Publishing. Retrieved from https://www.ncbi.nlm.nih.gov/books/NBK499834

Ball, J. W., Dains, J. E., Flynn, J. A., Solomon, B. S., & Stewart, R. W. (2019). *Seidel's guide to physical examination* (9th ed.). St. Louis, MO: Elsevier. Retrieved from https://www.clinicalkey.com/#!/browse/book/3-s2.0-C20160009889

Bickley, L. S. (2017). *Bates' guide to physical examination and history taking.* (12th ed.). Philadelphia, PA: Wolters Kluwer. Retrieved from https://meded.lwwhealthlibrary.com/book.aspx?bookid=1876

Bordoni, B., & Varacallo, M. (2018, January). *Anatomy, head and neck, sternocleidomastoid muscle*. Treasure Island, FL: StatPearls Publishing. Retrieved from https://www.ncbi.nlm.nih.gov/books/NBK532881

Carson, N. J., Katz, A. M., & Alegría, M. (2016). How patients and clinicians make meaning of physical suffering in mental health evaluations. *Transcultural Psychiatry, 53*(5), 595–611. doi:10.1177/1363461516660901

Dains, J. E., Baumann, L. C., & Scheibel, P. (2012). *Advanced health assessment & clinical diagnosis in primary care*. (4th ed.). St. Louis, MO: Elsevier/Mosby.

De Guzman, F. L. M., Moukoulou, L. N. N., Scott, L. D., & Zerwic, J. J. (2018). LGBT inclusivity in health assessment textbooks. *Journal of Professional Nursing, 34*(6), 483–487. doi:10.1016/j.profnurs.2018.03.001

Dillon, P. (2016). *Nursing health assessment: The foundation of clinical practice*. (3rd ed.). Philadelphia, PA: F. A. Davis.

Goetz, P., McHale, B. R., Gilmore, M., & Finn, M. (2016). Novice navigator: A case study on community outreach for head and neck cancers. *Journal of Oncology Navigation & Survivorship, 7*(1), 29–36.

Goolsby, M. J., & Grubbs, L. (Eds.). (2015). *Advanced health assessment: Interpreting findings and formulating differential diagnoses* (3rd ed.). Philadelphia, PA: F. A. Davis.

Hogan-Quigley, B., Palm, M. L., & Bickley, L. S. (2017). *Bates' nursing guide to physical examination and history taking*. (2nd ed.) Philadelphia, PA: Wolters Kluwer Health.

Kikkawa, I., Fujita, S., Nakama, S., Okami, H., & Hoshino, Y. (2008). A case of cervical kyphosis after a minor trauma. *European Journal of Orthopaedic Surgery & Traumatology, 18*(1), 9–13. doi:10.1007/s00590-007-0259-4

Kristoffersen, E. S., Aaseth, K., Grande, R. B., Lundqvist, C., & Russell, M. B. (2018). Psychological distress, neuroticism and disability associated with secondary chronic headache in the general population–the Akershus study of chronic headache. *Journal of Headache & Pain, 19*(1), 1–12. doi:10.1186/s10194-018-0894-7

McKee, G., Kearney, P. M., & Kenny, R. A. (2015). The factors associated with self-reported physical activity in older adults living in the community. *Age & Ageing, 44*(4), 586–592. doi:10.1093/ageing/afv042

Mona, L. R., Cameron, R. P., & Clemency Cordes, C. (2017). Disability culturally competent sexual healthcare. *American Psychologist, 72*(9), 1000–1010. doi:10.1037/amp0000283

Sambasivam, R., Liu, J., Vaingankar, J. A., Ong, H. L., Tan, M., Fauziana, R., ... Subramaniam, M. (2019). The hidden patient: Chronic physical morbidity, psychological distress, and quality of life in caregivers of older adults. *Psychogeriatrics, 19*(1), 65–72. doi:10.1111/psyg.12365

Scanlon, V., & Sanders, T. (2019). *Essentials of anatomy and physiology* (8th ed). Philadelphia, PA: F. A. Davis.

Shuman, A. G., McKiernan, J. T., Thomas, D., Patel, P., Palmer, F. L., Shaffer, B. T., ... Boyle, J. O. (2013). Outcomes of a head and neck cancer screening clinic. *Oral Oncology, 49*(12), 1136–1140. doi:10.1016/j.oraloncology.2013.09.007

Thompson, J. (2018). *Essential health assessment*. Philadelphia, PA: F. A. Davis.

3

ADVANCED HEALTH ASSESSMENT OF THE NOSE, MOUTH, AND THROAT

Jensen Lewis

(continued)

Overview of Anatomy and Physiology

NOSE

The nose is the organ of smell. It warms and moistens the inspired air and filters small foreign particles. It is a resonating chamber for speech and houses the first cranial nerve, the olfactory nerve. Its protective filtration and ciliary mechanisms are abundant. The nose includes the *external nose*, the visible portion of the respiratory system projecting from the face, and the *nasal cavities*, the internal aspect of the nose that is divided by the midline nasal septum.

The external nose's skeletal framework consists partly of bones and mainly of cartilage (Figure 3.1). The upper one-third of the nose is continuous with the skull. It is composed of the nasal process of the maxillary bones, the nasal process of the frontal bones, and the two nasal bones. The lower two-thirds of the nose is cartilaginous. It is attached to the margins of the nasal bones and maxillae and is composed of the lateral process of the septal cartilage, the major alar, and the minor alar cartilages. The nasal vestibules are the most anterior aspect of the nasal cavities. They are enclosed by cartilage and lined by skin and contains hair follicles. The two cavities of the external nose are divided by the nasal septum. The nasal cavities communicate anteriorly through the nares and posteriorly with the nasopharynx through the choana.

NASAL CAVITY

The nasal cavities are separated from each other by the nasal septum, from the mouth by the maxilla and palatine bones forming the hard palate, and from the cranium by parts of the nasal, frontal, sphenoid, and ethmoid bones. Inspired air enters through the nares and passes over squamous epithelium or mucous membranes to keep the nose moist. The mucous membranes are lined with hair cells, which also play a role as a barrier that provides protection from the invasion of infectious and allergenic pathogens. *Cilia* are embedded in the mucous layer and constantly work to sweep mucus backward and downward to the throat, reducing potentially hazardous exposure to the lungs. *Turbinates* are curved bony protuberances in the nasal cavity that

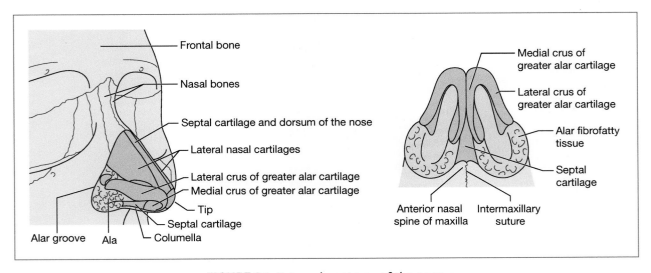

FIGURE 3.1 External anatomy of the nose.

act like shelves and create turbulence, slowing down airflow. The major function of the turbinates is to control airflow, allowing inhaled air to be warmed and moistened before reaching the lungs. The turbinates have airflow pressure and temperature-detecting nerve receptors that allow for congestion and decongestion in response to allergies, climatic conditions, or the changing needs of the body.

There are three turbinates in each nasal cavity: the inferior, middle, and superior turbinates. They divide each nasal cavity into four air channels: inferior meatus, middle meatus, superior meatus, and spheno-ethmoidal recess. Each meatus receives drainage from specific areas. The inferior meatus receives drainage from the nasolacrimal duct. The middle meatus receives drainage from the maxillary, anterior ethmoid, and frontal sinuses (Figure 3.2). The superior meatus receives drainage from the posterior ethmoid sinuses. The spheno-ethmoid recess receives drainage from some of the posterior ethmoid sinuses and the sphenoid sinuses.

NASAL SEPTUM

The nasal septum contains bone and hyaline cartilage. It is normally 2 mm thick. A deflection of the septum from midline can block or partially block the nasal cavities. A deviated septum is common; however, not all septal deviations are problematic.

BLOOD SUPPLY

The nose is well vascularized, allowing it to easily and effectively change the humidity and temperature of inspired air (Figure 3.3). The arterial supply to the nose is primarily divided into branches of the internal and external carotid arteries. Vessels originating from the *external carotid artery* include the sphenopalatine artery, greater palatine artery, superior labial artery, and lateral nasal arteries. The vessels that originate from the *internal carotid artery* are the anterior and posterior ethmoid arteries.

The arteries in the nose form anastomoses with each other. This is most prevalent in the anterior portion of the nose called *Kiesselbach's plexus* (Little's area). The anastomosis occurs between branches of the greater palatine, sphenopalatine, superior labial, and anterior ethmoidal arteries. This is the most common site for anterior epistaxis. The most common site for posterior

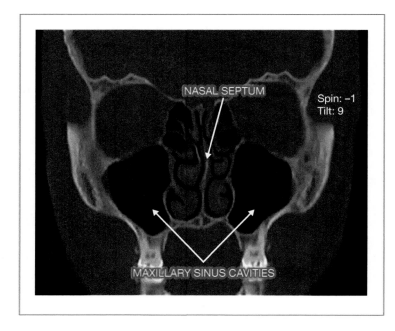

FIGURE 3.2 CT scan coronal view of the maxillary sinuses.

CT, computed tomography.

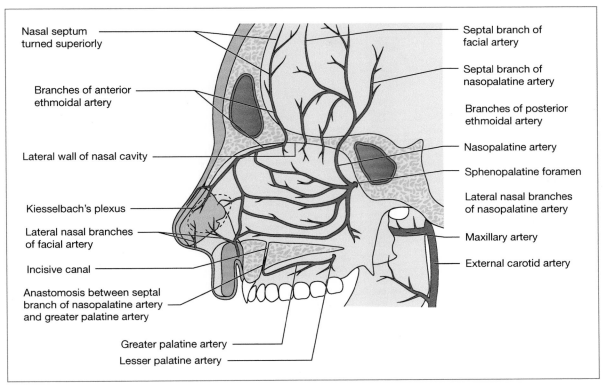

FIGURE 3.3 Arteries of the nasal cavity.

epistaxis is *Woodruff's plexus*, an anastomosis of the sphenopalatine artery and posterior pharyngeal artery.

The veins in the nose follow the path of the arteries. In some people, there are veins that join with the sagittal sinus that represent a potential pathway by which infection can spread from the nose into the cranial cavity.

LYMPHATIC DRAINAGE

Lymphatic drainage from the nose runs via the facial vessels into the neck nodes of levels I and II. The anterior one-third of the nose drains to the submental and submandibular nodes and the posterior two-thirds of the nose and sinuses drain to the retropharyngeal nodes and superior deep cervical nodes (Figure 3.4).

INNERVATION

The nasal cavity contains the following cranial nerves: olfactory nerve, trigeminal nerve, and facial nerve.

- Cranial nerve I—Olfactory: Carries the sense of smell from the olfactory mucosa in the roof of the nose back to the brain.

- Cranial nerve V—Trigeminal: Sensation in the face and motor functions, such as biting and chewing (Figure 3.5).

  o Ophthalmic branch (V_1)—Sensation to the superior aspect of the nasal cavity via the anterior ethmoidal nerve.

  o Maxillary branch (V_2)—Sensation to most of the nasal cavity via the nasopalatine and lateral nasal nerves.

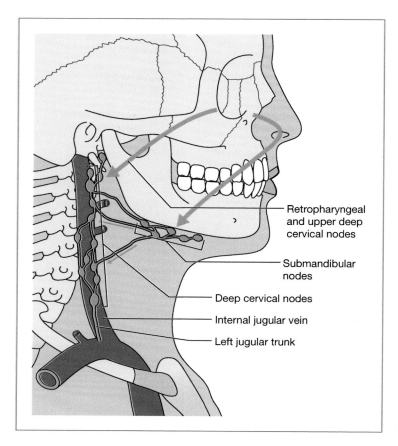

FIGURE 3.4 Lymphatic drainage of nasal cavity.

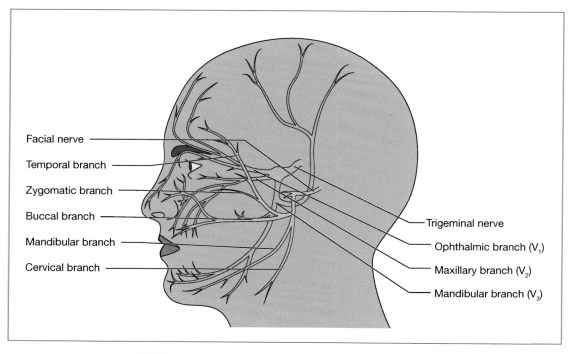

FIGURE 3.5 Trigeminal nerve and facial nerve branches.

- Cranial nerve VII—Facial: Emerges from the pons of the brainstem; controls the muscles of facial expression and functions in the conveyance of taste sensations from the anterior two-thirds of the tongue (see Figure 3.5).

- Visceral motor innervation to the nose

NASOPHARYNX

The *nasopharynx* is a noncollapsible tube in the upper part of the pharynx that connects with the nasal cavity above the soft palate (Figure 3.6).

- It continues anteriorly through the nasal cavity (choana).

- The floor of the nasopharynx is the soft palate.

- The roof of the nasopharynx is closely related to the base of the skull.

- The nasopharynx slopes downward and back and becomes contiguous with the posterior wall of the pharynx.
  - The posterior pharyngeal wall overlies the retropharyngeal space.
    - Infections in this space are deep neck infections and can cause potential for airway compromise.

- The eustachian tubes are present in the lateral aspects of the nasopharynx.
  - Nasopharyngeal masses, including hypertrophic adenoids, have the potential to block or obstruct the eustachian tubes.

- Adenoid tissue (pharyngeal tonsils) is located in the superior recess of the nasopharynx.
  - Adenoid tissue is lymphatic tissue in the posterior nasal cavity.
  - Adenoid tissue usually starts shrinking after the age of 5 and by adolescence often disappears.

- Fossa of Rosenmuller or lateral pharyngeal recess:
  - Deep recess posterior to the eustachian tube orifice in the nasopharynx
  - This is a clinically significant area for nasopharyngeal cancers.

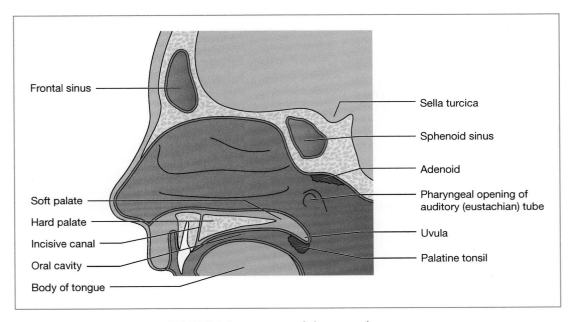

FIGURE 3.6 Anatomy of the nasopharynx.

PARANASAL SINUSES

There are four *paranasal sinuses:* the ethmoid sinuses, the sphenoid sinuses, the maxillary sinuses, and the frontal sinuses. The sinuses are named based off the bone in which they are found. They are lined with the same mucosa as the internal aspect of the nose. They open into the nasal cavity and are innervated by branches of the trigeminal nerve.

MOUTH AND THROAT

The *oral cavity* sits below the nasal cavities. It is bordered by the cheeks and lips.

PALATE

The palate forms the roof of the oral cavity and floor of the nasal cavity. It consists of both a hard and a soft palate. The soft palate has a structure called the uvula and is continuous with the palatoglossal and palatopharyngeal folds. It ensures that food moves inferiorly rather than up into the nose (velopharyngeal insufficiency).

BLOOD SUPPLY

Branches of the maxillary artery, the sphenopalatine and greater palatine artery, are the vascular makeup of the hard palate. The soft palate's vascular supply consists of the lesser palatine artery, the ascending palatine artery, and the palatine branch of the ascending pharyngeal artery.

INNERVATION

The hard palate is innervated by the nasopalatine and greater palatine nerves. General sensory innervation for the soft palate is provided by the lesser palatine nerves.

TONGUE

The tongue consists of skeletal muscle. It is covered with sensory taste buds and other nerve endings that contribute to sensation.

BLOOD SUPPLY

The lingual artery, arising from the external carotid artery, is the main vascular supply to the tongue.

INNERVATION

The tongue contains the following cranial nerves: trigeminal nerve, facial nerve, glossopharyngeal nerve, and hypoglossal nerve.

Cranial nerve V—Trigeminal:

- Mandibular branch (V_3)—Lingual nerve
  - General sensation, excluding taste, to the anterior two-thirds of the tongue

Cranial nerve VII—Facial:

- Taste to the anterior two-thirds of the tongue

Cranial nerve IX—Glossopharyngeal:

- General sensation, including taste, to the posterior one-third of the tongue

Cranial nerve XII—Hypoglossal:

- Motor to the tongue

SALIVARY GLANDS

The three glands that produce saliva are the parotid, submandibular, and sublingual glands. The parotid gland secretes saliva into the oral cavity, via Stensen's ducts, opposite the second maxillary molar. The submandibular gland secretes saliva via Wharton's ducts adjacent to the lingual frenulum. The sublingual glands secrete saliva via ducts at the base of the tongue.

TEETH AND GINGIVAE

Adults have 32 total teeth, 16 in the maxilla and 16 in the mandible. Children have 20 teeth total. Teeth are numbered in a clockwise fashion starting with the upper right maxillary molar, tooth 1, to the upper left maxillary molar, tooth 16. Tooth 17 is the left third mandibular molar and tooth 32 is the right third mandibular molar (Figure 3.7). Adults have eight incisors, four canines, eight premolars, and 12 molars.

OROPHARYNX

The *oropharynx* is posterior to the oral cavity. It is superior to the epiglottis and inferior to the soft palate. The *palatine* tonsils are located in the oropharynx. The palatine tonsils are collections of lymphoid tissue on each side of the oropharynx.

BLOOD SUPPLY

Arteries that supply the oropharynx include the ascending pharyngeal artery, the ascending palatine and tonsillar branches of the facial artery, and the maxillary and lingual arteries.

INNERVATION

Branches of the vagus and glossopharyngeal nerve are responsible for motor and sensory innervation of the oropharynx.

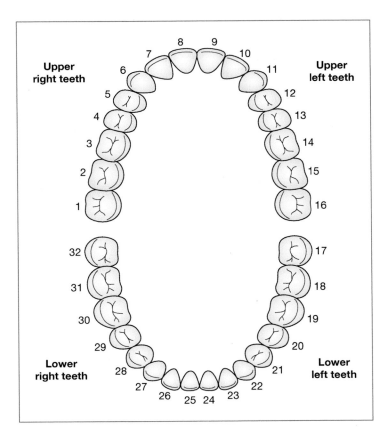

FIGURE 3.7 Numbering of adult teeth.

Screening Health Assessment and Normal Findings

NOSE

INSPECTION

Assessment of the nose should include inspection of the anterior and inferior surfaces of the nose. You should evaluate for any deformities or asymmetry of the nose. Observe for flaring. To inspect the nasal vestibule, slight pressure should be placed on the tip of the nose to widen the nares. Using a penlight, the vestibule can be evaluated for edema, erythema, and discharge. Testing for nasal obstruction involves occluding one side and asking the patient to breathe in. Breathing should be noiseless.

Using an otoscope or nasal speculum and penlight, the interior of the nose can be inspected. Tilt the patient's head back and carefully inspect the turbinates and septum. Avoid contacting the sensitive nasal septum. Inspect for septal deviation or perforation. Evaluate the color of the nasal mucosa covering the turbinates and septum. Inspect for rhinorrhea. Evaluation of the nasopharynx requires a nasal endoscopy or nasopharyngoscope.

PALPATION

The external nose should be palpated to evaluate for any step-off deformities indicative of a nasal fracture. Palpate the frontal sinuses by using your thumbs to press up under the bony brow on each side of the nose. Press up under the zygomatic processes to palpate the maxillary sinuses. *Note*: Tenderness over the frontal and maxillary sinuses, alone, does not indicate sinusitis. Sinusitis symptoms include nasal congestion, rhinorrhea, sore throat, and cough.

MOUTH AND THROAT

INSPECTION

With a penlight, inspect the lips, looking for fissures or angular cheilitis. The color of the lips should be noted as should the presence of any ulcers or cracking. Any dental appliances should be removed for a complete oral exam. After the patient clenches his or her teeth, the gingiva and teeth should be inspected, evaluating for any obvious ulcers or dental abscesses/caries. The teeth should be counted. Inspect the oral mucosa, looking for ulcers, white patches, or nodules. Inspect the palate. Inspect the sides and undersurface of the tongue. Evaluate the floor of the mouth and Wharton's ducts. Evaluate the buccal mucosa and Stensen's ducts. Inspect the oropharynx by asking the patient to say "ah" and depressing the tongue with a tongue blade. The palate and uvula should rise symmetrically. Inspect the palatine tonsils and corresponding tonsil grade (Table 3.1).

TABLE 3.1 Tonsil Grades and Definitions	
Grade	**Definition**
Grade 0	Surgically absent or entirely in fossa
Grade 1+	Occupy <25% of oropharynx
Grade 2+	Occupy <50% of oropharynx
Grade 3+	Occupy <75% of oropharynx
Grade 4+	Occupy >75% of oropharynx

PALPATION

Using gloves, the oral cavity should be palpated, evaluating for masses and other abnormalities. The tongue, floor of mouth, buccal mucosa, and tonsils should all be palpated, evaluating for occult malignancies. Gauze should be used to gently pull the tongue forward and then to each side in order to evaluate the lateral aspects of the tongue.

PERCUSSION

The teeth should be percussed, evaluating for any tenderness.

Focused Health Assessment and Abnormal Findings

When a patient presents to the provider with a focused chief complaint in the nose, mouth, or throat, the following health assessment techniques with their rationales would be performed.

NOSE

INSPECTION

Look for any edema or erythema of the external nose. A depression of the nasal bridge, known as saddlenose deformity, can occur following septal fracture or chronic septal inflammation. Respiratory distress may present with nasal flaring. The "allergic salute," a transverse crease at the junction between the cartilage and bone of the nose, indicates allergic rhinitis. Test for patency by having the patient occlude one side of his or her nose and breathe in. Assess for a septal hematoma if the patient presents after trauma. *Note*: Septal hematomas are medical emergencies that need to be treated immediately.

Inspect the nasal mucosa for changes in color or signs of discharge. Bluish gray, boggy turbinates indicate allergies. Polyps may be visible. Assess for ulcers or masses. Persistent complaints warrant ear, nose, and throat referral for specialized testing using nasopharyngoscopy/nasal endoscopy.

PALPATION

Palpate the nose, evaluating for step-off deformities, especially after trauma. Assess for induration or fluctuance.

MOUTH AND THROAT

INSPECTION

The lips should be closely evaluated for dryness or cracking, especially at the corners of the mouth (angular cheilitis). This may be seen with vitamin deficiencies. Angioedema may present with lip edema. Inspect the buccal mucosa for Fordyce spots, sebaceous glands on the buccal mucosa and lips. This is a normal variant. The tongue should protrude midline. Deviation to one side indicates atrophy and hypoglossal nerve impairment. *Note*: The tongue deviates away from the injured side of the hypoglossal nerve.

Geographic tongue, superficial denuded circles exposing the tips of the papillae, is a normal variant. Hairy tongue may be a result of antibiotic therapy. The oral cavity should be carefully inspected for masses or ulcers, especially when patients present complaining of pain or bleeding. The hard palate may reveal a torus palatinus, a bony overgrowth on the palate that is a normal variant. Inspect the tonsils for crypts or tonsiloliths. Make note of the size of the tonsils. Inspect for exudates or ulcers indicating infection. A thorough oral exam is imperative in all patients, but especially those with a smoking history.

PALPATION

The tongue should be thoroughly palpated to evaluate for masses. The dorsum of the tongue as well as the lateral borders of the tongue should be deeply palpated. The tongue should have a smooth, even texture. The floor of the mouth should be palpated, evaluating for induration or edema. This could signify a deep space neck infection such as Ludwig angina.

Holistic Assessment

When patients present with complaints regarding the nose, mouth, and throat, it is important to elicit a complete chief complaint by asking open-ended questions. The nose, mouth, and throat are intimately related to the rest of the body and obtaining an accurate, complete history will help with a differential diagnosis. Attention should be paid to the onset of the problem as well as the duration. A detailed past medical, family, and social history should be obtained for every patient. Smoking is an important risk factor in the head and neck.

SAFETY

Patients presenting with anosmia are at a significant safety risk pertaining to fire. With the inability to smell smoke, patients must be sure that they have working smoke detectors at all times. They must be able to read product dates to be sure they are not consuming expired food.

Patients presenting with dysphagia are at risk for aspiration. Those with difficulty swallowing should be evaluated by a speech and language pathologist in order to be sure that appropriate mechanisms are in place to reduce the risk of aspiration pneumonia.

DISTRESS

Patients complaining of anosmia will likely have an altered sense of taste. This can be very distressing for patients. The psychological well-being of all patients should be taken into account. Patients with a new diagnosis of oral cancer will have significant distress related to their diagnosis. Patients should be counseled on diet and exercise, especially when dysphagia related to the diagnosis occurs.

NUTRITION AND EXERCISE

Patients with obstructive sleep apnea need to be counseled on the need for adequate diet and exercise to achieve weight loss. Patients who have oropharyngeal carcinoma will need to supplement diet and possibly have a feeding tube placed to use while undergoing treatment.

FINANCIAL IMPLICATIONS

A thorough history should include financial implications due to morbid diagnoses.

SPIRITUAL CONSIDERATIONS

Ask the patient how he or she deals with difficult times, and if the patient has a support system. Self-care is a must.

CASE STUDY

DOCUMENTATION

Chief complaint: Nasal congestion, rhinorrhea

History of the present illness: Onset 5 days ago. Has progressively gotten worse. Complains of nasal congestion and rhinorrhea. Rhinorrhea is white. No blood. Pseudoephedrine (Sudafed) has worked to relieve the congestion but returns quickly. No cough. No sore throat.

REVIEW OF SYSTEMS

Constitutional: No complaints of fevers, chills, night sweats, or weight loss

Integumentary: No rashes

Neurological: No headache or blurred vision

Ear, nose, and throat: Nasal congestion, rhinorrhea. Denies epistaxis. No sore throat or dysphagia. No voice change.

PHYSICAL EXAMINATION

General: No acute distress, mouth breathing

Head and face: Normocephalic, atraumatic

Ears: Tympanic membrane translucent without signs of middle ear effusion. Mobile on pneumatoscopy.

Nose: Erythematous, edematous inferior turbinates, bilaterally. Mucoid rhinorrhea. No purulence.

Oropharynx: Tonsils 2+ without exudates or erythema. No purulent postnasal drip.

Diagnosis: Acute upper respiratory infection

ICD-10-CM Diagnosis Code: J06.9 Acute Upper Respiratory Infection, Unspecified

Assessment of Special Populations

 PEDIATRIC POPULATION

The external nose should have a symmetric appearance and be positioned on the midline of the face. Chromosomal disorders may present with a saddle-shaped nose. Small amounts of clear discharge will likely be seen in crying infants when examining the internal nose. If infants have any difficulty breathing through their nose, a catheter should be placed to rule out choanal atresia. Exam of the sinuses is generally unnecessary in infants as they are underdeveloped.

Evaluate for cleft palate or lip. Calluses may form on the upper lips from sucking. It is easier to evaluate the oropharynx when an infant is crying. Between 6 weeks and 6 months of age, drooling is common. If the tongue does not protrude beyond the alveolar ridge, the patient is suffering from ankyloglossia. The frenulum should be divided to help with suckling and with speech as the infant ages. You should evaluate the patient's suck by placing a gloved finger into the mouth.

Children will most often resist nasal and oral examinations. It may be beneficial to hold off on these until the end of the exam. It may help to have the patient sit on a parent's lap during the evaluation to ensure a secure feeling. You may need to immobilize the patient if he or she is unable to sit still even on a parent's lap. Allowing the patient to play with the tongue depressor and penlight may foster a rapport and allow you to examine the oral cavity completely.

 ELDERLY POPULATION

The mucosa of the nose may become dryer as the patient ages. Lips will also be dryer. The tongue may be fissured. Pay close attention to the patient's dentition to evaluate for caries.

 PREGNANT POPULATION

Increased vascularity of pregnancy will cause edema and erythema of the nose and pharynx. This can lead to nasal congestion. Increased estrogen may lead to an increase in secretions. Nosebleeds may be common.

Diagnostic Reasoning

Common Differential Diagnoses: Nose	
Diagnosis	**Key History or Physical Examination Differentiators**
Allergic rhinitis	Clear rhinorrhea with boggy turbinates; possible polyps; sneezing
Cerebrospinal fluid leakage	Unilateral watery discharge after head trauma or sinus surgery; salty or metallic taste in mouth
Epistaxis	Bloody discharge; crusting anterior septum

(continued)

Common Differential Diagnoses: Nose (*continued*)	
Diagnosis	**Key History or Physical Examination Differentiators**
Foreign body	Unilateral, thick, purulent discharge
Sinusitis	Nasal congestion, purulent rhinorrhea, sore throat, cough; rare headache
Upper respiratory infection	Mucoid or purulent discharge
Vestibulitis	Erythema, tenderness to anterior septum and nasal vestibule; purulent crusting

Common Differential Diagnoses: Mouth and Throat	
Diagnosis	**Key History or Physical Examination Differentiators**
Angioedema	"Watery" edema of the lips, floor of mouth, tongue, palate
Angular cheilitis (Figure 3.8)	Cracked lips at the corners; vitamin deficiency
Diphtheria	Gray "pseudomembrane"; sore throat
Fordyce spots (Figure 3.11)	Numerous small, yellow-white, raised lesions
Leukoedema	Diffuse filmy grayish surface with white streaks, wrinkles, or milky alteration
Measles (Figure 3.10)	Koplik spots—white lesions on buccal mucosa opposite 1st and 2nd molars
Peritonsillar abscess	"Hot-potato voice"; bulging soft palate; uvular deviation
Peutz–Jeghers syndrome (Figure 3.9)	Round, oval, bluish gray macules on lips/buccal mucosa
Phenytoin use	Gingival hyperplasia
Ranula	Obstructed sublingual gland; soft, mobile, unilateral floor of mouth edema
Strep pharyngitis	Tonsillar exudates, lack of cough, anterior cervical lymphadenopathy, fever (Centor criteria)
Torus mandibularis	Bony protuberance along the lingual surface of the mandible—normal variant
Torus palatinus	Bony protuberance at the midline—normal variant
Viral tonsillitis/Pharyngitis	Tonsillar or pharyngeal ulcers with clean base

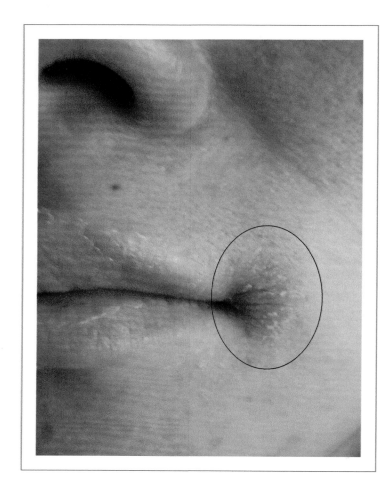

FIGURE 3.8 Angular cheilitis.
Source: Courtesy of James Heilman.

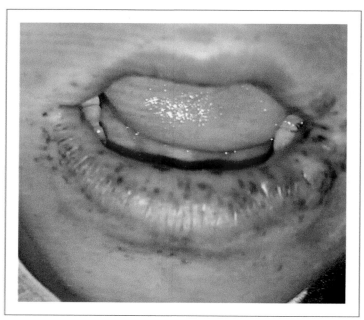

FIGURE 3.9 Peutz–Jeghers syndrome.
Source: Courtesy of Massryy.

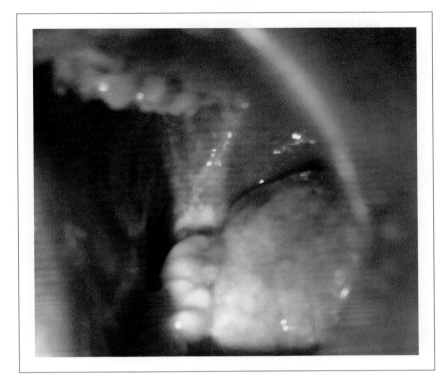

FIGURE 3.10 Koplik spots seen in measles.
Source: Dctrzl. (2019).

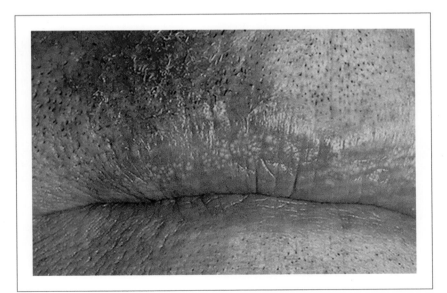

FIGURE 3.11 Fordyce spots.
Source: Courtesy of Perene.

BIBLIOGRAPHY

Andreeff, R. (2016). Epistaxis. *Journal of the American Academy of Physician Assistants*, *29*(1), 46–47. doi:10.1097/01.jaa.0000473373.47749.5f

Jeghers, H., Mckusick, V. A., & Katz, K. H. (1949). Generalized intestinal polyposis and melanin spots of the oral mucosa, lips and digits. *New England Journal of Medicine*, *241*(26), 1031–1036. doi:10.1056/nejm194912292412601

Madani, M., Berardi, T., & Stoopler, E. T. (2014). Anatomic and examination considerations of the oral cavity. *Medical Clinics of North America*, *98*(6), 1225–1238. doi:10.1016/j .mcna.2014.08.001

Ng, M. L., Warlow, R. S., Chrishanthan, N., Ellis, C., & Walls, R. (2000). Preliminary criteria for the definition of allergic rhinitis: A systematic evaluation of clinical parameters in a disease cohort (I). *Clinical Experimental Allergy*, *30*(9), 1314–1331. doi:10.1046/j.1365-2222.2000.00853.x

Patel, R. (2017). Nasal anatomy and function. *Facial Plastic Surgery*, *33*(01), 3–8. doi:10.1055/s-0036-1597950

Rosenfeld, R. M., Piccirillo, J. F., Chandrasekhar, S. S., Brook, I., Kumar, K. A., Kramper, M., … Corrigan, M. D. (2015). Clinical practice guideline (Update): Adult sinusitis. *Otolaryngology–Head and Neck Surgery*, *152*(2 Suppl.), S1–S39. doi:10.1177/ 0194599815572097

4

ADVANCED HEALTH ASSESSMENT OF THE EYES AND EARS

Kristen Marie Guida

CHAPTER CONTENTS

(continued)

DIAGNOSTIC REASONING: EYE

    Common Differential Diagnoses: Ocular Complaints

OVERVIEW OF ANATOMY AND PHYSIOLOGY OF THE EAR

    External Ear

    Middle Ear

    Inner Ear

SCREENING HEALTH ASSESSMENT AND NORMAL FINDINGS OF THE EAR

    Health History

    Physical Examination

    Hearing Acuity

FOCUSED HEALTH ASSESSMENT AND ABNORMAL FINDINGS OF THE EAR

    Abnormalities of the External Ear

    Abnormalities of the Ear Canal

    Abnormalities of the Tympanic Membrane

HOLISTIC HEALTH ASSESSMENT OF THE EAR

CASE STUDY: EAR

ASSESSMENT OF SPECIAL POPULATIONS: EAR

    Gestational Population

    Pediatric Population

    Young Adult Population

    Elderly Population

    Patients With Disabilities

    Veteran Population

DIAGNOSTIC REASONING: EAR

    Common Differential Diagnoses: Ear

Overview of Anatomy and Physiology of the Eye

Out of the five senses, people rely most on their vision. Visual receptors contained within the human eye allow us to perceive illumination as well as generate comprehensive optical images. During the first 8 weeks of gestation, the eye forms. Congenital malformation can occur with fetal exposure to maternal infection or ingestion of drugs. Vision develops over a greater time period and is reliant on nervous system development and maturation. Visual acuity in a full-term infant is less than 20/400, making them hyperopic. Peripheral vision is present at birth, whereas central vision develops over time. The lacrimal gland produces lacrimation by 2 to 3 weeks of age. The development of binocular vision is complete by 4 months. Color differentiation adequately develops by the age of 6 months. The eyes develop and grow simultaneously with the head and brain. Adult visual acuity is attained at approximately 4 years of age.

The external eye is composed of the palpebrae, conjunctiva, lacrimal gland, eye muscles, and the bony skull orbit (Figure 4.1). The adjunct structures of the eye include the palpebrae or eyelids, the superficial epithelium of the eye, and the structures associated with the regulation of production, secretion, and removal of lacrimation or tears (Figure 4.2).

PALPEBRAE

The palpebrae act as a protective mechanism, keeping the surface of the eye free from debris and well lubricated as the palpebrae open and close (blinking; Figure 4.3). The eyelids can close tightly to preserve the sensitive surface of the eye. The free margins of the upper and lower palpebrae are separated by the palpebral fissure, but the two are connected at the medial canthus and the lateral canthus. Eyelashes line the palpebral margins, serving to protect the surface of the eye from foreign bodies such as debris and insects.

EYELASHES

The eyelashes are short, thick, curved, and more numerous on the upper eyelid (approximately 150 in the upper lid and 75 in the lower). Eyelashes are generally darker than the scalp hairs, do not gray with age, and are replaced every 100 to 150 days. The hair follicles are arranged in two or three rows along the anterior edge of the eyelids and do not possess erector pili muscles. The eyelashes are associated with large sebaceous glands of Zeis, which open

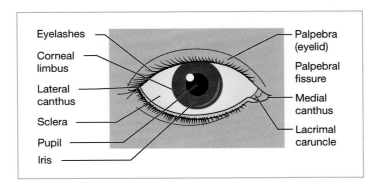

Eyelashes
Corneal limbus
Lateral canthus
Sclera
Pupil
Iris

Palpebra (eyelid)
Palpebral fissure
Medial canthus
Lacrimal caruncle

FIGURE 4.1 External anatomy and accessory structures of the eye.

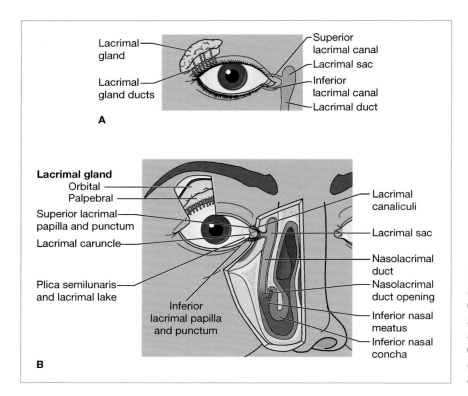

FIGURE 4.2 The lacrimal apparatus of the eye. (**A**) External anatomy and anterior view of the lacrimal apparatus of the eye. (**B**) External anatomy and dissection of the lacrimal apparatus of the eye.

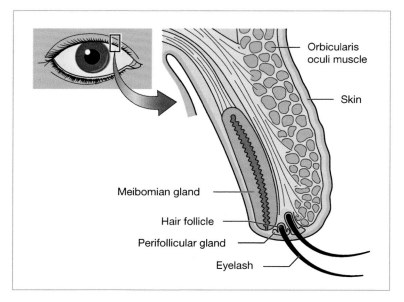

FIGURE 4.3 Glands associated with the palpebrae.

into each follicle. Along the inner margin of the lid, Meibomian glands secrete a lipid-rich product that helps to keep the eyelids from affixing together. At the medial canthus, the lacrimal caruncle contains glands producing the thick secretions that contribute to the naturally occurring mucous discharge known as rheum, sometimes found after a good night's sleep.

PALPEBRAL CONJUNCTIVA

The skin covering the visible surface of the palpebrae is very thin. The conjunctiva is the epithelium covering the inner surfaces of the eyelids and the outer surface of the eye. It is a mucous membrane covered by a specialized stratified squamous epithelium. The palpebral conjunctiva covers the inner surface of the eyelids, and the ocular conjunctiva, or bulbar conjunctiva, covers the anterior surface of the eye, extending to the edges of the transparent cornea. The cornea is covered by a very thin and delicate squamous corneal epithelium that is continuous with the ocular conjunctiva.

LACRIMAL GLAND

The lacrimal gland found in the temporal region of the superior palpebrae produces lacrimation or tears (see Figure 4.2). Lacrimation helps reduce friction, remove debris, prevent bacterial infection, and provide nutrients and oxygen to portions of the conjunctival epithelium. A constant supply of fluid washes over the surface of the eye, keeping the ocular conjunctiva and cornea moist and clean.

EXTRAOCULAR EYE MOVEMENT

There are six eye muscles that support movement of the eye: the superior, inferior, medial, and lateral rectus muscles and the superior and inferior oblique muscles (Figure 4.4). Three cranial nerves are responsible for the movement of the extraocular muscles (Table 4.1). Cranial nerve VI, the abducens nerve, innervates the lateral rectus muscles, which abducts the eye. Cranial nerve IV, the trochlear nerve, innervates the superior oblique muscle, and cranial nerve III, the oculomotor nerve, innervates the rest: superior, inferior, medial rectus, and the inferior oblique muscles.

INTERNAL EYE STRUCTURES

The internal eye is composed of three separate areas. The cornea comprises the anterior outer surface and the sclera forms the posterior outer portion (Figure 4.5).

The eye is a hollow sphere with the interior divided into two cavities. The large posterior cavity is also called the vitreous chamber because it contains the gelatinous vitreous body. The smaller anterior cavity is subdivided into two chambers,

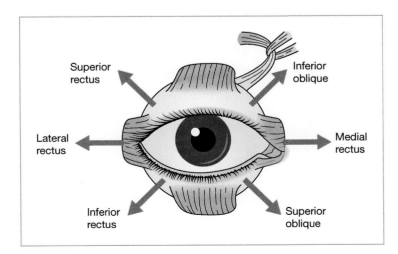

FIGURE 4.4 Extraocular eye movement. Six eye muscles support movement of the eye: the superior, inferior, medial, and lateral rectus muscles and the superior and inferior oblique muscles.

TABLE 4.1
Extraocular Muscles and Cranial Innervation

Muscles	Innervation	Primary Function
Superior rectus	CN III (oculomotor)	Elevation, maximal on lateral gaze
Inferior rectus	CN III (oculomotor)	Depression, maximal on lateral gaze
Medial rectus	CN III (oculomotor)	Adduction
Lateral rectus	CN VI (abducens)	Abduction
Superior oblique	CN IV (trochlear)	Depression, maximal on medial gaze
Inferior oblique	CN III (oculomotor)	Elevation, maximal on medial gaze

CN, cranial nerve.

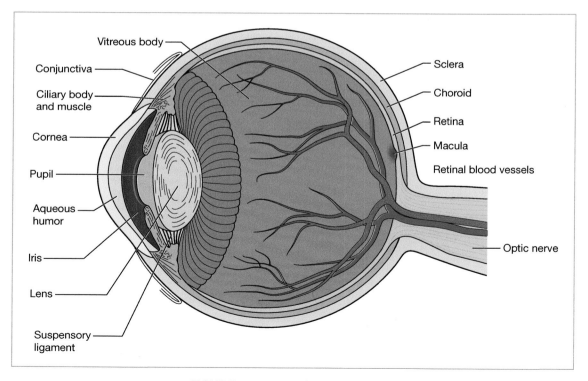

FIGURE 4.5 Internal eye structures.

the anterior and posterior. The shape of the eye is stabilized in part by the vitreous body and the clear aqueous humor that fills the anterior cavity. Within the anterior cavity, aqueous humor circulates, passing from the posterior to the anterior chamber via the pupil of the eye.

The sclera covers most of the ocular surface. The sclera, which is the white of the eye, consists of a dense fibrous connective tissue containing both collagen and elastic fibers. The cornea is transparent and is structurally continuous with the sclera. The cornea consists primarily of a dense matrix containing multiple layers of collagen fibers. There are no blood vessels in the cornea and the superficial epithelial cells must obtain oxygen and nutrients from the tears that flow across their free surfaces. The lens lies behind the cornea and is held in place by suspensory ligaments that originate on the ciliary body of the choroid. The primary function of the lens is to focus the visual image on the retinal photoreceptors. It does so by changing its shape.

The iris, which is visible through the transparent corneal surface, contains blood vessels, pigment cells, and two layers of smooth muscle fibers (Figure 4.6). The pupil, or central opening, of the iris changes diameter when these muscles contract. One group of smooth muscle fibers forms a series of concentric circles around the pupil. The diameter of the pupil decreases when these pupillary constrictor muscles contract.

The retina contains photoreceptors that respond to light, which generate nerve impulses that travel along the optic nerve to the brain, where a visual image is created.

There are two types of photoreceptors: rods and cones (Figure 4.6). Rods are light sensitive and enable us to see in dimly lit rooms, at twilight, or in pale moonlight. Cones provide us with color vision.

The highest concentration of cones is found in the central portion of the macula lutea, an area called the fovea (Figure 4.7A). The optic disc is a circular region just lateral to the fovea. The optic disc is the origin of the optic nerve CN II. These areas can be assessed with an ophthalmoscope during the examination of the eye (Figure 4.7B).

VISUAL PATHWAY

The visual pathway (Figure 4.8) commences as light passes through the translucent components of the eye (cornea, lens, aqueous humor, and vitreous

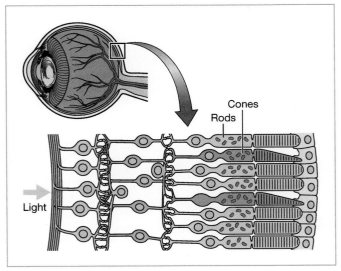

FIGURE 4.6 Inner eye structures: rods and cones.

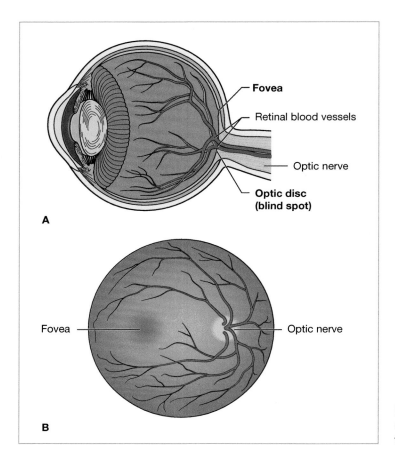

FIGURE 4.7 Inner eye structures: fovea and optic disc. (**A**) Anatomy. (**B**) As visualized through an ophthalmoscope.

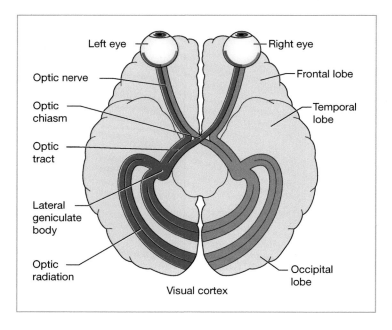

FIGURE 4.8 Visual pathway.

body) and reaches the retina. Images in the brain are interpreted as the retina transforms the light into neuronal impulses that move through the optic nerve and optic tract to the brain. The retinal image is originally inverted and reversed right to left as it travels through the lens. An image in the upper temporal visual field of the right eye will reflect onto the lower nasal portion of the retina. The optic chiasm is the point at which the optic nerves from each eye cross over to the opposite side. The right optic tract has only nerve fibers from the left half of each retina. As a consequence, the right side of the brain sees images only from the left side of view and vice versa.

FIELDS OF VISION

The field of vision or visual field is the area or range in which objects are visible to the stationary eye (fixed gaze; Figure 4.9). The visual field of each eye can be partitioned into four quadrants: upper nasal, lower nasal and upper temporal, and lower temporal. The nasal quadrants are slightly smaller than the temporal quadrants, and these visual fields overlap, resulting in a slightly different view of the same visual field. This allows for depth perception, as well as binocular and peripheral vision.

VISUAL REFLEXES

Pupillary constriction in response to light is known as the pupillary light reflex. Upon exposure to light, whether consensually or indirect, the pupillary light reflex can be elicited. Exposure to light in one eye causes the pupil in the contralateral eye to constrict concurrently. In order to prevent excess light exposure, a subcortical reflex is mediated by cranial nerve III to protect the specialized photoreceptor cells of the retina.

The ciliary muscles, which are innervated by cranial nerve III, contract, causing a curvature of the lens; this is also known as accommodation. It is a reflex that allows the eye to focus on near objects. This results in the pupils accommodating themselves to objects at close range by constricting and to those farther away by dilating. This reflex cannot be directly observed but can be indirectly assessed when pupillary constriction and convergence (movement toward) of the eyes occur simultaneously.

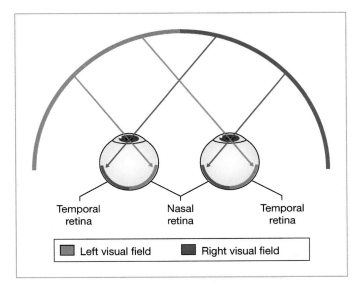

FIGURE 4.9 Fields of vision.

Screening Health Assessment and Normal Findings of the Eye

When conducting a health assessment and physical exam, it is important to elicit a complete health history by querying the patient on the following elements.

HISTORY OF THE PRESENT ILLNESS

- Palpebrae: Recurrent hordeola, ptosis, pruritus, lesions, or masses
- Visual difficulties:
  - One eye/both eyes
  - Near/far vision, peripheral vision, central vision
  - Floaters
  - Diplopia, adequacy of color vision, halos around lights
- Pain/Swelling:
  - Loss of vision with eye pain
  - Duration of eye pain
  - Sensation: Burning, stabbing, crushing, throbbing, itching, or something stuck in eye
- Exudate:
  - Green, yellow, clear, mucous, or purulent
  - Constant tearing or watering
  - Palpebrae stuck together
- Medication history: Eye drops or preparations, exposures, contacts, antibiotics, glaucoma, or ocular agents

PAST MEDICAL HISTORY

- History of eye, laser, or cataract surgery
- Ocular trauma/retinal detachment: Events leading to the trauma

- Chronic illness: Diabetes, glaucoma, allergies, atherosclerotic heart disease, hypertension, HIV, collagen vascular diseases, thyroid dysfunction, or inflammatory bowel disease
- Medications: Beta-blockers, plaquenil, antihistamines, antipsychotics, antidepressants, or antiarrhythmics

FAMILY HISTORY

- Nearsightedness, farsightedness, amblyopia, or strabismus
- Retinoblastoma or cancer of the retina
- Glaucoma, diabetes, macular degeneration, or hypertension
- Color blindness, retinal detachment, cataract formation, or retinitis pigmentosa

SOCIAL HISTORY

- Seasonal/medicinal allergies: Associated symptoms
- Occupational exposures:
  - Foreign body exposure, gas, irritants, or high-speed machinery
  - Use of protective ocular wear
- Hobbies or sports that could result in eye trauma: Riding a motorcycle, squash, fencing, or racquetball
- Use of contacts/glasses:
  - Appropriate prescription and date of last optometrist exam
  - Proper handling of contacts and recommended duration of wear
- Hazardous activities: Use of eye protection
- Cigarette smoking: Current or past

PEDIATRIC POPULATION

- Birth:
  - Preterm/full term
  - Exposure to oxygen or ventilator
  - Diagnosis of retinopathy, prematurity, intracranial hemorrhage, or cerebral palsy
- Failure of infant to gaze at mother or other objects; failure to blink to bright lights
- Absence of red eye reflex: White area in the pupil of a photograph or on examination; inability of eye to reflex light properly
- Excessive discharge or tearing
- Strabismus: Frequency, time of day, and duration
- Itching/frequent rubbing of the eyes, frequent hordeola, or inability to see objects
- Poor progress in school not related to intellectual ability; having to sit at the front of the room

PREGNANT WOMEN

- Gestation: Weeks
- Postpartum status
- Current diagnosis of hypertension or diabetes
- Use of ophthalmic eye drops
- Pregnancy-induced hypertension (PIH), diplopia, scotomata, or amaurosis fugax

ELDERLY POPULATION

- Nocturnal eye discomfort/pain
- Difficulty completing tasks without lenses
- Dry eyes
- Development of brown spots on the sclera
- Change in visual acuity: Central vision, distortion of central vision, glare, presence of halos, or floaters
- Excessive tearing

PHYSICAL EXAMINATION

SUGGESTED EQUIPMENT FOR AN OCULAR EXAM

- Ophthalmoscope
- Penlight
- Cotton-tipped applicator
- Snellen eye chart
- E chart
- Rosenbaum near-vision pocket screening card
- Amsler grid
- Vision occluder

VISUAL INSPECTION OF EXTERNAL EYES

Next, the provider will conduct a visual inspection of the external eyes. The provider will inspect the eyes, observing for any asymmetry, ptosis, exudate, and erythema (Figure 4.10). Eyelashes and eyebrows should be inspected for equal hair distribution. Unequal hair distribution could denote an underlying endocrine disorder. Visual inspection should continue with the provider holding a raised finger 12 inches from the patient's nose. The provider should instruct the patient to follow his or her finger with the eyes by keeping his or her head straight. The provider will move a finger in a downward fashion, observing for symmetrical eye movement, assessing sclera (should appear white), and evaluating blinking of the eyes. The patient should next be instructed to raise his or her eyelids. The palpebrae should cover the superior curve of the iris.

LACRIMAL GLAND

The provider should perform a visual inspection of the outside of the lacrimal gland of both eyes, at the upper palpebrae. Visual inspection includes noting any erythema, exudate, edema,

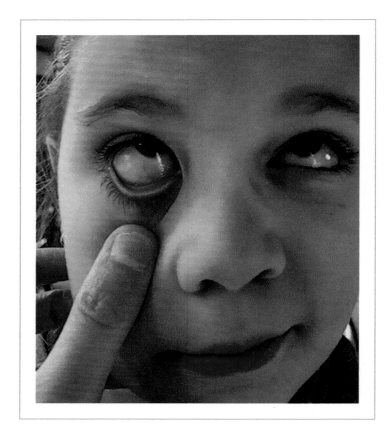

FIGURE 4.10 Visual inspection of the external eye.

or lacrimation. Abnormal findings would be the presence of exudate, erythema, or tenderness. Infection or obstruction should be suspected in the setting of inflammation. Wearing gloves, the provider should palpate the lacrimal gland at the inner canthus.

EXTRAOCULAR EYE MOVEMENTS

Ocular movement is controlled and coordinated by six muscles. Testing of these six muscles is performed by assessing corneal light reflex, cover/uncover test, and cardinal fields of gaze. This assesses function of cranial nerves III, IV, and VI.

CORNEAL LIGHT REFLEX (HIRSCHBERG TEST)

The provider has the patient focus by looking straight ahead. Holding a penlight approximately 14 inches from the patient's eyes, the provider shines the penlight into the center of each of the corneas (Figure 4.11). The reaction should be equal muscle response. If the provider observes corneal light reflex asymmetry, it could be indicative of a neurological cause and may warrant further evaluation and treatment.

COVER/UNCOVER TEST

The provider has the patient focus on an object beyond the provider. The patient places the occluder over the left eye for several seconds (Figure 4.12). As the patient is performing this task, the provider is observing the uncovered eye for movement. Have the patient switch to the right eye and repeat. Next, have the patient focus on an object held close to the eye. Coordinated movement with both eyes is considered normal. Nystagmus is an abnormal finding and should not be present. Marginal eye muscle weakness may cause misalignment or drifting of the eyes.

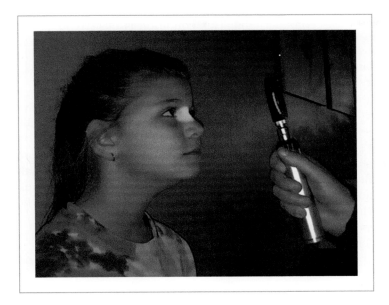

FIGURE 4.11 Hirschberg test.

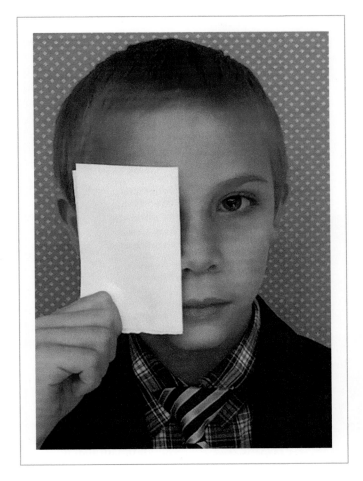

FIGURE 4.12 Cover/uncover test.

CARDINAL FIELDS OF GAZE

As the patient remains in a seated position, he or she is instructed to keep his or her head straight and follow the provider's finger with his or her eyes (Figure 4.13). The provider is evaluating the patient's ocular movement in assessing the superior, inferior, lateral, and medial rectus ocular muscles as well as the superior and inferior obliques. The provider returns to the midline before assessing each field. Movement of the eyes through these six fields should be smooth and coordinated. The final movement would be to assess for convergence, which has the patient focusing on the provider's finger as the provider brings it 6 inches from the patient's nose. The eyes should converge.

ANTERIOR STRUCTURES OF THE EYE

With fingers on the palpebra, the provider should assess the conjunctiva (Figure 4.14). The patient is instructed to look down and up. It is important to pay close attention to the bulbar conjunctiva, assessing for foreign bodies, erythema, exudate, or edema. Small blood vessels should be visible within the conjunctiva and it should be white. If there is the presence of palpebra swelling or edema, and exudate, it may be suggestive of bacterial conjunctivitis. This condition is best treated with ocular anti-infective drops. Upon visual inspection, the sclera should appear white. Icteric sclera, or blue sclera, are abnormal physical exam findings and warrant further investigation.

Next, the provider should assess the upper inner palpebra by asking the patient to gaze down while the eyelashes are pulled gently downward and forward to break the suction between the palpebra and the globe. Next, evert the palpebra on a small cotton-covered applicator. Ask the patient to look up while applying downward pressure against the eyelid (Figure 4.15).

CORNEA

The cornea can be assessed by shining a penlight directly over each eye. The corneal surface should appear smooth, free of debris or ulceration, and shiny. The cornea is avascular and blood vessels should not be present. Cranial nerve V (trigeminal nerve) controls corneal sensitivity. Assessment of cranial nerve V is tested by touching a wisp of cotton to the cornea (Figure 4.16). The anticipated reaction is to blink, which requires intact sensory fibers of cranial nerve V and motor fibers of cranial nerve VII (facial nerve). A decreased corneal sensation is often associated with herpes simplex infection.

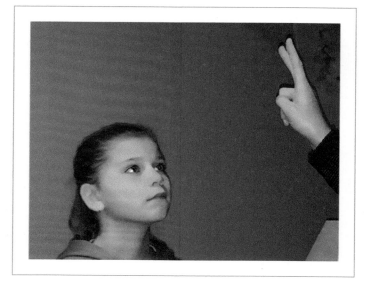

FIGURE 4.13 Assessment of cardinal fields of gaze.

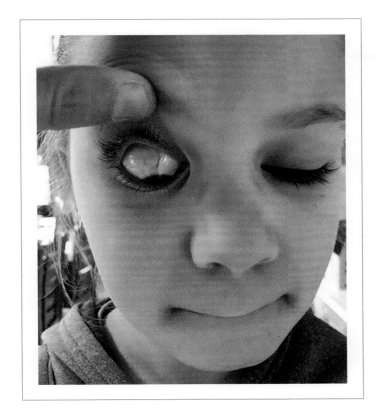

FIGURE 4.14 Assessment of sclera.

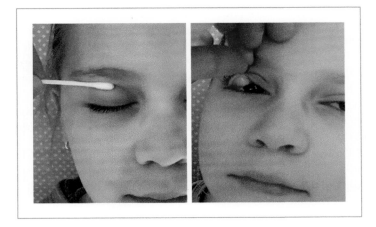

FIGURE 4.15 Eversion of the upper eyelid for inspection.

IRIS

The iris should be visually inspected next. The provider should shine the penlight in each eye, paying close attention to the vascularity, color, and texture (should be smooth). Melanoma should be a consideration if there is variation of the pigment or raised areas. As such, a referral should be made for further work up and evaluation by an optometrist.

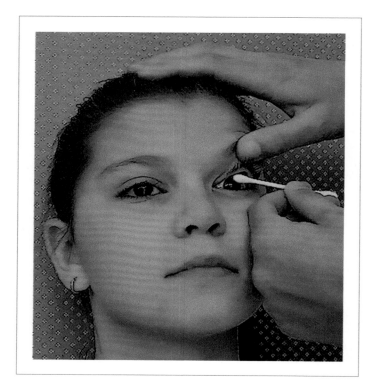

FIGURE 4.16 Testing corneal sensitivity by touching a wisp of cotton to the cornea.

PUPIL

Pupillary response is an important ocular assessment. The provider darkens the room and observes the size and shape of both pupils. Continuing with the penlight, the provider moves the light from the side to the center of the right pupil and back to the side. The provider should observe the direct light response including constriction of the pupil, speed of response, and size of the right pupil (Figure 4.17). The provider repeats the same procedure with the right pupil, but this time looks for consensual response in the left eye. The provider performs this entire exam on the left pupil.

In testing for accommodation, the patient should focus on an object beyond the provider. Next, the provider should ask the patient to focus on the penlight, which should be held 5 inches from the patient's nose. Note the pupils' size and ability to converge. The pupillary size ranges from 2 mm to 6 mm. Response should be brisk and equivalent. Ability for accommodation, far to near, measures cranial nerve III. A miotic response (pupil 2 mm) or

mydriatic response (>6 mm) suggests medications such as sympathomimetic or cranial nerve III paralysis from carotid artery insufficiency. A pupil that is irregularly shaped could indicate removal of an iridectomy or cataract. Optic nerve damage or injury, or a brain lesion, can cause a vacillating response to light.

The lens is positioned behind the pupil. When shining a penlight on the pupil, the lens should appear clear/transparent.

POSTERIOR STRUCTURES OF THE EYE

The ability to visualize the posterior structures of the eye requires utilization of an ophthalmoscope (Figure 4.18). In a darkened room, have the patient focus on an object in the distance. Shine the light (lens set at O) of the ophthalmoscope at a 15-degree angle in the patient's eye. Stay 12 inches from the patient; the light of the ophthalmoscope reflects off the retina. The diopter wheel should be moved from 0 to +, or black numbers, to bring ocular

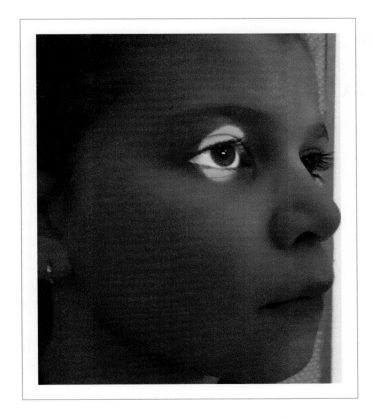

FIGURE 4.17 Assessment of pupillary response.

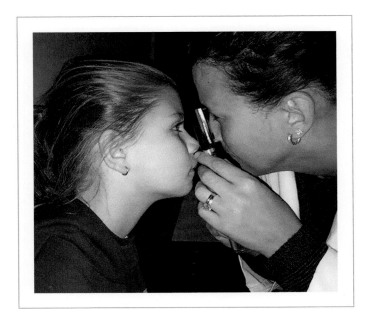

FIGURE 4.18 Use of an ophthalmoscope.

structures into focus. To visualize the optic disc, move in closer to the patient, approximately 1 inch from the patient's eye. Move the diopter to the negative or red numbers. The optic disc is best visualized toward the nasal side of the retina. Assess the retina for color and lesions. Pay close attention to the optic disc describing the size, margins, color, and shape. Perform this exam on both eyes. The optic disc should appear pinkish with a yellow-white center. Cup-to-disc diameter is about 1:3. Four major vascular branches should be evident.

MACULA

The macula is visualized by moving the ophthalmoscope from the optic disc over about 2 disc diameters. The macula is not easily identifiable because it is not sharply delineated. The fovea centralis is located central to the macula and is

light sensitive. While a healthy macula will appear darker, the fovea centralis will appear like a point with a reflective center.

ASSESSMENT OF VISUAL ACUITY

Assessment of visual acuity tests the second cranial nerve. Using a Snellen eye chart (Figure 4.19), have the patient stand 20 feet away. If the patient wears eyeglasses, have him or her remove them and use the vision occluder to cover one eye. The patient is asked to read as many lines on the chart as possible. If the patient is unable to read the largest print at 20 feet, ask him or her to move closer and note the distance, in feet, from the chart. Repeat this procedure with the opposite eye. The test is also performed with the patient wearing glasses. Results are charted as visual

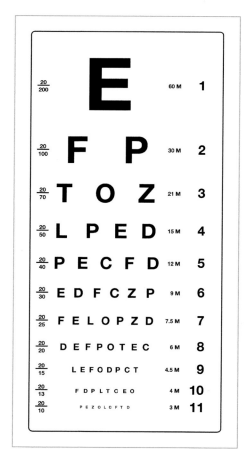

FIGURE 4.19 Snellen eye chart.

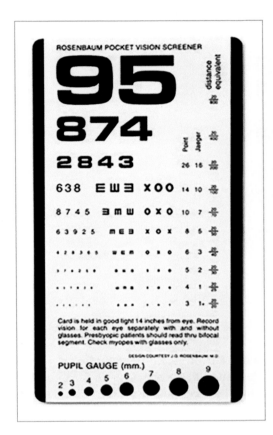

FIGURE 4.20 Rosenbaum pocket eye vision card.

acuity corrected (with glasses) and uncorrected (without glasses). To score visual acuity, use the number at the end of the last line that the patient is able to read. Normal visual acuity is considered 20/20 vision in each eye. When utilizing a Snellen eye chart, it is not uncommon for a patient to have myopia or nearsightedness. Visual acuity may also be different in each eye. The Snellen eye chart can also be useful for assessing color vision, by having the patient identify the six primary colors present on the chart.

The Rosenbaum card is used to test for farsightedness (Figure 4.20). The patient is positioned comfortably in a chair or on the exam table, given the card, and instructed to hold the card 14 inches from the face. The patient is instructed to read the smallest line possible.

ASSESSMENT OF VISUAL FIELDS

Cranial nerve II is assessed by testing visual fields and the degree of peripheral vision (Figure 4.21). The patient sits in a chair 2 to 3 feet in opposition from the provider. The provider asks the patient to cover his or her left eye as the provider covers his or her right eye. The patient should focus on the provider's uncovered eye. The provider then places his or her hand within the patient's line of vision at the level of the nose. The provider moves two fingers to the superior, inferior, oblique, and temporal angles. These angles follow four imaginary quadrants. The provider asks the patient to say "Yes" when the patient can visualize the movement of fingers in his or her visual field. Then both the provider and the patient switch covering eyes,

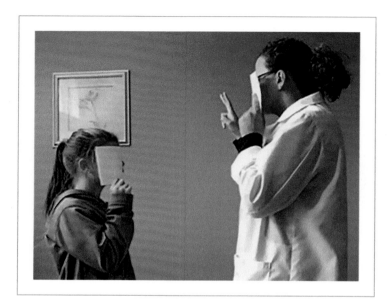

FIGURE 4.21 Assessment of cranial nerve II.

with the patient now covering his or her right eye and the provider now covering his or her left eye. The process is then repeated. If the patient is unable to visualize the provider's fingers during assessment of visual fields, it could represent an underlying health concern such as cerebrovascular accident, retinal detachment, macular degeneration, or glaucoma.

Focused Health Assessment and Abnormal Findings of the Eye

When assessing vision with a Snellen vision screen and the individual's visual acuity falls below 20/200, even with the help of glasses or contact lenses, the individual is considered to be legally blind. Common causes of blindness include accidental injuries, cataracts, corneal scarring, diabetes, glaucoma, retinal detachment, and hereditary factors.

Arcus senilis: Caused by lipid deposits and is commonly seen around the cornea as a gray-white arc or circle around the limbus (Figure 4.22).

Blepharitis: Inflammation of the palpebrae (Figure 4.23). The palpebrae has the appearance of red, scaly, and greasy flakes with crusted lid margins. Blepharitis can be caused by seborrheic dermatitis or a staphylococcal infection of the lid edge.

Cataract: A cataract often has a pearly gray appearance and occurs when the lens loses its transparency (Figure 4.24). Causes include drug reactions, injuries, and radiation. Senile cataracts are the most common type. The most frequently performed surgery in the geriatric population is cataract surgery. Removal of cataracts and replacement with a synthetic lens allow individuals to appreciate the detail and beauty that nature has to offer. Chronological age should not be a deterrent for not performing cataract surgery.

Chalazion: The assorted glands contiguous to the eye are exposed to occasional invasion and infection by bacteria. An infection affecting the Meibomian gland usually results in a cyst, or chalazion. A painful localized swelling, known as a sty (Figure 4.25),

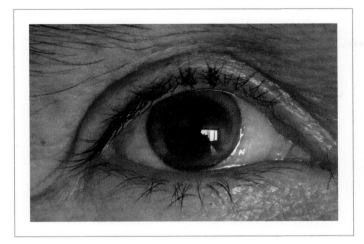

FIGURE 4.22 Arcus senilis. Note the gray-white arc or circle can be seen around the limbus.
Source: Courtesy of Afrodriguezg.

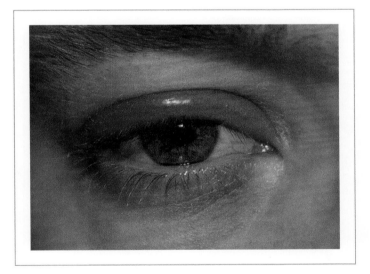

FIGURE 4.23 Blepharitis. Inflammation of the palpebrae.

occurs when there is an infection in a sebaceous gland of one of the eyelashes, a Meibomian gland, or one of the many sweat glands open to the surface between the follicles.

Color blindness: Persons who are unable to differentiate certain colors have a form of color blindness. This is a consequence of one or more classes of cones being nonfunctional.

Conjunctivitis: Also known as pink eye; results from damage to and irritation of the conjunctival surface, which results in dilation of the blood vessels beneath the conjunctival epithelium. This condition may be caused by pathogenic infection (Figure 4.26) or by an allergen (Figure 4.27), as well as physical or chemical irritation of the conjunctival surface.

Corneal injury: The cornea has a limited ability to repair itself; therefore, any injuries to the cornea should be treated promptly to prevent loss of vision (Figure 4.28). Corneal damage can result in blindness even if the rest of the eye—photoreceptors included—are picture-perfect.

Cotton wool spot: Visualized during funduscopic examination. They are poorly defined, yellow areas caused by infarction of the nerve layer of the retina. It may be related to vascular disease as a consequence of hypertension or diabetes mellitus.

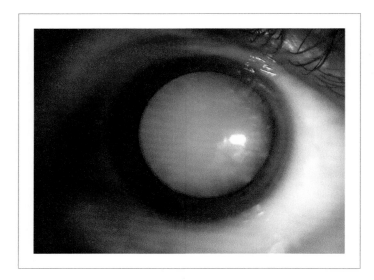

FIGURE 4.24 Pearly gray appearance of a cataract.

Source: Courtesy of Imrankabirhossain.

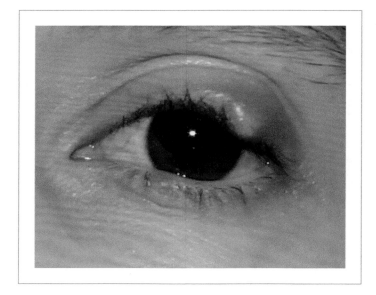

FIGURE 4.25 Chalazion.

Dacryoadenitis: An infection of the lacrimal gland with associated edema, erythema, and pain. Causes include infectious mononucleosis, measles, mumps, and traumatic injuries.

Dacryocystitis: An infection that results in blockage of the lacrimal sac and duct. It occurs at the inner canthus toward the nose; subsequently, people will present with localized erythema, swelling, pain, and warmth. There is lacrimation present.

Manual pressure applied to the sac produces purulent exudate from the puncta.

Detached retina: The photoreceptors are completely dependent on the distribution of oxygen and nutrients from blood vessels in the choroid. When a retina detaches, the neural retina becomes separated from the pigment layer. This condition can result from a sudden impact to the eye or from a variety of other factors. Unless the

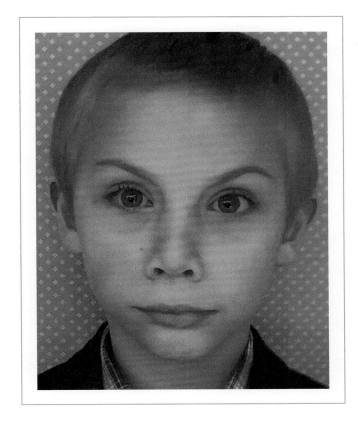

FIGURE 4.26 Patient with bacterial conjunctivitis.

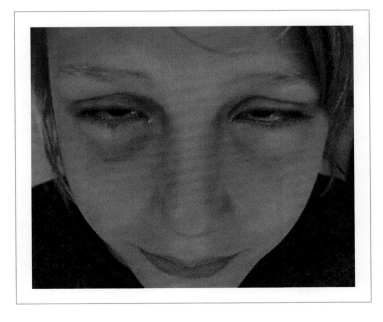

FIGURE 4.27 Allergic conjunctivitis with allergic shiners.

two layers of the neural tunic are reattached, the photoreceptors will degenerate and vision will be lost.

Ectropion: Occurs as a result of atrophy of elastic and fibrous tissues that may cause the lower lid to droop away from the eye. As a consequence, this can compromise eye structures as tears cannot drain appropriately. Constant rubbing of lashes can cause corneal irritation.

Entropion: Results from turning inward of the lower lid (Figure 4.29). It may irritate the eye from friction of the eyelashes. Can be a consequence of aging, but can occur from trauma.

Estropia: An inward turning of the eye.

Exophthalmos: A protrusion of the globes forward secondary to an increase in the volume of the orbital content. It can be bilateral or unilateral. Graves' disease is the most common cause.

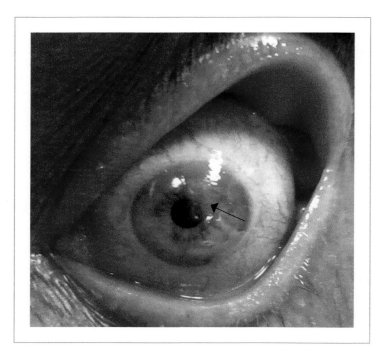

FIGURE 4.28 Corneal injury.
Source: Courtesy of James Heilman.

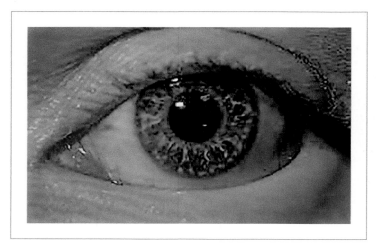

FIGURE 4.29 Entropion.

In unilateral exophthalmos, a retro-orbital tumor must be considered, even though thyroid ocular disease is the most common cause of unilateral proptosis as well. Retraction of the upper lid and exposure of the sclera above the iris may embellish the appearance of exophthalmos.

Exotropia: An outward turning of the eye.

Glaucoma: If left untreated, it can result in blindness. Testing for glaucoma includes measuring the intraocular pressure in the anterior chamber, where it pushes against the inner surface of the cornea. A tiny blast of air is bounced off the surface of the eye and measured; measuring the deflection allows the practitioner to measure intraocular pressure. Normal intraocular pressures range from 12 to 21 mmHg. If aqueous humor cannot enter the canal of Schlemm, the fluid pressure rises, distorting soft tissues within the eye.

Hordeolum: Caused by a staphylococcal infection of the hair follicles at the lid margin, resulting in an erythematous, painful, swollen pustule at the palpebral margin (Figure 4.30).

Hyphema: Can be a consequence of a spontaneous hemorrhage, scleral rupture, or major intraocular trauma. Results from blood in the anterior chamber (Figure 4.31).

Hypopyon: Purulent matter is visualized within the anterior chamber (Figure 4.32). It can occur with iritis as well as inflammation of the anterior chamber.

Impaired ocular movement: Deviations in ocular movement imply diverse degrees of nerve damage:

- If the patient cannot move the eye downward and inward, it is suggestive of a cranial nerve IV issue.
- If the patient cannot move the eye laterally, it is suggestive of a cranial nerve VI issue.
- If the patient has variations with ocular movements, it is suggestive of a cranial nerve III issue.

Increased intracranial pressure: Can lead to optic muscle paralysis. A horizontal gaze deviation may be present if there is damage to the cerebral cortex, or motor center damage. A vertical gaze deviation may be present if the patient suffered midbrain trauma or tumors. If one eye is looking in an upward gaze and one eye is in a downward gaze, suspect a lesion in the pons.

Iritis: Requires immediate referral. Typical patient complaints include photophobia, throbbing pain, blurred vision, and a constricted pupil. On physical exam, there are findings of a deep, dull red halo encircling the iris and cornea (Figure 4.33). The pupil may be irregular from swelling of the iris.

Macular degeneration: Includes a blurry border of the macula and pigmented or hole-like center.

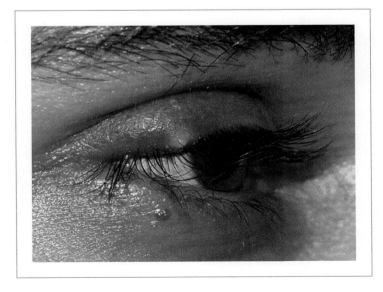

FIGURE 4.30 Hordeolum.

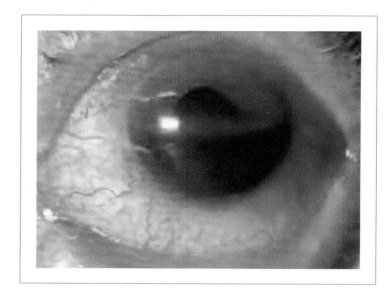

FIGURE 4.31 Hyphema.
Source: Courtesy of Rakesh Ahuja.

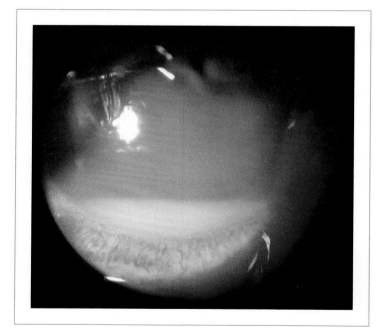

FIGURE 4.32 Slit lamp view of hypopyon.
Source: Courtesy of Imrankabirhossain.

A hallmark feature of macular degeneration is a loss of central vision (Figure 4.34A and B). Early laser treatment may improve the condition.

Myopia: Individuals who are nearsighted.

Nystagmus: It is an involuntary eye movement that can have the eyes moving rapidly from side to side. It can be the result of a visual pathway trauma, brainstem issue, or intoxication.

Papilledema: Triggered by increased intracranial pressure. Funduscopic exam findings include blurred disc margins, hemorrhages, and absent venous pulsations, with venous stasis, erythema, and disc elevation.

Periorbital edema: Palpebrae are swollen and edematous (Figure 4.35), and can be seen with allergies, crying, heart failure, hypothyroidism, local infections, and renal failure.

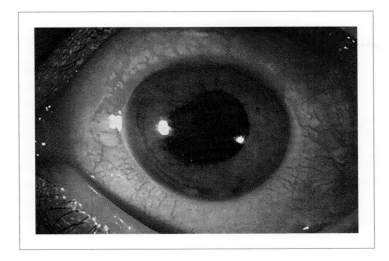

FIGURE 4.33 Iritis.

Source: Courtesy of Jonathan Trobe.

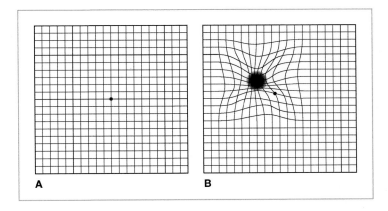

A   B

FIGURE 4.34 Loss of central vision with macular degeneration. (**A**) Amsler Grid. (**B**) Amsler Grid as seen by a patient with macular degeneration.

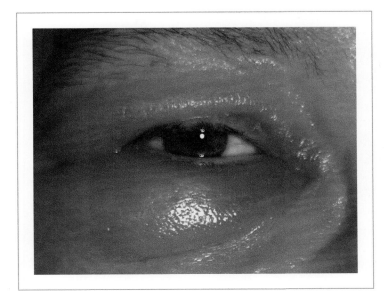

FIGURE 4.35 Periorbital edema.

Presbyopia: Individuals who have presbyopia are said to be farsighted.

Pseudostrabismus: A child may have the appearance of strabismus; however, it is related to the epicanthic fold. This can be a normal variant for a young child.

Pterygium: This condition may obstruct eyesight as it covers the pupil (Figure 4.36). It occurs when the bulbar conjunctiva grows in a triangular fashion toward the center of the cornea. It can result from chronic exposure to a hot, dry, sandy climate, which stimulates the growth of a pinguecula into a pterygium.

Strabismus: A true disparity of the eye, evidenced by constant misalignment (Figure 4.37). Thought to be caused by amblyopia.

Subconjunctival hemorrhage: Can result from coughing, childbirth, increased intraocular pressure, labor, sneezing, straining with stool, trauma, or weightlifting. The conjunctiva looks unsettling, as there is an erythematous patch on the sclera (Figure 4.38), but it is usually not serious.

Traumatic injury to the eye socket: Can lead to a degree of injury to the cranial nerve. Botulism, herpes zoster, syphilis, or a vitamin deficiency could lead to altered ocular movements.

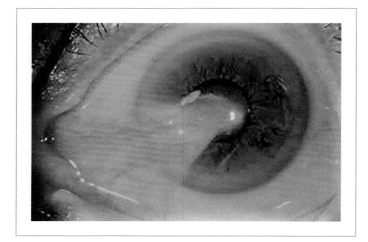

FIGURE 4.36 Pterygium.

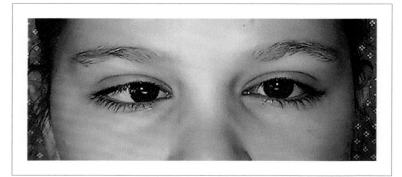

FIGURE 4.37 Strabismus.

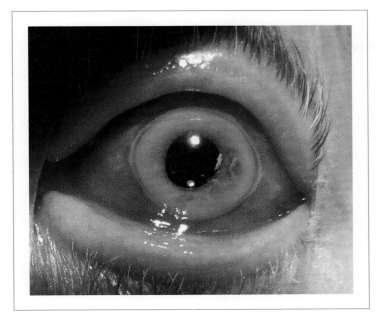

FIGURE 4.38 Subconjunctival hemorrhage.
Source: Courtesy of James Heilman.

Holistic Health Assessment of the Eye

In performing a holistic assessment of a patient it is important to assess the patient's overall well-being. As a healthcare provider, it is important to assess for patient safety. If the patient is working in a high-risk occupation, is he or she wearing appropriate protective eye wear? If the patient works in an environment with noise pollution, is he or she wearing appropriate ear protection such as ear plugs or ear muffs? Is the patient wearing a helmet while riding a bicycle or motorcycle? Protective eye wear?

Does the patient follow a specific diet? Is he or she consuming enough beta-carotene? Is the patient eating a healthy well-balanced diet? Does the patient take any supplements or vitamins? Does he or she see a naturopathic provider? Does the patient use alternative and complementary therapies such as acupuncture, chiropractors, or yoga? Does the patient routinely exercise?

What is the patient's living situation? Does he or she provide care for others such as grandparents, parents, spouse, children, in-laws, nieces or nephews, or foster children?

Does the patient have any financial concerns? Is he or she worried about making ends meet and not being able to pay the bills? Perhaps the patient cannot afford his or her eyeglasses or contact lenses. Does the patient need financial assistance or counseling? Perhaps a referral to a social worker?

Are there particular spiritual beliefs that the patient ascribes to? If so, how does this impact his or her care? Are there other concerns that the patient would want to discuss during his or her visit?

Are there sources of stress in the patient's life? Are there marital issues, issues with children, problems at work, or anything else that he or she wants to discuss?

Does the patient wear headphones or ear buds? If so, is he or she listening at an acceptable level?

CASE STUDY: EYE

Naomi is a 75-year-old married female who had fallen down a couple of stairs.

SUBJECTIVE

Naomi states that she was carrying some laundry upstairs when she lost her footing and fell down three stairs. She hit the side of her eye and face on the banister. She presents with pain in her right cheek and eye. There is no bleeding. Does report difficulty opening right eye.

OBJECTIVE

- **General:** 75-year-old female in no apparent distress. Conversing in full sentences. Is alert, oriented, and answering questions appropriately.

- **Head, Eyes, Ears, Nose, Throat:** Right palpebrae are swollen and ecchymotic. Right eye is 2 mm with a bright red patch over the lateral aspect of the globe. There is no active bleeding of the eye, iris is intact, and anterior chamber is clear. The left conjunctiva is clear, sclera anicteric, white, cornea, and iris intact and the anterior chamber is clear. Pupils equal, round, reactive to light, and accommodation (PERRLA). Pupils Right 4/1 = 4/1 Left. Vision intact by Rosenbaum pocket card. 20/40 each eye with corrective lenses. Right cheek is swollen and erythematous, no laceration.

ASSESSMENT

- Subconjunctival hemorrhage right eye
- Right cheek ecchymosis
- Facial pain related to fall

Assessment of Special Populations: Eye

Palpebral fissures can highlight racial differences. Those of Asian descent are identified by characteristics of their eyes and have narrowed palpebral fissures. Non-Asians with narrowed palpebral fissures may have trisomy 21 or Down syndrome. Those individuals with darker retinal pigmentation and color of the iris may have a culturally based variability. Those possessing darker irides often have darker retinas behind them. Those with light retinas may suffer ocular pain or headaches in an environment with too much light, but generally have better night vision.

 PEDIATRIC POPULATION

Performing an ocular exam on infants can be challenging as they often shut their eyes tightly when eye examination is attempted. It may be arduous to separate the palpebrae, and often they will evert when too much energy is exerted. The provider should be positioned behind the caregiver who is holding the infant over a shoulder. With a crying infant, there may be a moment that the infant's eyes open. This will afford you the opportunity to learn a bit about the eyes, their evenness and extraocular muscular balance, and presence or absence of a light reflex. The infant may start crying again, but assessment has been achieved.

Commence with a visual inspection of the infant's external eye structures. Observe the size of the eyes, paying close attention to small or differently sized eyes. Inspect the palpebrae for presence of epicanthal folds, swelling, and position. To detect epicanthal folds, look for a vertical fold of skin nasally that covers the lacrimal caruncle. Prominent epicanthal folds are an expected variant in Asian infants, but they may be suggestive of Down syndrome or other genetic anomalies in children of other ethnic groups. Observe the alignment and slant of the palpebral fissures of the infant's eyes. Draw an imaginary line through the medial canthi and extend the line past the outer canthus of the eyes. The medial and lateral canthi are usually horizontal. When the outer canthi are above the line, an upward, or Mongolian, slant is present. When the outer canthi are below the line, a downward, or anti-Mongolian, slant is present.

Examine the level of the palpebrae covering the eye. To detect the sun-setting sign, rapidly lower the infant from upright to supine position. Look for sclera above the iris. This sign may be an expected variant in newborns; however, it also may be observed in infants with hydrocephalus and brainstem lesions.

Observe the distance between the eyes, looking for a wide spacing, or hypertelorism, which can be linked with craniofacial defects including some with developmental delays. Pseudostrabismus, the false appearance of strabismus caused by a flattened nasal bridge or epicanthal fold, is an expected variant in Asian and Native American/American Indian infants, as well as in some whites. By 1 year of age, pseudostrabismus generally disappears. To distinguish pseudostrabismus from strabismus, use the corneal light reflex. An asymmetric light reflex may indicate a real strabismus or hypertelorism.

Inspect the conjunctiva, sclera, pupil, and iris of each eye. Inspect and compare corneal sizes for symmetry. Congenital glaucoma may be seen with enlarged corneas. As a consequence of birth trauma, the newborn's palpebrae may be edematous or swollen. However, if the edema or swelling is accompanied by drainage and conjunctival inflammation, it may represent opthalmia neonatorum.

Any discharge, erythema, hemorrhages, or granular appearance outside the newborn period may be indicative of an infection, allergy, or trauma. Examine each iris and pupil for any abnormality in shape. Congenital anomalies may be associated with a coloboma, or keyhole pupil. Brushfield spots, which can be seen as white specks scattered in a lined pattern about the entire border of the iris, strongly suggests Down syndrome or developmental delays.

Vision is grossly examined by observing the infant's preference for looking at certain objects. An infant should be able to focus on and track a light or face through 60 degrees.

The optical blink reflex can be elicited by shining a bright light at the infant's eyes. The provider should note the prompt closing of the eyes and dorsiflexion of the head.

The corneal reflex is performed the same as it is in adults.

Unless there is a compelling need, a funduscopic examination is generally deferred until the infant is 2 to 6 months of age. It is difficult to perform on a newborn or young infant, as well as with the visual problems of prematurity. If there was a need to perform dilation, it can safely be done. Dilation of the eyes for effective visualization of the fundi can be safely achieved in the nursery by using weak solutions of mydriatics. For infants with blue irides, very little of a weak solution is necessary; one drop in each eye is usually sufficient. With darker colored irides, a second drop a few seconds later may be indicated. Cyclopentolate hydrochloride 0.5% is a common mydriatic.

During a physical exam, it is important that the provider elicit the red reflex bilaterally in every newborn. If qualified to do so, dilate the pupils if necessary. Observe for any opacities, dark spots, or white spots within the circle of red glow. Opacities or interruption of the red reflex may indicate congenital cataracts or retinoblastoma or other serious intraocular pathology. If there are any concerns, refer to an ophthalmologic specialist.

The visual inspection of the external eye on the young child is performed in the same manner as described for the infant. At approximately the age of 3, visual acuity is tested using a Snellen E eye chart. In order to be meaningful, it takes cooperation of the child and caregiver. To use the Snellen E eye chart, have one provider point to the line on the chart and another aid the child with covering one eye. As with adults, the child should stand 20 feet (6 m) away. Prior to administering the exam, allow the child to practice following the instructions. The child should be instructed to point his or her finger or arm in the same direction as the legs of the E. Should the child have difficulty complying with these directions, a handout with a large E on it can be provided to the child with directives to turn the E to match the letter indicated on the chart. Each eye should be tested separately. If the child wears corrective lenses, his or her vision should be tested with and without eyeglasses and recorded independently.

Visual acuity may be observed in younger children by viewing their activities. Afford an opportunity for the child to play with toys in the exam room. As the child is stacking, building, or placing objects inside of others, observe his or her behaviors. If the tasks are performed well, the child should not have any visual difficulties in one eye. Table 4.2 delineates the expected visual acuity of young children.

When you are analyzing the visual acuity in a child, any difference in the scores between the eyes should be documented. A two-line difference (e.g., 20/60 and 20/40) may be indicative of amblyopia.

Examination of extraocular movements and cranial nerves III, IV, and VI in children is performed the same as with adults. When examining a child, the provider may encounter challenges of the child

not sitting still or cooperating. The provider may have to hold the child's head still or use an alluring object such as a stuffed animal for the child to cooperate and follow through the six cardinal fields of gaze. If the child is obliging, peripheral vision can be tested; the young child may choose to be seated on the parent's lap while his or her tests are completed.

Resolve is often needed to gain the child's cooperation for the funduscopic examination. A young child is often unable to keep a fixed gaze and focus on a distant object. The provider should place the young child supine on the exam table, with his or her head near one end. Standing at that end of the table, the provider should then use the right eye to examine the child's left eye and vice versa. Do not attempt to hold the child's eye forcibly, as it will only lead to confrontation. Recall that all retinal findings will appear upside down. Rather than move the ophthalmoscope to visualize all retinal fields, inspect the optic disc, the fovea, and the vessels as they happen by. The best results are generally when the child sits on the caregiver's lap. If this position is utilized, examine the child in the same fashion as an adult.

PREGNANT POPULATION

As a consequence of physiologic and hormonal influences, the eyes undergo several changes during pregnancy. Hypersensitivity and a change in visual acuity are some of the changes that can occur. During pregnancy, women who wear contacts may find it difficult because of an increased level of lysozyme within tears, which results in a greasy sensation with resultant blurred vision. For this reason, it is recommended that women not change their lens prescription during pregnancy, but rather wait until several weeks after delivery. During the third trimester, mild corneal edema and thickening associated with blurred vision may occur.

Retinal exam in the pregnant woman can help discriminate between chronic hypertension and PIH. Findings with a long-standing history of hypertension include angiosclerosis, exudates, hemorrhage, and vascular tortuosity. In a patient with PIH, conversely, there is a segmental arteriolar narrowing with a wet, glimmering appearance indicative of edema.

TABLE 4.2 Visual Acuity of Young Children	
Age	Visual Acuity
3 years	20/50 or better
4 years	20/40 or better
5 years	20/30 or better
6 years	20/20

This finding is not exclusive to pregnant women. Hemorrhages and exudates are rare. Detachment of the retina may occur with spontaneous reattachment after hypertension is successfully controlled.

Because of systemic absorption, cycloplegic and mydriatic agents should be avoided unless there is a need to evaluate for retinal disease. Use of nasolacrimal occlusion after instillation of topical eye medications may reduce systemic absorption.

PATIENTS WITH DISABILITIES

Patients with disabilities need to have optimal vision to compensate for associated physical limitations. Therefore, patients with disabilities need to have as thorough an examination of vision as other individuals and treatment provided accordingly.

VETERAN POPULATION

The provider should ask the patient if they served in the military. If so, the dates and capacity in which they served (e.g., pilot, ground forces, medical services) should be ascertained. Based upon this information, the provider will be aware of what potential hazards or chemicals of warfare the patient may have been exposed to.

Diagnostic Reasoning: Eye

Common Differential Diagnoses: Ocular Complaints

Issue	Assessment	Cause/Differential Diagnosis
Blurry vision	• Neurological findings • Related to medications • Head injury	Eye injury or injury to head; related to astigmatism, hyperopia, myopia; glaucoma, cataracts, migraine, uveitis, keratitis, iritis, or related to medications such as benzodiazepines
Burning sensation	• Pruritus to eyes • Sensation of foreign body present • Contact with anyone with bacterial conjunctivitis	Allergies, blepharitis, conjunctivitis, foreign body, refractory error
Changes with red eye reflex	• Red reflex asymmetrical • Leukocoria present	Strabismus can have findings of asymmetrical red eye reflex. Leukocoria is seen with retinoblastoma, cataracts, or retinal detachment.

(continued)

Common Differential Diagnoses: Ocular Complaints (*continued*)		
Issue	**Assessment**	**Cause/Differential Diagnosis**
Conjunctival inflammation	• Discharge from the eye present: watery, thin, thick, and/or purulent • Blurry vision, diplopia, presence of spots, or floaters • Orbital pain • Presence of contact lenses	Allergies, corneal abrasion, bacterial or viral conjunctivitis, presence of foreign body, iritis, keratitis, uveitis; smoking cannabis
Dacryoadenitis	• Swelling, tenderness at site of lacrimal gland	Pain in the eye at the upper lateral aspect at site of lacrimal gland
Desiccated eyes	• Recent illness • Contact lens use • Medications	Dehydration, exopthalmos, use of medications such as anticholinergics, diuretics, diphenhydramine
Diplopia	• Duration, timing, onset • Head injury, recent trauma • Potential change in medications	Amblyopia, congenital cataracts, traumatic injury
Discolored	• Eyelid erythematous or edematous • Associated periorbital ecchymosis • Conjunctival hemorrhage • Recent eye trauma or injury	Eye trauma, hyphema, bilateral periorbital ecchymosis (raccoon eyes, also known as Battle's sign) can be indicative of basilar skull fracture.
Drainage	• Erythematous conjunctiva • Tenderness or edema • Purulent discharge • Pain or edema at inner canthus • Discharge or crusty drainage • Pyrexia • URI symptoms • Outbreaks of conjunctivitis at school, day care, or place of employment • Contact lens use	Allergic conjunctivitis (clear drainage), viral conjunctivitis (mucous drainage), bacterial conjunctivitis (purulent with crusting upon awakening), dacryocystitis; URI, blepharitis, keratitis, hordeolum

(continued)

Common Differential Diagnoses: Ocular Complaints (*continued*)

Issue	Assessment	Cause/Differential Diagnosis
Edema	• Pyrexia, inflammation, erythema of the palpebral fissure, periorbital edema, drainage • Drainage; eyelashes matted with associated drainage	Blepharitis, conjunctivitis, periorbital or orbital cellulitis, nephrosis, nephritis, systemic lupus erythematous
Eyelid inflammation	• Pruritus, irritation, dry eyes, and/or associated pyrexia	Allergies, blepharitis, conjunctivitis, dry eyes, or foreign body
Excessive blinking	• Allergies, dry eyes, pruritus, sensation of foreign body • Contact lens use	Corneal abrasion, foreign body, irritation, infection, or tic
Eye protrusion/bulging	• Onset, timing, duration • Pain • Dry eyes • Bleeding, hemorrhaging	Exophthalmos, ocular trauma
Eye twitching	• Contractions of orbicularis oculi muscle (due to cranial nerve VII lesions, eye irritation, fatigue, or stress)	Blepharospasm
Foreign body	• Gritty sensation, pain, scratchy sensation • Recent injury • Contact lens use	Foreign body, blepharitis, corneal abrasion, conjunctivitis
Headache	• Visual changes, floaters, spots, photophobia, nausea, and/or vomiting, progressive or sudden loss of vision. • Any medications • Recent funduscopic exam (papilledema) • Recent head injury • URI symptoms or pyrexia	Hyperopia, myopia, migraine, increased intracranial pressure (cerebral edema, hydrocephalus, tumor, idiopathic, pseudotumor cerebri), viral illness, sinusitis

(*continued*)

Common Differential Diagnoses: Ocular Complaints (*continued*)		
Issue	**Assessment**	**Cause/Differential Diagnosis**
Increased lacrimation	• Color is the conjunctiva • Any sensation of foreign body in the eye	Allergic rhinitis, blepharitis, conjunctivitis, dry eyes, foreign body
Intractable crying	• Age of patient • Signs of recent injury	Foreign body
Nasal discharge	• Onset, quality, quantity, and duration of discharge • Purulence, clear mucus • Pyrexia, pruritus, cough, congestion, or watery eyes • Allergies • Medications	Allergic rhinitis, sinusitis, URI, periorbital or orbital cellulitis
Nystagmus	• Onset, duration, frequency • Recent neurological examination • Relevant past medical history	Albinism, congenital blindness, Down syndrome, idiopathic nystagmus, optic nerve diseases, ocular structural abnormalities, retinal diseases
Pain	• Onset, duration, location, quality • Pyrexia • History of recent injury • Complaint of associated edema, erythema, or swelling	Corneal abrasion, blepharitis, foreign body, migraine, eye injury, eye trauma, head trauma, iritis, keratitis, periorbital or orbital cellulitis, sinusitis, uveitis
Photophobia	• Onset, duration, quality, any associated symptoms • Ocular pain • Influenza, pyrexia, or headache	Blepharitis, cataracts, corneal abrasion, glaucoma, bacterial or viral meningitis, migraine, iritis, keratitis, uveitis
Pruritus	• Ocular discharge • Burning sensation • Dry eyes	Allergies, blepharitis, conjunctivitis, dry eyes, foreign body

(continued)

Common Differential Diagnoses: Ocular Complaints (*continued*)

Issue	Assessment	Cause/Differential Diagnosis
Ptosis	• Onset, duration • Associated amblyopia, astigmatism, and strabismus • Recent neurological examination	Congenital ptosis, ocular tumor, neurological disorder; lesions, adipose tissue, or periorbital edema; muscular disorders such as multiple sclerosis; neurological disorders such as paralysis, cerebral vascular accident, neuronal disruption
Pyrexia	• URI symptoms, drainage from the eye, palpebral edema, injected conjunctiva • Vaccinations status	Periorbital or orbital cellulitis, uveitis, viral conjunctivitis. Influenza, mumps, rubeola, rubella, and varicella all have ocular manifestations.
Subconjunctival hemorrhages	• Onset, duration • Recent injury • Relevant past medical history • Immunizations status • Medications	Blood dyscrasias, eye trauma, ruptured ocular globe, chest trauma, meningococcemia, measles, scarlet fever, shaken baby syndrome
Vertigo	• Onset and duration • Any associated symptoms • Pyrexia or vomiting	Cardiac causes, dehydration, vertigo, cerebellar disease
Visual changes	• Recent changes in visual acuity • Diplopia or blurred vision • Hemianopsia • Flashing lights, floaters, or spots • Ocular pain • Increased lacrimation • Recent neurological exam	Blepharitis, cataracts, central nervous system disorder (brain tumor, bacterial meningitis), glaucoma, keratitis, migraine, ocular trauma, periorbital or orbital cellulitis, retinal detachment, retinal hemorrhage, uveitis (floaters, spots)

URI, upper respiratory infection.

Overview of Anatomy and Physiology of the Ear

Equilibrium and hearing are senses that are derived from the inner ear, which is a receptor complex located in the petrous portion of the temporal bone of the skull. The hair cells, or receptors, are simple mechanoreceptors (Figure 4.39). The inner ear is composed of a complex structure coupled with the different arrangement of accessory structures that accounts for the abilities of the hair cells to respond to different stimuli, and thus provide input for two different senses:

- Equilibrium, or sense of balance, informs an individual of the position of the body in space by monitoring gravity, linear acceleration, and rotation.
- Hearing enables the detection and interpretation of sound waves

EXTERNAL EAR

The external ear includes the cartilaginous pinna, or auricle, that surrounds the external auditory meatus. The pinna acts to protect the opening of the external auditory meatus and provides directional sensitivity to the ear. Sounds emanating from behind are blocked by the pinna; sounds emanating from the side or front are collected and channeled into the external auditory canal of the temporal bone. The external auditory canal ends at the tympanic membrane. The tympanic membrane is a thin, delicate, semitransparent sheet that separates the external ear from the middle ear.

The pinna and narrow external auditory canal provide some protection from accidental injury

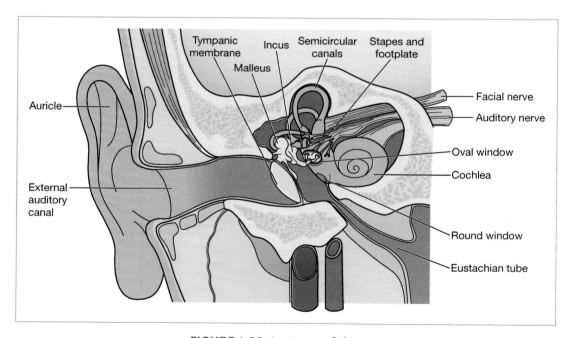

FIGURE 4.39 Anatomy of the ear.

to the tympanic membrane. Ceruminous glands line the external auditory canal and secrete a wax material. Additionally, many small outwardly projecting hairs help deny access to foreign objects or insects. Cerumen is known as the waxy secretion of the ceruminous glands, which helps to slow the growth of microorganisms in the external auditory canal and reduces the chances for an auricular infection.

MIDDLE EAR

Air fills the middle ear, or tympanic cavity. The tympanic membrane separates the external auditory canal, but it connects with the superior portion of the pharynx. This is an area known as the nasopharynx, coupled with the mastoid air cells via a small number of variable communications. The auditory tube or Eustachian tube, also known as the pharyngotympanic tube, connects with the pharynx. This tube, about 4 cm long, consists of two portions. The narrow connection to the middle ear is strengthened by cartilage. The nasopharynx opening is relatively broad and cone shaped. The Eustachian tube serves to equalize the pressure both inside as well as outside the eardrum. The anatomy can also, unfortunately, allow microorganisms to travel from the nasopharynx into the tympanic cavity. Otitis media, which is a middle ear infection, can result from invasion by microorganisms.

The middle ear consists of three tiny ear bones, collectively called the auditory ossicles. The ear bones connect the tympanic membrane with the receptor complex of the inner ear. The three auditory ossicles are the malleus, the incus, and the stapes. The malleus (which is hammer shaped) attaches to the interior surface of the tympanum at three points. The middle bone, the incus (anvil shaped), attaches the malleus to the inner stapes (stirrup shape). The oval window of the inner ear is almost completely filled by the base of the stapes.

Tympanic vibrations convert incoming sound waves into mechanical movements. Sound conduction occurs when the auditor ossicles act as levers to transmit those vibrations to the fluid-filled chamber of the inner ear. With this amplification, faint sounds can be heard. However, if repeatedly exposed to loud noises, that degree of amplification can be impacted and manifested as hearing loss.

INNER EAR

The receptors of the inner ear provide the senses of equilibrium and hearing. The membranous labyrinth, which is a collection of fluid-filled tubes and chambers, houses the receptors of the inner ear. Endolymph is a fluid, with electrolyte concentrations different from those of other body fluids, found within the membranous labyrinth.

The membranous labyrinth is surrounded and protected by a shell of dense bone known as the bony labyrinth. The bony labyrinth's inner contours closely mirror the contours of the membranous labyrinth, and its outer confines are fused with the surrounding temporal bone. The perilymph is a liquid whose properties closely resemble those of cerebrospinal fluid, which flows between the bony and membranous labyrinths. The bony labyrinth can be subdivided into the vestibule, the semicircular canals, and the cochlea.

The semicircular canals encircle the semicircular ducts. Rotation of the head stimulates the receptors in the semicircular ducts. The bony cochlea contains the cochlear duct of the membranous labyrinth. Located within the cochlear duct are receptors that provide the sense of hearing.

Screening Health Assessment and Normal Findings of the Ear

HEALTH HISTORY

EARACHE OR PAIN IN THE EARS

- Location, duration, pain to palpation
- Character: Throbbing, crushing, stabbing, sharp, constant, dull, affected by positioning of the head
- Reoccurrence of pain
- Sore throat, rhinorrhea, sinus pain, dental pain, or cold-like symptoms
- Fevers, chills, or night sweats
- Trauma to the ears
- Anything that makes the pain better or worse

EAR INFECTIONS

- Frequency
- Tympanostomy tubes inserted
- Exudate or discharge from the ear(s): Color, consistency, and odor
- For children:
  - Day care
  - Age of first ear infection
  - Smoking in the home
  - Hearing issues
  - Begin babbling around 6 months of age
  - Puts items in ears
- For adolescents:
  - Play contact sports—if so, use of appropriate protective equipment

HEARING LOSS

- Onset: Slow or rapid
- Perception that people are shouting

- Hearing issue most notable: At a party, listening to TV, casual conversation, or talking on the phone
- Sounds appear muffled, such as underwater
- Recent air travel
- Family history of hearing loss
- Impact on daily life
- Occupation: Exposed to loud noises, such as with heavy machinery or work at an airport

TINNITUS

- Ringing or buzzing in the ears
- Any medications

VERTIGO

- Felt the room spinning or perceived that they themselves were spinning
- Felt dizzy or unsteady on feet

SELF-CARE

- Ear-cleaning method and tools
- Last hearing checkup
- Hearing aid use: duration, age of batteries

PHYSICAL EXAMINATION

SUGGESTED EQUIPMENT FOR AN OTOSCOPIC EXAM

- Tuning forks in 512 Hz, 1,024 Hz
- Otoscope, with pneumatic attachment and fresh batteries as well as a functional light

A visual inspection of the size and shape of the ears should be performed. The pinna should be free and clear of lesions, masses, and exudate. The skin should be consistent with the patient's ethnicity.

Palpation is performed to the pinna, tragus, and mastoid process. The patient should not feel any pain.

Visual inspection of the external auditory meatus includes assessing for swelling, redness, or exudate, which should not be present. Cerumen may be present. If there is a large amount, it could impede the ability to view the tympanic membrane and bony landmarks.

THE OTOSCOPIC EXAMINATION

When performing an otoscopic exam, it is important to choose the appropriate size speculum to attach to the otoscope, so that it will safely fit into the ear canal. The patient should be instructed to gently tilt his or her head away from you toward the opposite shoulder. Holding it gently but firmly, pull the pinna up and back (on older children and adults; on an infant and child under 3, pull the pinna down); this helps to better visualize the tympanic membrane.

The provider should grasp the otoscope "upside down" along the fingers and position the dorsal aspect of the hand along the patient's cheek, braced to secure the otoscope. This helps to prevent forceful insertion. Should the patient suddenly move his

or her head, this technique also helps to stabilize the hand and act as a protecting mechanism to prevent local trauma.

While monitoring the insertion technique, the provider should cautiously introduce the speculum slowly along the axis of the canal and place an eye up to the otoscope (Figure 4.40). It is important to avoid touching the inner bony section of the canal wall as it is covered by a thin epithelial lay and is sensitive to pain. Occasionally, it is difficult to see anything but canal wall. If the view is obscured, try to reposition the patient's head, apply more traction on the pinna, and re-angle the otoscope to look forward toward the patient's nose.

Slight rotation of the otoscope may be required to visualize the tympanic membrane. Finally, complete the otoscopic examination prior to the hearing test. Impacted cerumen within the ear canals may give a false perception of pathologic hearing loss.

THE EXTERNAL CANAL

Inspect the external canal for any erythema, edema, exudate, foreign bodies, and lesions. With exudate, if any is present, observe the color and odor. (To avoid cross contamination with possibly infected exudate from one ear to another, be sure to clean the discharge

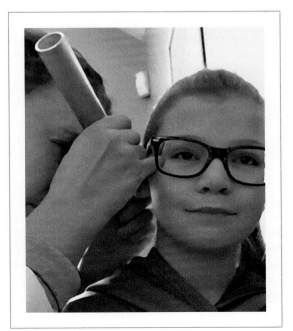

FIGURE 4.40 Otoscopic examination.

from the speculum.) As part of the visual inspection in a patient with hearing aids, observe for any irritation on the canal wall from ill-fitting ear molds.

THE TYMPANIC MEMBRANE

Thoroughly explore the landmarks of the tympanic membrane. The normal tympanic membrane is shiny and translucent, with a pearl-gray color. The cone-shaped light reflex is prominent in the anteroinferior quadrant, which is the reflection of the illumination from the otoscope. Through the translucent tympanic membrane, portions of the malleus are visible: the umbo, manubrium, and short process. At the border, the annulus looks whiter and denser.

The tympanic membrane is uniform, yet slightly drawn in at the center. When the patient holds his or her nose and swallows, or performs the Valsalva maneuver, the tympanic membrane quivers. These maneuvers allow the provider to assess drum mobility. Caution is advised with an aging patient, as this technique may disrupt the equilibrium. Also avoid insufflation to the middle ear in a patient with an upper respiratory infection (URI), as it may force infective material into the middle ear.

Inspect the tympanic membrane and the entire circumference of the annulus for perorations. A normal tympanic membrane is intact. As a consequence of repeated ear infections over time, some patients may have scarring. This manifests as a dense white patch on the tympanic membrane.

HEARING ACUITY

As the health history is being conducted, the physical exam is also commencing. The initial interview helps you screen for a hearing impairment. Is the patient able to hear conversational speech? An audiometer gives a precise quantitative measure of hearing by assessing the patient's ability to hear sounds of varying frequency. This medical device may not be available to the provider; if a formal hearing screen is required, consideration can be given for a referral to audiology.

VOICE TEST

The voice test is performed one ear at a time. The provider asks the patient to mask hearing in the other ear by placing a hand over it to prevent sound transmission around the head. This patient should not be able to view the provider's lips; this impedes the patient's ability to compensate for a hearing loss by lip reading. Stand approximately 1 to 2 feet from the patient and whisper two-syllable words such as, "Saturday, recliner, airplane, football, ninety-nine." Normally the person repeats each word correctly after you say it.

TUNING-FORK TESTS

Tuning-fork tests measure hearing through air conduction (AC) or bone conduction (BC), through which the sound reverberates from the cranial bones to the inner ear. The AC route through the ear canal and middle ear is usually the more sensitive route. To activate the tuning fork, the provider should hold it by the stem and strike the tines softly on the back of the hand. Striking the tuning fork with fingers make the tone too loud, and it takes a long time to diminish.

The Weber test is valuable when a patient reports hearing better with one ear over another ear. Place a vibrating tuning fork on the top of the middle of the patient's head and ask if the pitch sounds the same in both ears, or better in one (Figure 4.41). Normal findings are considered when the Weber test is negative. The patient should hear the pitch from the vibrating tuning fork through BC through the top of the middle of the head, and it should sound equally in both ears.

The Rinne test compares AC and BC sound. Place the stem of the vibrating tuning fork on the patient's mastoid process and ask him or her to alert you when the sound is no longer heard (Figure 4.42A). Quickly upend the tuning fork so the vibrating end is near the external ear canal; the patient should still hear a sound (Figure 4.42B). Normally the sound is heard twice as long by AC (next to ear) as by BC (through mastoid process). A normal response would be a positive Rinne test, or AC>BC. Repeat in the other ear.

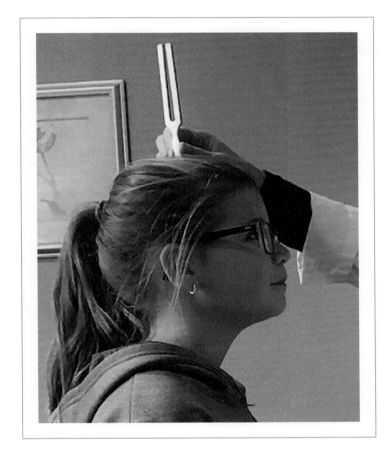

FIGURE 4.41 The Weber test. Tuning fork is placed on the top middle of the patient's head.

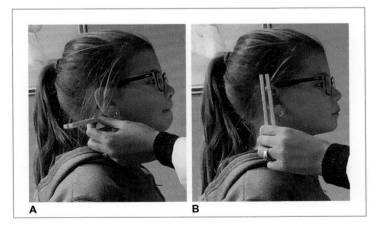

FIGURE 4.42 Rinne test. (**A**) Stem of tuning fork is placed on the patient's mastoid process. (**B**) Tuning fork upended so that the vibrating end is near the external ear canal.

Focused Health Assessment and Abnormal Findings of the Ear

ABNORMALITIES OF THE EXTERNAL EAR

Microtia and atresia: A diminutive undeveloped auricle appears as a vertical bowed ridge with the presence of atresia (absence or closure) of the ear canal with associated hearing loss (Figure 4.43).

Frostbite: Occurs following exposure to extreme cold. Appears as reddish blue discoloration and swelling of the auricle. May present with vesicles or bullae may develop, and the person feels pain and tenderness.

Otitis externa: The outer ear is severely painful with movement of the pinna and tragus. There is associated redness and swelling of the pinna and canal as the result of an infection of the outer ear (Figure 4.44). There is scant purulent discharge; also, there may be scaling, pruritus, pyrexia, and enlarged tender regional lymph nodes. Hearing is normal or slightly diminished. Common in hot humid weather; also called swimmer's ear. The external canal becomes filled with water and as a consequence swells; skinfolds trap water and result in an ensuing infection.

Sebaceous cyst: Commonly found behind the ear lobule, in the postauricular fold. Often appears as a small nodule with central black punctum, which may indicate a blocked sebaceous gland. If infected, it is painful.

Tophi: Usually a sign of gout. Typically presents with hard, nontender, small whitish-yellow nodules in or near the helix or antihelix. Often contain greasy chalky material of uric acid crystals.

Carcinoma: Typically presents with pain and swelling of the canal, as well as an ulcerated crusted nodule with indurated base that fails to heal. May intermittently bleed. May occur in external canal and show chronic discharge that is either serosanguineous or bloody. Must refer for biopsy.

ABNORMALITIES IN THE EAR CANAL

Excessive cerumen: Excessive cerumen is generated or is obstructed secondary to constricted tortuous canal or due to poor cleaning habits. May be evident as a circular ball partially obscuring

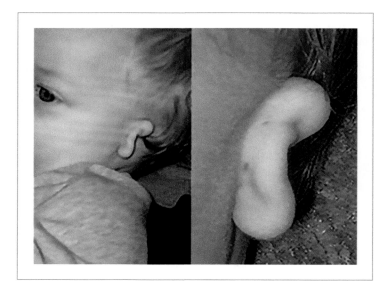

FIGURE 4.43 Microtia.

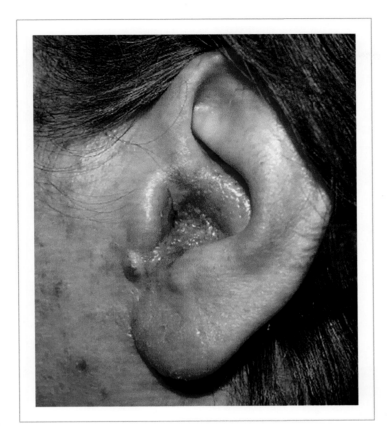

FIGURE 4.44 Otitis externa.
Source: Courtesy of CNX OpenStax.

the tympanic membrane or totally occluding the external canal (Figure 4.45). Hearing remains intact even when the external ear canal is 90% to 95% obscured. But when the remaining 5% to 10% is totally obstructed, the patient reports complaints of fullness or sudden hearing loss.

Otitis externa: A patient may complain of pain and tenderness. Otoscopic examination reveals inflammation with severe swelling of the ear canal. The ear canal is reduced to a fraction of its normal size.

Osteoma: Osteoma is a rounded single, hard nodule that obscures the tympanic membrane that is attached to the inner third, bony part of the ear canal (Figure 4.46). Usually nontender; the surrounding skin appears normal.It is benign, but the patient requires referral to an ear, nose, and throat (ENT) specialist for removal.

Foreign body: Oftentimes it is the pediatric population that presents after having complaints of ear

pain; upon physical examination, there is the presence of a foreign body. Children commonly place beads, beans, corn, small stones, sponge, rubber, and cotton from cotton-tipped applicators into their ear canals. Additionally, insects both live and deceased have been extracted from the ear canal.

Exostosis: Exostosis is more common than an osteoma. In the ear canal, there are multiple nodules that are small, bony, hard, and rounded, consisting of hypertrophic bone covered with normal epithelial tissue found bilaterally. They arise near the tympanic membrane but usually do not obstruct the view. They may occur more frequently in cold-water swimmers. The condition needs no treatment, although it may cause an accumulation of cerumen, which blocks the canal.

Furuncle: Furuncle is an infected hair follicle that is extremely painful and erythematous. It can occur on the cartilaginous aspect of the ear canal,

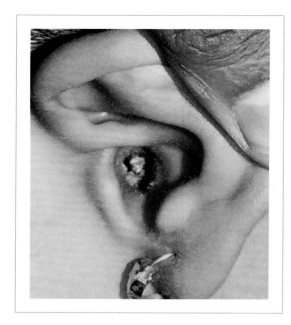

FIGURE 4.45 Excessive cerumen.
Source: Courtesy of Annand2022.

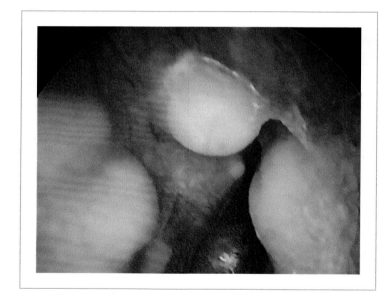

FIGURE 4.46 Osteoma.
Source: Courtesy of Didier Descouens.

as well as on the tragus. May also be associated with regional lymphadenopathy.

Polyp: Arises in ear canal from mucosal or granulomatous tissue; erythematous and bleeds easily; typically immersed in purulent, foul drainage; may be indicative of chronic auricular disease. Benign, but need to refer to an ENT specialist for removal.

ABNORMALITIES OF THE TYMPANIC MEMBRANE (TABLES 4.4 AND 4.5)

Retracted drum: With this condition, bony landmarks appear more pronounced and well defined (Figure 4.47). The handle of the malleus has a shorter

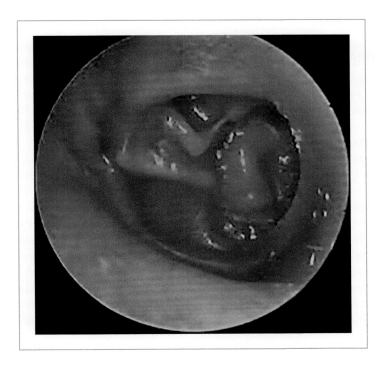

FIGURE 4.47 Retracted tympanic membrane.

TABLE 4.4
Tympanic Membrane Problems Based on Pneumatic Exam

Mobility	Condition
Bulging TM, nonmobile	Purulent fluid or fluid in middle ear
Retracted TM, nonmobile	Blocked Eustachian tube, (+)/(–) middle ear effusion
(+) Mobility with (–) pressure	Blocked Eustachian tube, (+)/(–) middle ear effusion
Small areas of hypermobility	Atrophic TM, or healed perforated TM

TM, tympanic membrane.

TABLE 4.5
Tympanic Membrane Problems Based on Otoscopic Exam

Color of Tympanic Membrane	Condition
Blue or red TM	Blood in middle ear
Dull TM	Fibrotic
Erythema	Middle ear infection, persistent crying
Pale yellow TM	Serous fluid in middle ear
Thick white plaques/flecks	Healed irritation
White TM	Middle ear infection
Air bubbles	Serous fluid in middle ear

TM, tympanic membrane.

appearance and is more horizontal than usual. Short process is very pronounced. The light reflex is absent or distorted. The drum is dim and lusterless and is motionless. These physical exam findings signify negative pressure and a middle ear vacuum due to an obstructed Eustachian tube and serous otitis media.

Serous otitis media: Often caused as a consequence of a blocked Eustachian tube. The resultant otoscopic exam finding is an amber-yellow appearing tympanic membrane that is suggestive of serum in the middle ear (Figure 4.48). It transudates to relieve negative pressure as a result of an obstructed Eustachian tube. There may be evidence of an air/fluid level with a subtle black dividing line, or air bubbles visible behind the tympanic membrane. Patients often report symptoms such as a feeling of fullness in their ear, transient hearing loss, and popping sound with swallowing. Also called secretory otitis media, middle ear effusion, or glue ear.

Acute purulent otitis media: Acute purulent otitis media is present when the middle ear fluid is infected. On otoscopic examination, there is an absent light reflex as a consequence of the increasing middle ear pressure. Erythema, edema, and a bulging of tympanic membrane are first noted in the superior part of the tympanic membrane. The patient will often complain of earache, fever, and difficulty sleeping. Second, if untreated, it will progress to an erythematous bulging of the entire tympanic membrane. Patients often will report profound pulsating pain and fever, as well as transient hearing loss. Pneumatic otoscopy reveals hypomobility of the tympanic membrane (Figure 4.49).

Perforated tympanic membrane: If left untreated, the acute otitis media may lead to rupture of the tympanic membrane from increased intra-auricular pressure. Perforations also occur from traumatic injuries (such as a slap or punch to the ear). Generally, the perforation appears as an oval or round darkened area on the tympanic membrane (Figure 4.50). *Central* perforations occur in the pars tensa. *Marginal* perforations occur at the annulus. Marginal perforations are called attic perforations when they occur in the superior part of the tympanic membrane, the pars flaccida.

Cholesteatoma: Cholesteatoma follows a marginal perforation from years ago and is the consequence of a malignant overgrowth of epidermal tissue. Upon otoscopic examination, the tympanic membrane appears pearly white and cheesy (Figure 4.51). Over time, this manifestation of the

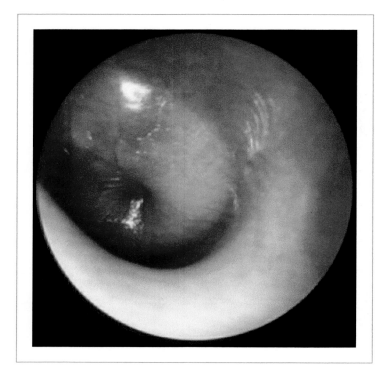

FIGURE 4.48 Serous otitis media.

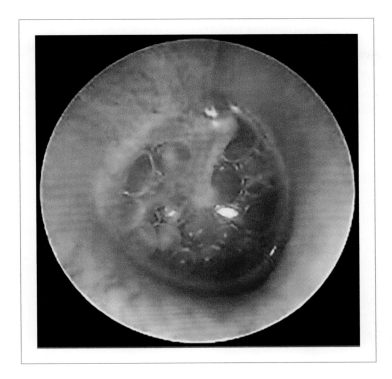

FIGURE 4.49 Acute purulent otitis media. Note distinctive air bubbles.

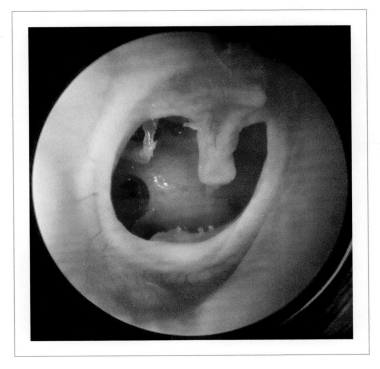

FIGURE 4.50 Perforated tympanic membrane.

Source: Courtesy of Michael Hawke.

growth of cholesteatoma can erode bone and produce hearing loss.

Tympanostomy tubes: Tympanostomy tubes are polyethylene tubes that are surgically inserted into the tympanic membrane (Figure 4.52). They are placed to alleviate middle ear pressure and to promote drainage of chronic or recurrent middle ear infections. The tympanostomy tubes spontaneously extrude in 6 months to 1 year.

Scarred tympanic membrane: Upon otoscopic examination, the practitioner will note dense white patches on the tympanic membrane. These white

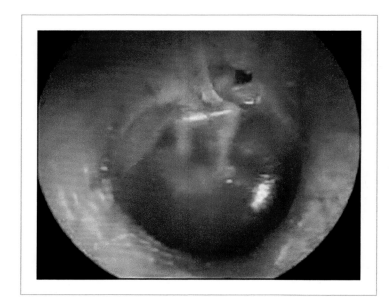

FIGURE 4.51 Cholesteatoma.

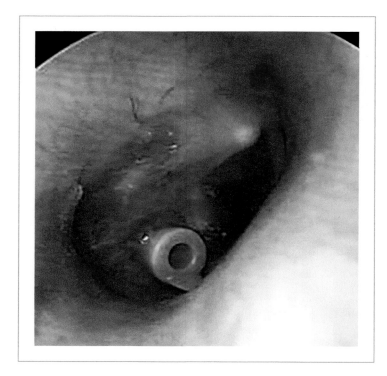

FIGURE 4.52 Tympanostomy tube.

patches are the sequelae of repeated ear infections. Despite the appearance of the tympanic membrane, hearing is not necessarily impacted.

Hemotympanum: If this condition is seen on otoscopic exam, it is an indication of the presence of blood in the middle ear (Figure 4.53). This

condition is typically seen in patients who have suffered head trauma, such as a skull fracture.

Bullous myringitis: Can present as a sudden onset of severe pain. Physical exam findings reveal small vesicles present on the tympanic membrane (Figure 4.54). If these rupture, they can be evidenced

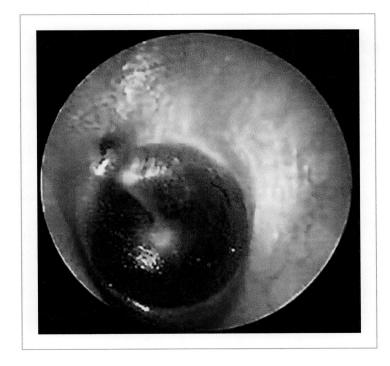

FIGURE 4.53 Hemotympanum.

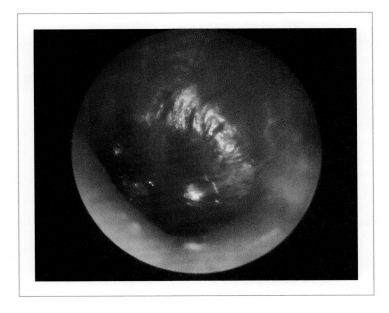

FIGURE 4.54 Bullous myringitis.

Source: Courtesy of B. Wellescik.

by bloody otorrhea. May be seen in patients with mycoplasma pneumonia and viral infections.

Fungal infection: Collection of black or white specks on the tympanic membrane or canal wall. Can be suggestive of a fungal or yeast infection.

Nystagmus: If the body is turning or spinning rapidly, the eyes will fix on one point for a moment, then jump ahead to another in a series of short, jerky movements. If the brain stem or inner ear is damaged, this type of eye movement can occur even when the body is stationary. This condition is known as nystagmus, and occurs when an individual has trouble controlling eye movements.

Holistic Health Assessment of the Ear

It is important for the healthcare provider to assess the patient in a holistic fashion. If the patient is an infant, it is important to ask the caregivers about healthcare practices and beliefs and infant feeding, bathing, and cleansing.

- Do they use cotton swabs to clean the infant's ears?

- Is the infant bottle fed or breastfed? If the infant receives a bottle, does the caregiver hold the infant while giving the bottle, or does he or she prop the bottle?

- While feeding, does the provider lay the infant flat or keep the infant upright? Is there any smoking in the home? Does the infant go to day care?

When assessing the patient, it is important to ascertain any hearing issues:

- Are family members reporting that the patient has the volume up louder than others?

- Is a referral to an ENT specialist warranted, based on physical exam findings? If so, are there financial concerns?

- Does the patient need a referral to audiology? Can the patient afford hearing aids?

CASE STUDY: EAR

SAMPLE CLINICAL PROBLEM

Jameson is a 4-month-old infant brought to the provider's office by his mother because he "was up all night crying, and is warm."

PAST HISTORY

Jameson is the only child to Mr. and Mrs. G. Mrs. G. received regular prenatal care. Jameson was born at 39 weeks' gestation; labor and delivery were uneventful. Jameson weighed 3,500 grams at birth and was discharged home 2 days after delivery. Jameson was fed with formula via bottle. All of Jameson's

(continued)

(continued)

well-infant visits have been normal and are up-to-date. Jameson is up-to-date on his vaccinations. Jameson has had one previous episode of otitis media, but otherwise Jameson is healthy.

SOCIAL HISTORY

Jameson lives with his parents in a duplex. Jameson's dad drives a truck for a living. Jameson's mother stays home and provides care to two other neighborhood toddlers. Both of Jameson's parents smoke cigarettes.

SUBJECTIVE

Two days prior to the office visit, Mrs. G. placed Jameson down in his crib for a nap. She gave him a bottle filled with apple juice. He woke up crying. Jameson stopped crying when held, but remained fussy. He would not eat his baby food. A rectal temperature was taken and was 38.1°C. Jameson cried all night. Mrs. G. administered one dose of acetaminophen during the night, which quieted Jameson for a brief duration.

OBJECTIVE

Vital Signs: Temperature 38.5°C (tympanic), pulse 155, respirations 38, weight 8.5 kg (90th percentile for weight), height 30 inch (97th percentile)
General: Alert, interactive, crying, and fussy. Developmentally appropriate
Skin: Warm and dry, and without lesions or rashes
Head: Anterior fontanel flat, posterior fontanel patent, flat
Eyes: Sclera white, anicteric. Conjunctiva clear and without exudate. Red reflex present bilaterally
Ears: Both tympanic membranes injected, erythematous, and bulging. No light reflex, no mobility on pneumatic otoscopy
Mouth/Throat: Pink/moist mucosa. No lesions or exudate. Tonsils (+2)
Neck: Supple and without cervical lymphadenopathy
Heart: Regular rate and rhythm, no murmurs
Lungs: Unlabored respirations, breath sounds clear and equal bilaterally
Abdomen: Protuberant abdomen, soft, and nontender. Positive bowel sounds in all four quadrants

ASSESSMENT

- Otitis media, unspecified, bilateral

- Pain related to inflammation in tympanic membranes

- High risk for ear infection secondary to supine bottle feeding, exposure to secondhand smoke, group childcare

- Knowledge deficit (parents) related to lack of exposure to risk factors for otitis media

Assessment of Special Populations: Ear

GESTATIONAL POPULATION

In the four week of gestation, the inner ear starts to develop. Damage to the organ of Corti and impaired hearing may result if there is maternal rubella infection during the first trimester. Anatomically, the infant's Eustachian tube is relatively shorter and wider, and its position is more horizontal than the adult's, making it easier for pathogens from the nasopharynx to migrate through the middle ear.

PEDIATRIC POPULATION

The most common illness in children is otitis media, which is a middle ear infection. Otitis media can be a consequence of an obstructed Eustachian tube, or transference of secretions from the nasopharynx into the middle ear. Down syndrome, infant prematurity, and bottle-fed babies in a supine position are those that are at an increased risk for otitis media. Feeding an infant in the supine position causes the effects of gravity. While the infant is drinking the bottle, he or she tends to attract the nasopharyngeal secretions into the middle ear. Breastfeeding aids to inhibit this issue. Parents are encouraged to not lie the infant flat, or prop a bottle up for feeding. Parents are encouraged to hold the infant upright against their arm as the infant is feeding.

As a consequence of acute otitis media, persistent middle ear effusion can have significant impacts on hearing, speech/language, and cognitive development, leading to delays. Patients who suffer persistent episodes of otitis media should be referred to an ear, nose, and throat provider, as the patient may require myringotomy tubes.

Cerumen has a genetic component resulting in two types: (a) dry cerumen, which is gray, flaky, and frequently becomes a thin, removable mass in the ear canal, and (b) wet cerumen, which is honey brown to dark brown and moist.

In childhood, the lumen is surrounded by lymphoid tissue that increases, thus making the lumen easily occluded. The infant is at greater risk for middle ear infections than the adult secondary to these factors.

YOUNG ADULT POPULATION

A common cause of conductive hearing loss in young adults between 20 and 40 years old is known as otosclerosis. Over time, there is hardening that causes the foot plate of the stapes to become affixed in the oval window. The transmission of sound is impeded, thus resulting in progressive hearing loss.

ELDERLY POPULATION

In the aging adult, cilia that line the ear canal become stiff and coarse, impeding sound waves traveling toward the tympanic membrane. As a result, this condition may cause decreased hearing. Cerumen can also accumulate and oxidize, further reducing hearing. Atrophy of the apocrine glands leads to the cerumen becoming drier and impacted within the external ear canal. Also, an older person with a life history of frequent ear infections may have noticeable scarring on the tympanic membrane, which also contributes to hearing loss.

Impacted cerumen is a common but reversible cause of hearing loss in older people. Those undergoing removal of impacted cerumen reported that 75% had significantly improved hearing.

Hearing loss that occurs with aging is known as presbycusis. It can occur in people living in a quiet environment. Over time it is caused by nerve degeneration in the inner ear or auditory nerve, resulting in a gradual sensorineural loss. Typical age of onset is in the fifth decade, and then it slowly progresses. The individual may notice a loss of high-frequency tone; it is more difficult to hear consonants than vowels. Words may sound garbled. Impaired sound localization is also an issue. Loud environments accentuate communication dysfunction, making it harder for the individual to hear.

PATIENTS WITH DISABILITIES

Patients with disabilities need to have optimal hearing to compensate for limitations associated with physical limitations. Therefore, patients with disabilities need to have as thorough an examination of vision as other individuals and treatment provided accordingly.

VETERAN POPULATION

The provider should ask the patient if they served in the military. If so, the dates and capacity in which they served (e.g., pilot, ground forces, medical services) should be ascertained. Based upon this information, the provider will be aware of what potential hazards or chemicals of warfare the patient may have been exposed to.

Diagnostic Reasoning: Ear

Common Differential Diagnoses: Ear

Symptom	Assessment	Condition
Large ears	Ears that are larger than 10 cm vertically	Macrotia
Pain	Erythema, pain, swelling, tenderness to touch +/− exudate	Otitis externa Furuncle
Pain with movement (mastoid process)	Pain at the posterior auricular node	Mastoiditis Lymphadenitis
Painful discoloration	Red/blue discoloration	Frostbite
Pruritus, dry, flaking, scaling skin	Dry scaling skin over the ears, may have pruritus over the otitis externa	Eczema Contact dermatitis Seborrhea
Skin over the ears that is reddened, excessively warm	Erythema, warmth	Inflammation
Small ears	Ears that are smaller than 4 cm vertically	Microtia

BIBLIOGRAPHY

Albert, D. M., Miller, J. W., Azar, D. T., Blodi, B. A. (2008). *Albert & Jakobiec's principles and practice of ophthalmology* (3rd ed.). Philadelphia, PA: Saunders Elsevier.

Centers for Disease Control and Prevention. (n.d.). Hearing loss in children: Types of hearing loss. Retrieved from http://www.cdc.gov/ncbddd/hearingloss/types.html

Dedhia, K., Kitsko, D., Sabo, D., & Chi, D. H. (2013). Children with sensorineural hearing loss after passing the newborn hearing screen. *JAMA Otolaryngology–Head & Neck Surgery, 139*(2), 119–123. doi:10.1001/jamaoto.2013.1229

Denniston, A. K., & Murray, P. I. (2014). *Oxford handbook of ophthalmology* (3rd ed.). Oxford, England: Oxford University Press.

Katz, J., Chasin, M., English, K., Hood, L. J., & Tillery, K. l. (2015). *Handbook of clinical audiology* (7th ed.). Philadelphia, PA: Wolters Kluwer Health.

Jarvis, C. (1996). *Physical examination and health assessment* (2nd ed.). Philadelphia, PA: W. B. Saunders.

Kane, R. L., Ouslander, J. G., Abrass, I. B., & Resnick, B. (2013). *Essentials of clinical geriatrics* (7th ed.). New York, NY: McGraw-Hill.

Leigh, R. J., & Zee, D. S. (2015). *The neurology of eye movements* (5th ed.). New York, NY: Oxford University Press.

Malekzadeh, S. (Ed.). (2015). *Otolaryngology lifelong learning manual* (3rd ed.). New York, NY: Thieme.

Morris, J. G., & Grattan-Smith, P. J. (2015). *Manual of neurological signs*. Oxford, England: Oxford University Press. doi:10.1093/med/9780199945795.003.0173

Muse, C., Harrison, J., Yoshinaga-Itano, C., Grimes, A., Brookhouser, P. E., Epstein, S., . . . Martin, B. (2013). Supplement to the JCIH 2007 position statement: Principles and guidelines for early intervention after confirmation that a child is deaf or hard of hearing. *Pediatrics, 131*(4), E1324–E1349. doi:10.1542/peds.2013-0008

Olver, J., Cassidy, L., Jutley, G., & Crawley, L. (2014). *Ophthalmology at a glance* (2nd ed.). Chichester, England: Wiley-Blackwell.

Riordan-Eva, P., & Augsburger, J. J. (Eds.). (2018). *Vaughan & Asbury's general ophthalmology* (19th ed.). New York, NY: McGraw Hill.

5

ADVANCED HEALTH ASSESSMENT OF SKIN, HAIR, AND NAILS

Lindita Vinca

(continued)

HOLISTIC ASSESSMENT
   Specific Health History
   Safety
   Distress
   Nutrition and Exercise
   Financial Implications
   Spiritual Considerations

CASE STUDY

ASSESSMENT OF SPECIAL POPULATIONS
   Elderly Population
   Pediatric Population
   Pregnant Population
   Patients With Disabilities

DIAGNOSTIC REASONING
   Common Differential Diagnoses: Hair
   Common Differential Diagnoses: Skin
   Common Differential Diagnoses: Nails

Overview of Anatomy and Physiology

The skin is the largest organ of the body and makes up approximately 16% of the total adult body weight. The skin has many substantial functions; however, its main function is to act as a barrier to protect the body from noxious external factors and to keep the internal systems unharmed. The skin's other responsibilities include the containment of its complex adnexal structures, such as hair follicles, nails, glands, and specialized sensory structures, all of which function in protection, homeostasis, and the transmission of sensation. The integumentary system is assembled by the skin and its derivative structures. The skin is composed of three layers: the epidermis, dermis, and subcutaneous tissue (Figure 5.1). The epidermis is the outermost layer that consists mainly of keratinocytes. The keratinocytes function to synthesize keratin, which is a long, threadlike protein with a protective role. The dermis is the middle layer that provides structural integrity;

its primary components are made up of collagen, elastin, and extrafibrillar matrix. The hypodermis (also known as the subcutaneous layer) is the layer directly below the dermis and serves to support the skin to the underlying fascia (fibrous tissue) of the bones and muscles. The subcutaneous layer consists of well-vascularized, loose, areolar connective tissue and adipose tissue, which functions as a method of fat storage and provides insulation for the integument.

EPIDERMIS

The epidermis is a continually renewing layer that gives rise to derived structures, such as pilosebaceous apparatuses, nails, and sweat glands. It is a stratified squamous epithelium that measures approximately

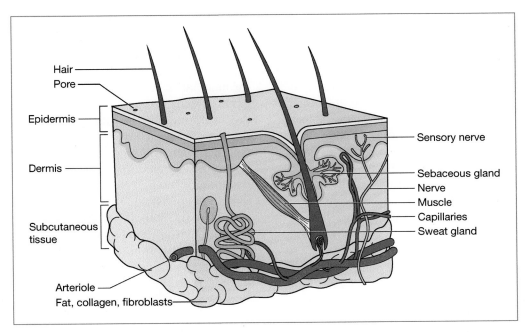

FIGURE 5.1 Anatomy of the skin. Epidermis consists of the top layer of the skin, which serves as the protective barrier and is divided into four layers. The dermis makes up the middle layer of the skin composed of blood appendages, vessels, and nerves. The subcutaneous fat lies below the dermis.

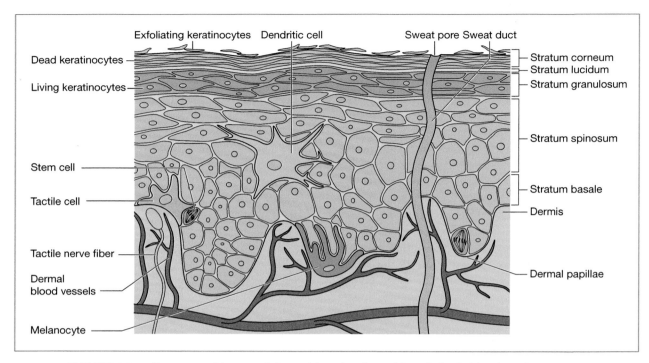

FIGURE 5.2 Cell types and layers of the epidermis. The epidermis is divided into four layers: basal cell, stratum spinosum, stratum granulosum, and stratum corneum. Basal layer is responsible for cell division and the process of cell differentiation. Stratum spinosum is abundant in keratinocytes. Stratum granulosum involves the process of differentiation that gives rise to cells that provide the granular layer with further structural support. Stratum corneum is the superficial layer composed of dead cells that protect the skin from microbes.

0.1 mm thick, although the thickness is greater (0.8–1.4 mm) on the palms and soles. The epidermis is responsible for acting as the protective barrier and its main cells consist of keratinocytes and dendritic cells. The epidermis stores a number of other cells such as melanocytes, Langerhans cells, and Merkel cells. The epidermis is divided into four layers in ascending order: basal cell, stratum spinosum, stratum granulosum, and stratum corneum (Figure 5.2).

BASAL CELL LAYER

The basal cell layer (*stratum germinativum*) is made up of undifferentiated and proliferating basal cells. Skin stem cells are located in the basal layer in the interfollicular epidermis, and they give rise to keratinocytes. All of the keratinocytes are produced from this layer of cells that are constantly going through mitosis in order to generate new cells. The existing cells are pushed superficially away from the stratum germinativum while the new cells are formed. The basal layer is the primary location for cell division and the process of cell differentiation. Melanocytes make up 5% to 10% of the basal cell community. These cells produce the melanin cells that are responsible for skin pigmentation. Melanin gives hair and skin its color, and also facilitates the protection of living cells of the epidermis from ultraviolet (UV) radiation damage. Merkel cells are also found in the epidermis; they function as a receptor in which the primary function is to stimulate sensory nerves that the brain perceives as touch. Fingerprints form where the cells of the basal layer meet the papillae of the underlying dermal layer, resulting in the formation of the ridges on your fingers that are known as fingerprints, a process that occurs in the growing fetus.

STRATUM SPINOSUM

The stratum spinosum lies above the basal layer and is primarily composed of keratinocytes, which differentiate from the basal cells beneath them. The keratinocytes produce keratin that makes up eight to 10 layers of the stratum spinosum as a result of cell division from the stratum germinativum. The stratum spinosum derives its name from the "spines," or intercellular bridges, that develop between the keratinocytes. This layer forms spiny protruding cell processes that join the cell by structures called desmosomes. The desmosomes interlock with each other to enhance the bond between the cells.

STRATUM GRANULOSUM

The stratum granulosum is the process of differentiation that continues with further changes to the keratinocytes, giving the cells a grainy appearance. The cells become flatter because their cell membranes thicken due to the additional keratin. The cells contain distinctive dark granules that are composed of keratohyalin. Keratohyalin contains two proteins, one of which is called profilaggrin. This protein is the precursor to filaggrin. Filaggrin plays an important role in the collection of keratin filaments in the stratum corneum. Involucrin (from the Latin for "envelope") is another protein that plays a crucial role in the formation of the cell envelope of the stratum corneum. Granular layer also contains cells known as lamellar granules that contain polysaccharides, glycoproteins, and lipids. These cells extrude into the intercellular space and ultimately are the cells that provide the "cement" that supports the stratum corneum cells and holds them together.

STRATUM CORNEUM

The stratum corneum is the most superficial layer of the epidermis and is the layer exposed to the outside environment. There are usually 15 to 30 layers of cells in the stratum corneum that are stacked in vertical layers due to the production of increased keratinization. The stratum corneum is a dry, dead layer of cells that supports the prevention of the penetration of microbes. This layer also provides a mechanical protection against abrasion and prevents dehydration of the underlying tissues. The cells in this layer shed periodically and are replaced by cells that are pushed up from the stratum granulosum. The entire layer is replaced during a period of about 4 weeks.

EPIDERMAL CELLULAR COMPONENTS

The cells of the epidermis consist of the melanocytes, Merkel cells, and Langerhans cells (Figure 5.3). Melanocytes are responsible for synthesizing melanin. Merkel cells serve as mechanoreceptors that are found in the basal layer. Langerhans cells' primary role is identifying foreign antigens found in the epidermal tissue.

MELANOCYTES

Melanocytes are pigment-rich dendritic cells found in the basal layer and derived from the neural crest, which is found in skin, hair, the uveal tract of the eye, leptomeninges, and the inner ear. Melanocytes absorb UV radiation and protect the skin from UV-induced mutations. The dendrites extend into the stratum spinosum and serve as passage ways through which pigment granules are transferred to their neighboring keratinocytes. The granules are termed melanosomes, and the pigment within is melanin, which is synthesized from tyrosine. Melanosomes are found situated above the nucleus to protect the DNA. The difference in skin pigmentation depends on the number and size of melanosomes and their distribution in the skin (Figure 5.4). In heavily pigmented skin, melanosomes are larger in size with greater production and more abundant when compared to melanosomes in lightly pigmented skin. Sunlight stimulates melanocytes to increase pigment production and circulate their melanosomes more extensively.

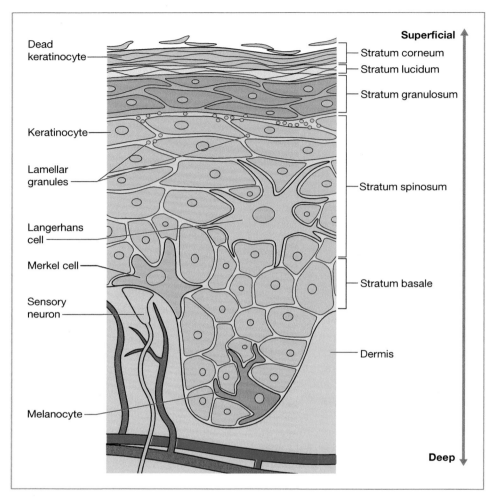

FIGURE 5.3 Cells of the epidermis: melanocytes, Merkel cells, and Langerhans cells.

MERKEL CELLS

Merkel cells are ectoderm-derived cells found in the basal layer that function as mechanoreceptors. These cells are oval-shaped, slow-adapting, and located in sites of high-tactile sensitivity that are attached to basal keratinocytes by desmosomal junctions. Merkel cells are typically found in the digits, lips, regions of the oral cavity, and the outer sheath of the hair follicle. Merkel cells in certain regions such as fingertips result in smaller and more densely packed receptive fields as well as greater tactile resolution and responsiveness to stimuli.

LANGERHANS CELLS

Langerhans cells are involved in recognizing and presenting foreign antigens to specific T lymphocytes. They are bone marrow–derived dendritic cells with monocyte–macrophage lineage found in stratum spinosum. These cells constitute 3% to 5% of cells of the total epidermal cell population and maintain nearly constant numbers and distributions in a

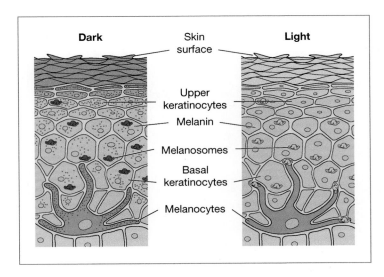

FIGURE 5.4 Melanocyte production. Melanocytes are found in the basal layer; they synthesize melanin and are derived from the neural crest, which is found in hair, the uveal tract of the eye, leptomeninges, the inner eye, and skin.

particular area of the body. In addition to the epidermis, Langerhans cells are found in squamous epithelia, such as the oral cavity, esophagus, vagina, and lymphoid organs. The cells must recognize and process soluble antigens found in the epidermal tissue. In the beginning stages of life, the Langerhans cells are weak stimulators of unprimed T cells; however, they are able to ingest and process antigens. Once the cell has evolved into an effective activator of naïve T cells, activation via contact with the antigen will not stimulate phagocytosis but rather will provoke cell migration.

CUTANEOUS APPENDAGES

ECCRINE SWEAT GLANDS

Eccrine glands' most important function is to regulate the body temperature through evaporative heat loss (Figure 5.5). Eccrine glands are activated by emotional and thermal stimuli and are necessary for thermoregulation. They have generalized distribution, with the highest density in the palm and soles. The eccrine secretory unit consists of a coiled secretory section that drains into a long thin duct whose apical portion (acrosyringium) opens to the skin surface. The secretory coils contain two cell types within a single cell layer. The first cell type is the large clear cell responsible for the

gland's secretory function. The second cell type is the dark cell, of unknown function, with basophilic granules. Both cell types are surrounded by myoepithelial cells, which likely function to augment the transfer of sweat to the skin surface. The innervation of eccrine glands consists of postganglionic sympathetic fibers that have acetylcholine as the key neurotransmitter. The latter explains why hypohidrosis and subsequent hyperthermia can result from administration of medications with potential anticholinergic side effects. On the contrary, excess function of eccrine glands is due to an enhanced cutaneous sympathetic outflow in response to mental and thermal stimuli. The former results in the hyperhidrosis of the palms, soles, and axillae.

APOCRINE GLANDS

The apocrine glands are found in certain anatomic locations (axillae, anogenital region, periumbilical region, nipples, and vermilion border of the lip) and are larger than eccrine glands (Figure 5.5). They consist of a secretory portion, which is located in the deep dermis and subcutaneous fat, and a stretched duct that opens directly into the upper portion of the follicular canal (i.e., the acrosyringium). Sympathetic innervation, with acetylcholine as the terminal neurotransmitter, fine-tunes function, as does adrenergic stimulation. Apocrine

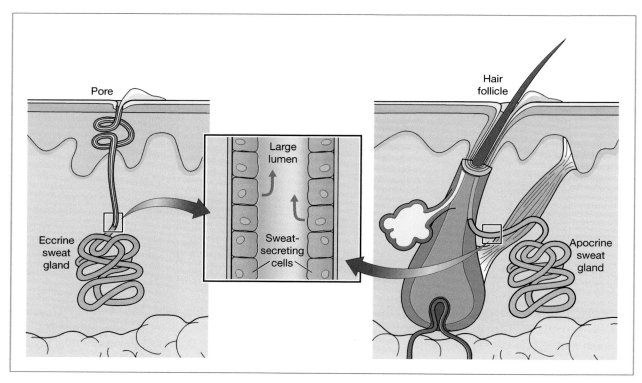

FIGURE 5.5 Structure of the eccrine and apocrine sweat glands. The eccrine glands control the regulation of body temperature through the activation of thermal and emotional stimuli. The apocrine glands continuously give off oily fluid found in the axillae, anogenital region, periumbilical region, nipples, and vermilion border of the lip. The secretory portion is located deep in the dermis and subcutaneous fat, in which the stretched duct opens directly into the upper portion of the follicular canal.

glands continuously give off very small amounts of an oily fluid. Apocrine sweat is sterile and odorless as it is secreted. The bacterial decomposition on the skin is responsible for an odor named bromhidrosis. Unsatisfactory body and textile hygiene will worsen the condition.

APOECCRINE SWEAT GLANDS

The apoeccrine sweat glands are found only in the adult axilla. The sweat gland develops during puberty from eccrine-like precursor cells. The relative percentage of axillary apoeccrine sweat glands is higher in patients with hyperhidrosis as compared to normohidrotic persons. Apoeccrine sweat is a clear fluid that has a secretory rate as much as 10 times that of the eccrine gland. Growth factors in

sweat may be involved in stimulating the differentiation of the apoeccrine glands.

SEBACEOUS GLANDS

Sebaceous glands produce sebum, which is an oily substance via holocrine secretion. The function of sebaceous glands is unknown; in fact, the skin of children and the palmar and plantar skin of adults function well without sebum. The cells themselves disintegrate, releasing sebum. Once produced, sebum is released into the infundibular portion of the hair follicle. Sebaceous glands are part of the pilosebaceous unit and are found wherever hair follicles are generally located (Figure 5.6). Ectopic sebaceous glands are found on mucous membranes, where they may form small yellow

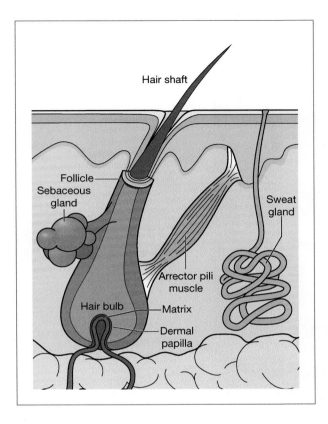

FIGURE 5.6 Structure of a pilosebaceous unit. Sebaceous glands produce sebum, which consists of an oily substance. Sebaceous glands are found on the scalp, upper back, chest, and face. The structure consists of hair, hair follicle, sebaceous gland, and the arrector pili muscle.

papules called Fordyce spots. Sebaceous glands are well developed on the scalp, face, upper back, and chest. There are three different types of pilosebaceous units: Vellus hair follicles are small sebaceous glands with a short, thin structure; sebaceous follicles are large sebaceous glands with midsized hair found on the face, chest, and back; and terminal hair follicles are fairly large hair follicles with thick long hairs.

The size and secretory activity of these glands are under androgen control. Androgens, specifically, appear to be the major factor that controls the development of the glands and the production of sebum. The level of sebum production at the completion of puberty remains perpetual through adulthood. Sebaceous follicles harbor bacteria and fungi, which comprise the normal flora. The major fungi are *Malassezia*, which is a yeast that is found in the most superficial desquamated cells. *Staphylococcus epidermis* and other micrococci are found in the pilosebaceous unit of the hair follicle. *Propionibacterium* is found deeper into the follicle where they tend to predominate.

DERMIS

STRUCTURE OF THE DERMIS

The dermis is a tough, but elastic, support structure that contains blood vessels, nerves, and cutaneous appendages (Figure 5.7). It supports structural integrity and ranges in thickness from 0.3 mm on the eyelid to 3.0 mm on the back. The dermis is approximately 15 to 40 times as thick as the epidermis. It is biologically active by communicating and regulating the functions of the cells by tissue regeneration. The dermis constitutes the majority

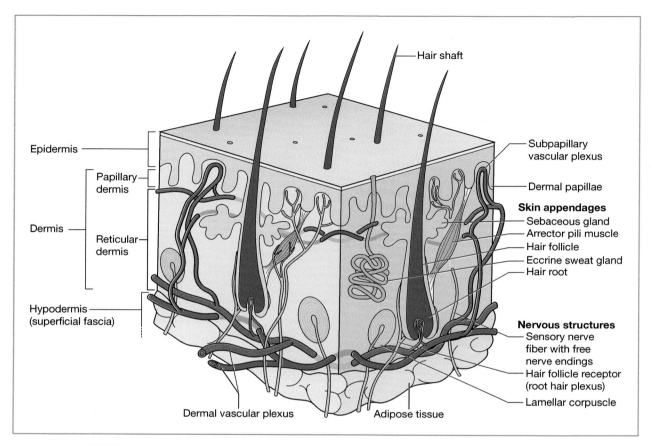

FIGURE 5.7 Structure of the dermis. The dermis is largely composed of collagen fibers. The cellular components of the dermis consist of mast cells, histiocytes, vascular channels, and nerves. The appendages of the skin are also found well into the dermal matrix.

of the skin and provides strength and resiliency. It protects the body from mechanical injury, binds water, aids in thermal regulation, and includes receptors of sensory stimuli. The dermal matrix is composed of three types of connective tissue: collagen, elastic tissue, and reticular fibers, which are produced by fibroblasts. The primary element of the dermis consists of the collagen fibers, with smaller amounts of the elastic fibers and matrix. The matrix mainly comprises the extracellular matrix and the ground substance made up of proteoglycans and gelatin. Fibroblasts, mast cells, macrophages, plasma cells, vascular channels, and nerves make up the dermal cellular components.

The layers of the dermis consist of the papillary and reticular layers. The *papillary layer* is made of loose, areolar connective tissue. Within the papillary layer are fibroblasts, small amounts of fat cells (adipocytes), and a great supply of blood vessels. Phagocytes are also found in the papillary layer and their fundamental role is to help fight bacteria or other infections that have violated the skin. The *reticular layer* is composed of dense, irregular connective tissue which is much more consolidated in comparison to the papillary layer. This layer is well vascularized and has a network of rich sensory nerves and a sympathetic nerve supply.

INTERSTITIAL COMPONENTS OF THE DERMIS

Collagen fibers account for 70% of the weight of dry dermis, which is extremely tenacious and particularly resistant to tension parallel to the fibers. Collagen's ability to maintain the dynamic strength of the skin is a critical characteristic. The collagen fibers form by thin fibril aggregation; the greater the number of fibrils, the thicker and more robust the fiber. Narrow collagen fibers are sparsely seen in the papillary layers and subpapillary layers; nonetheless, collagen bundles, with fully matured thick collagen fibers, are densely distributed in the reticular dermal upper layers. Elastic fibers, in contrast, play a role in maintaining elasticity but do very little to resist tearing of the skin. Elastic fibers are exceedingly elastic and are found in the dermis of the scalp, face, and the extensible organs such as arteries and tendons. The elastic fibers differ both structurally and chemically from collagen. The fibers are not as sturdy as collagen fiber; however, the deeper in the dermis, the thicker they are. Elastic fibers in the reticular layers are scattered among collagen bundles running parallel to the skin surface. Clearly, the closer to the surface of the papillary layer the elastic fibers, the thinner the network. The fibers are also connected to the lamina densa of glands, sweat ducts, smooth muscle, nerves, and blood vessels.

CELLULAR COMPONENTS OF THE DERMIS

MAST CELLS

Mast cells are specialized secretory cells derived from bone marrow and distributed in connective tissues throughout the body. Mast cells are abundant in the papillary dermis; however, they are also found in the subcutaneous fat. A large number of mast cells are found around blood vessels, especially postcapillary venules. The structure of a mast cell granule is round, oval, or angular membrane-bound containing histamine, heparin, serine proteinases, and certain cytokines. The surface of the cell contains hundreds or thousands of glycoprotein receptor sites for immunoglobulin E. Mast cells are categorized as type I and type II; type I,

or *connective tissue mast cells*, are located in the dermis and submucosa, and type II, or *mucosal mast cells*, are located in the respiratory tract mucosa and in the bowel. Mast cells accumulate in the skin because of abnormal proliferation, migration, and failure of apoptosis when mastocytosis occurs. Mast cells can be subjected to activation by antigens or allergens acting via the high-affinity receptor for immunoglobulin E, superoxides, complement proteins, neuropeptides, and lipoproteins. Mast cells express histamine, leukotrienes, prostanoids, proteases, and many cytokines after activation. These mediators that are released are crucial to the genesis of an inflammatory response. Mast cells are thought to play an active role in many conditions such as allergy, parasitic diseases, atherosclerosis, malignancy, asthma, pulmonary fibrosis, and arthritis.

HISTIOCYTES

Histiocytes are a type of macrophage that broadly distributes in the connective tissue and intermingles with fibroblasts on the outside of endocapillary cells. The structure of a histiocyte is a small circular nucleus and a large spindle- or star-shaped cell seen on light microscopy; furthermore, concave nuclei and the formation of pseudopodial protrusions are observed by electron microscopy. Golgi apparatus, smooth and rough endoplasmic reticuli, and lysosomes are found within the structure of a histiocyte. The histiocyte releases collagenase and lysosomal enzymes containing elastase to digest the interstitium. Histiocytes present foreign substances to T cells as an antigen postdegradation and phagocytoses.

VASCULAR CHANNEL AND NERVES OF THE DERMIS

The dermal vasculature consists of two intercommunicating plexuses: the *subpapillary* or *superficial plexus* composed of postcapillary venules found at the junction of the papillary and reticular dermis, and the *lower plexus* at the dermal-subcutaneous interface. Multiple branches of arteries allocated in the skin are joined in the dermal layer to form the subcutaneous plexuses. The arterioles ascend through the papillary layer, with a configuration of capillary loops in the dermal papillaries before reaching the venules that link to each other to arrange two types of plexuses. This extraordinary connection allows the blood to flow into the cutaneous veins. The deeper plexus is supplied by larger blood vessels and is more complex, surrounding adnexal structures. The peripheral regions of the eccrine glands are particularly rich in vascular networks that regulate blood flow volume as well as body temperature by perspiration.

In addition, hair follicles in the anagen (growth) stage are also largely supplied with blood vessels. Blood flow fluctuates significantly in response to thermal stress because of the regulation of the preoptic-anterior hypothalamus. Increased skin blood flow, vasodilation, and sweating are vital to heat dissipation during hot temperatures and exercise. In contrast, exposure to cold temperatures results in vasoconstriction in the skin, decreasing heat loss from the body to inhibit hypothermia (Figure 5.8). Therefore, a dysfunction of control of skin blood flow can consequently hinder the skin's ability to maintain normal body temperature.

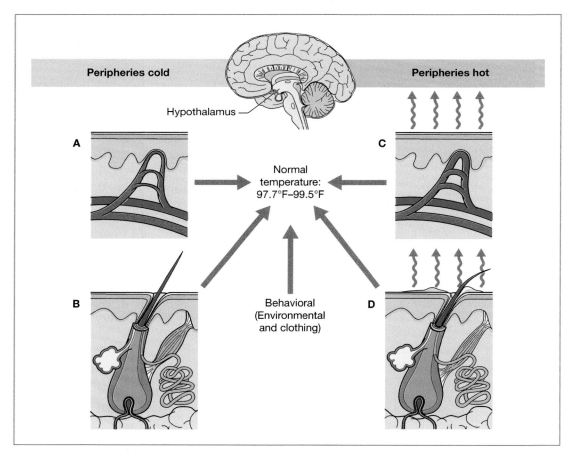

FIGURE 5.8 Variations in skin blood supply under warm and cold temperatures. This diagram depicts the intercommunicating plexuses of the hypothalamus. Blood flow vacillates in response to thermal stress due to the signaling of the preoptic-anterior hypothalamus. (**A**) Capillaries vasoconstrict to conserve heat. (**B**) Secretion of sweat ceases and hairs stand up, which traps an insulating layer of air. (**C**) Capillaries dilate near the skin's surface, losing heat. (**D**) Sweat glands begin secreting, which causes heat loss by evaporation.

Nerve bundles, in conjunction with arterioles and venules, are found in enormous quantity in neurovascular bundles of the dermis. The skin has a rich sensory innervation that pierces the fascia and ramifies in the subcutaneous tissue and dermis to arrange formation of the plexus. Meissner corpuscles that are organized in the dermal papillae are responsible for mediation of touch that is found on the ventral sides of the hands and feet. Meissner corpuscles occur in such a great amount on the hands, with the largest concentration in the fingertips. These corpuscles are particularly efficient in transducing information about the relatively low-frequency vibrations (30–50 Hz) that occur when textured objects are moved across the skin. Pacinian corpuscles are large encapsulated endings located in the subcutaneous tissue. Pacinian corpuscles adapt more briskly than Meissner's corpuscles and have a lower response threshold. The attributes suggest that Pacinian corpuscles are involved in the discrimination of fine surface textures or other moving stimuli that produce high-frequency vibration of the skin. They make up approximately 10% to 15% of the cutaneous receptors in the hand. Pacinian corpuscles located in interosseous membranes probably identify vibrations transmitted to the skeleton. They provide information primarily about the dynamic qualities of mechanical stimuli.

SUBCUTANEOUS TISSUE

A layer of subcutaneous fat lies between the dermis and the underlying fascia. The primary role of this layer is to help insulate the body from cold temperatures; it cushions deep tissues from blunt trauma and serves as a reserve source of energy for the body. Biologically active fat cells play a role in hormone communication, as evidenced by metabolic disturbances in obese children and adolescents with peripheral insulin resistance. A recent discovery is that adipose-derived stem cells aid in wound healing, hair follicle support/growth, and protection against photoaging. Aggregates of fat cells (lipocytes) are separated by fibrous septa that are traversed by blood vessels and nerves within the subcutaneous fat layer.

DERIVATIVES OF THE SKIN

HAIR

Hairs are found over the entire surface of the skin, except for palms, soles, glans penis, and vulval introitus (Figure 5.9). The human skin contains approximately 5 million hair follicles, with roughly 100,000 hair follicles of the scalp (plus those of the eyelashes and eyebrows) being the most apparent. There are three types of hair: lanugo, vellus, and terminal hairs. Lanugo hairs are fine and long, and formed in the fetus at 20 weeks' gestation. Vellus hairs are the short, fine, light-colored hairs that cover most body surfaces. Terminal hairs are longer, thicker, and darker, and are found on the scalp, eyebrows, eyelashes, and pubic, axillary, and beard areas. They originate as vellus hair; differentiation is stimulated at puberty by androgens. A hair follicle is thought to be an invagination of the epidermis, with a population of cells at the bottom known as the hair bulb. The hair bulb has cells that are replicating even more actively than the normal epidermal basal cells which constitute the hair matrix. Similar to the basal cells in the epidermis, the matrix cells first divide and then differentiate, eventually forming a keratinous hair shaft. Melanocytes are found in the matrix where they produce pigment, the amount of which determines the color of the hair. As the matric cells continue to divide, hair is pushed outward and exits through the epidermis at a rate of approximately 1 cm per month.

Hair growth in an individual follicle is cyclical, with a growth (anagen) phase, a transitional (catagen) phase, and a resting (telogen) phase (Figure 5.10). The lengths of the phases may differ from one area of the body to another; for example, on the scalp the anagen phase lasts for about 3 years. In comparison, the catagen

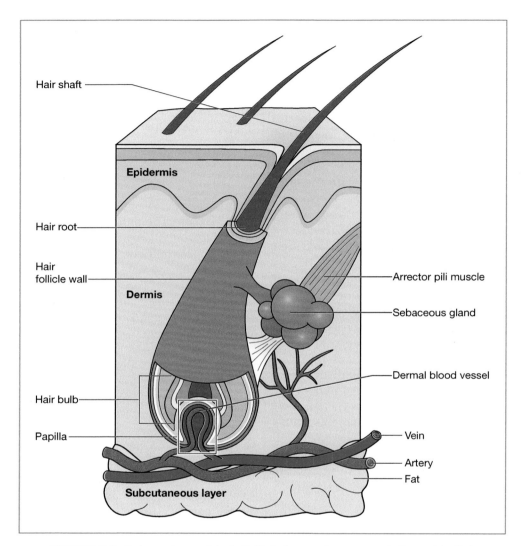

Hair shaft

Epidermis

Hair root

Hair
follicle wall

Dermis

Arrector pili muscle

Sebaceous gland

Dermal blood vessel

Hair bulb

Papilla

Vein

Artery

Fat

Subcutaneous layer

FIGURE 5.9 Hair anatomy. A hair follicle is a major reservoir for epithelial and melanocyte stem cells; it contains a unique pigmentary unit for hair shaft pigmentation and displays special innate, anti-infection defenses as well as an intraepithelial region of relative immune privilege.

phase may last for about 3 weeks and the telogen phase for about 3 months. The extent of the anagen phase ranges from person to person, confirming why some people can grow hair longer than others. At the term of the anagen phase, hair growth comes to a halt; the hair follicles will then begin the catagen and telogen phases. During the catagen and telogen phases, the matrix portion and the lower two-thirds of the hair follicle dwindle and the hair within the follicle is shed. Subsequently, a new hair matrix is formed at the bottom of the follicle and the cycle is repeated. Approximately 80% to 90% of scalp hair is in the anagen phase and 10% to 20% is in the telogen phase, thus accounting for a normal shedding of 25 to 100 hairs per day. Other sites on the body tend to have shorter anagen and longer telogen phases, causing most body hair to be shorter and remain in place for longer periods of time.

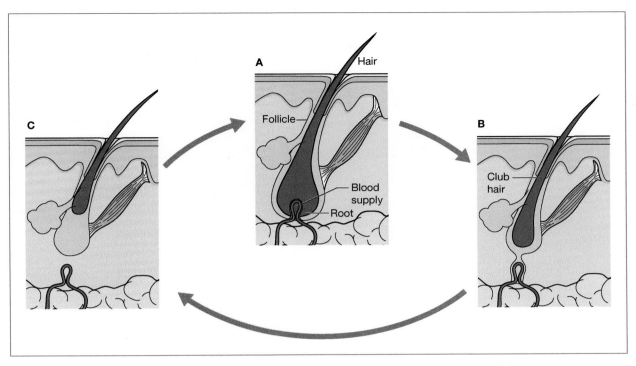

FIGURE 5.10 The hair growth cycle. The hair cycle consists of four phases: (**A**) Growth phase (anagen)—blood supply nourishes the follicle, enabling growth; (**B**) regression phase (catagen)—the hair follicle detaches from the blood supply; (**C**) resting phase (telogen)—the hair dies and falls out; and the last phase is shedding (exogen).

Hormonal factors controlling hair growth include estrogens, thyroid hormones, glucocorticoids, retinoids, prolactin, and growth hormone. Androgens (testosterone and its active metabolite, dihydrotestosterone) are the most impactful hormones that act directly on the androgen receptors in the dermal papilla. These hormones increase the size of hair follicles in androgen-dependent areas such as the beard area during adolescence. As we age, the androgen hormones can cause miniaturization of follicles in the scalp, resulting in androgen alopecia (male pattern baldness). Aside from scarring alopecia and rare congenital hair defects, hair loss and unwanted hair growth reflect alterations of hair follicle cycling and, thus, are considered reversible events. Several different physiological factors can impact the hair cycle and influence its course. Pregnancy is the prime example of the prolongation of the telogen phase and an increased amount of scalp hairs in the anagen phase. Once estrogen levels are balanced after delivery, telogen hairs are lost while anagen hairs simultaneously are converted to telogen, and this enormous number of telogen hairs will be lost in 3 to 5 months. Therefore, this type of hair loss is known as *telogen effluvium*, given the synchronous termination of anagen or telogen. Telogen effluvium is also observed after trauma, surgery, weight loss, severe stress, anemia, endocrine disorders, and malnutrition.

NAILS

The nail matrix contains dividing cells that mature, keratinize, and move forward to form the nail plate (Figure 5.11). The nail plate has a thickness of 0.3 to 0.5 mm and grows at a rate of 0.1 mm/24 h for the fingernails, with the toenails growing at a

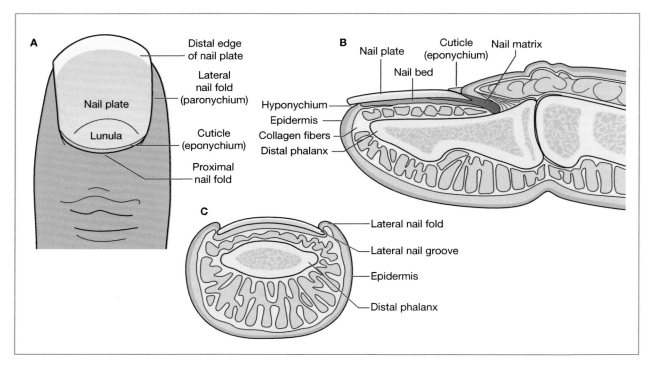

FIGURE 5.11 The anatomy of the nail. The nail is a rather complex architecture, with five distinct anatomic regions: the nail plate as a fully cornified structure, and four highly specialized epithelial tissues: the proximal nail fold; the nail matrix; the nail bed; and the hyponychium. (**A**) Dorsal, (**B**) sagittal, and (**C**) cross-section views of the nail.

slower rate. The nail apparatus develops from an ingrowth of the epidermis into the dermis. It gives rise to a plate formed by fully cornified, "dead" cells, the nail plate. Nails similar to hair are made of keratin, which is formed from a matrix of dividing epidermal cells. In comparison to hair, nails are hard and flat, and lie parallel to the skin surface. The proximal nail fold helps to protect the matrix. The stratum corneum that is produced in the nail fold forms the cuticle. The matrix generates the nail plate from its rapidly dividing, keratinizing cells. The majority of the matrix underlies the proximal nail fold; however, some digits extend under the nail plate, where it is grossly detectable as the white lunula. The epithelium of the nail bed produces a minimal amount of keratin, which ultimately evolves into a tightly adherent structure to the bottom of the nail plate. The pink color of a nail is related to the vascularity in the dermis of the nail bed. The *hyponychium* is the thickened epidermis that underlies the free margin of the nail. The dermis of the nail apparatus is a fibro-collagenous network lacking subcutaneous tissue and pilosebaceous units. The epithelia of the nail apparatus are the highly specialized nail matrix epithelium, the very thin nail bed epithelium, and the hyponychium, which continues into the epidermis of the palms and soles. Nails are conveniently placed anatomically at the ends of fingers and toes; they facilitate fine grasping and pinching maneuvers. Melanocytes are discernible in a high density in the nail matrix, although the presence of melanocytes in the nail bed is a controversial issue. Nail matrix melanocytes of darkly pigmented skin contain mature melanosomes and incorporate melanin, whereas those of lightly pigmented skin are usually in a "dormant" stage containing immature melanosomes.

Screening Health Assessment and Normal Findings

INSPECTION OF THE SKIN

An assessment of the integumentary system consists of inspection of color variations, skin integrity, and skin lesions (Figure 5.12). The inspection of general skin coloration and the amount of pigment in the skin accounts for the intensity of color as well as hue. Normal findings include evenly colored skin tones without unusual or prominent discoloration. Small amounts of melanin are common in white skins, while large amounts of melanin are common in olive and in darker skins. Carotene accounts for a yellow cast. A blue coloring may be a signal of cyanosis, a sign of illness. While inspecting skin coloration, allow the opportunity to note any odors emerging from the skin. Skin may have slight to no odor with perspiration,

depending on activity. Inspect localized parts of the body, noting any color variations, while keeping in mind that some clients have sun-tanned areas, freckles, or white patches known as vitiligo. Color variation is attributed to different amounts of melanin in certain areas. A generalized loss of pigmentation is seen in albinism. In dark-skinned patients, a normal variant is lighter-colored palms, soles, nail beds, and lips. Freckle-like or dark streaks of pigmentation are also common in the sclera and nail beds of dark-skinned patients as well. White-skinned patients have darker pigmentation around the nipples, lips, and genitalia. A normal finding in Asians, Native Americans, African Americans, and some whites are Mongolian spots, which can be found on the lower back, buttocks, or even on the upper back, arms, thighs, or abdomen. Mongolian spots are bluish, bruise-like markings that usually fade by 2 years

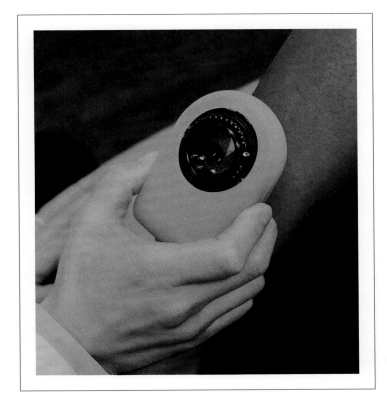

FIGURE 5.12 Skin inspection. Inspection of the skin includes color variations, skin integrity, and skin lesions.

of age. Inspection of the skin integrity includes carefully checking the skin in pressure point areas (i.e., sacrum, hips, elbows) for skin breakdown. Normal findings of intact skin integrity would consist of nonreddened areas. Skin inspection should also include the observation of skin lesions and the detection of abnormalities. Normal findings include smooth skin without lesions or stretch marks (striae), healed scars, freckles, moles, or birthmarks.

PALPATION OF THE SKIN

Palpate the skin to assess for texture using the palmar surface of your three middle fingers (Figure 5.13). Typically, the skin should be smooth and even. If lesions are noted during palpation, observe for drainage or other characteristics. Include measurements of skin lesions with a centimeter ruler during skin examination. Skin is normally thin; however, calluses (rough, thickened epidermis) are often seen on areas of the body that are exposed to constant pressure.

Skin surfaces tend to vary from moist to dry depending on the area assessed. Recent activity or a warm environment may cause increased moisture. Assessment of skin temperature should include the dorsal surface of the hands. Skin is normally a warm temperature. The palpation of the skin is necessary to assess for mobility and turgor, which involves skin pinching (Figure 5.14). Normally, skin pinches easily and returns to its normal state immediately. *Mobility* refers to how easily the skin can be pinched. *Turgor* refers to the skin's elasticity and how quickly the skin returns

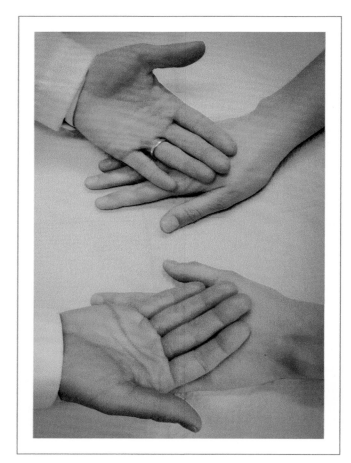

FIGURE 5.13 Palpating to assess temperature and moisture. Palpation of the skin typically incudes the assessment of texture, consistency, temperature, and integrity. The temperature is assessed with the provider's palmar surface of the hands.

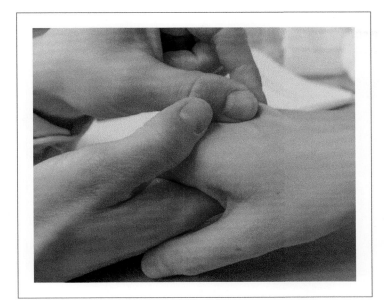

FIGURE 5.14 Assessment of skin turgor. The assessment of skin turgor is the act of the provider pinching the skin of the dorsal aspect of the hand. In a normal state of hydration, the skin returns to its original form immediately after assessment.

to its original shape after being pinched. Skin of the lower extremities in the normal heathy patient rebounds and does not remain indented when pressure is released.

INSPECTION AND PALPATION OF THE HAIR

Inspection of the hair includes the scalp and the hair. Inspection of hair should involve the amount and distribution of scalp, axillae, and pubic hair. Observe for unusual growth elsewhere on the body. Varying amounts of terminal hair cover the scalp, axillary, body, and pubic areas according to the normal gender distribution and hormonal influence. Fine vellus hair covers the entire body except for the soles, palms, lips, and nipples. Normal male pattern balding is symmetric. Natural hair color, as opposed to chemically colored hair, varies among patients from pale blond to black to gray or white. The color is determined by the amount of melanin present. The scalp should be clean and dry, although sparse dandruff may be visible. Hair is normally smooth, firm, and somewhat elastic. As we age, hair becomes coarser

and drier. Individuals of the African descent often have very dry scalp, and dry, fragile hair.

INSPECTION AND PALPATION OF THE NAILS

An assessment of the integumentary system consists of the inspection of the nails. Inspection should include the assessment for grooming, cleanliness, color, markings, and shape. The nails should be clean and manicured. Nails are pink toned with some longitudinal ridging, which is a normal variant. Dark-skinned patients may have freckles of pigmented streaks in their nails. The shape of the nail is normally at a 160-degree angle between the nail base and the skin.

The palpation of the nail is done to assess for texture and consistency (Figure 5.15). Normally, nails are hard and basically immobile. Darker-skinned patients may have thicker nails. The nail should be smooth and firm during skin palpation. Testing for capillary refill in the nail beds is done by pressing the nail tip briefly and monitoring for color change (Figure 5.16). A normal finding of capillary refill includes a pink tone that returns immediately post nail pressure release.

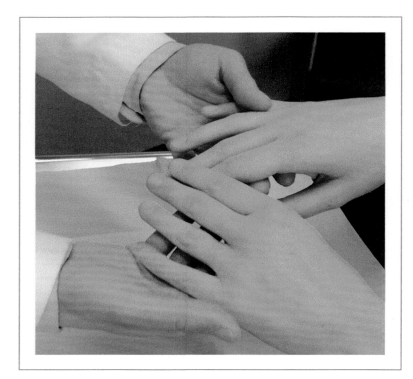

FIGURE 5.15 Nail inspection. The assessment includes grooming, cleanliness, color, markings, and shape. The nail plate is transparent and has a slightly convex shape. The normal nail plate has a smooth surface.

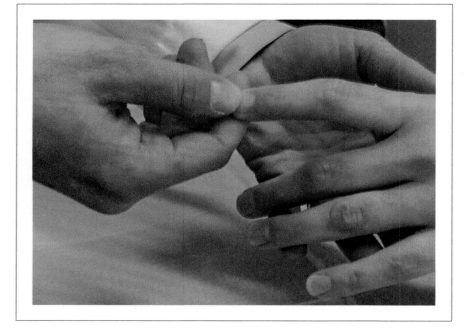

FIGURE 5.16 Nail palpation to assess for capillary refill. The provider presses on the nail tip and releases while monitoring for color change. Normal response would include the immediate return of the pink tone post nail pressure release.

Focused Health Assessment and Abnormal Findings

INSPECTION OF THE SKIN

While inspecting the skin, the provider must observe for abnormal findings and document location, description, configuration, texture, color, size, and shape. The description of abnormal findings is critical in the integumentary examination in order to yield a clinical diagnosis or differential diagnoses. The inspection of pallor, which is loss of color, is typically seen in arterial insufficiency and decreased blood supply, as well as anemia. Chalk-white depigmented macules or patches that are well-circumscribed are indicative of vitiligo.

Vitiligo is an acquired, idiopathic disorder that is usually asymptomatic and lesions can range in size from millimeters to centimeters (Figure 5.17). While any part of the body can be affected, vitiligo often exhibits distinct patterns including symmetric involvement of the face, upper chest, hands, ankles, axillae, groin, and around orifices. The inspection of color variations, such as albinism, represents loss of pigmentation. Patients with albinism are at substantially higher risk for UV radiation–induced carcinogenesis.

Cyanosis is an example of an abnormality that causes white skin to appear blue-tinged, particularly in the nail bed, perioral, and conjunctival areas. Dark skin patients present with blue and dull discoloration in the same anatomical locations as white-skinned patients. Central cyanosis (oral mucosa) may result from cardiopulmonary disease and peripheral cyanosis may be indicative of local disease related to vasoconstriction. Jaundice in light- and dark-skinned people is characterized by yellowing of the skin or whites of the eyes related to liver disease or blood disorder.

Acanthosis nigricans is a term used to describe areas of dark, velvety discoloration of the skin that is localized to body folds and creases, which is more commonly seen on the posterior neck with patients who have insulin resistance or diabetes (Figure 5.18). In the process of skin inspection, the provider must observe for any abnormal odor emanating from the skin. A strong odor of perspiration or foul odor may represent a disorder of the sweat glands. Putrid odor may be related to poor hygiene practices, which may warrant patient education or need for nursing services, depending on the patient's age and state of health.

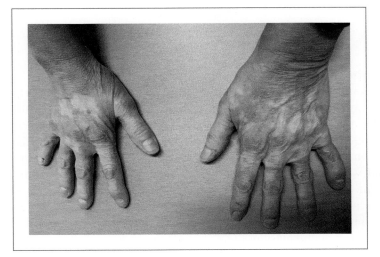

FIGURE 5.17 Vitiligo of the hands and forearms. Vitiligo is an acquired, idiopathic disorder characterized by circumscribed depigmented macules and patches. Functional melanocytes disappear from involved skin by a mechanism(s) that has not yet been identified.

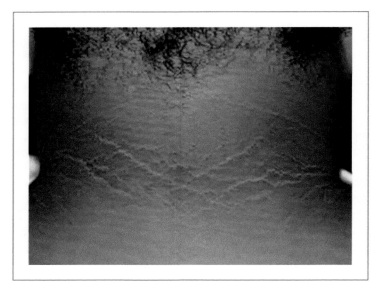

FIGURE 5.18 Acanthosis nigricans. The photo of the posterior neck depicts a patient with a hyperpigmented, velvety discoloration of the skin consistent with acanthosis nigricans. The pathogenesis of the skin disease is unknown, although it is consistently found in those who suffer from insulin resistance or diabetes.

Erythema is an abnormality that may be seen during a skin inspection and symbolizes inflammation. Erythema is the redness of the skin or mucous membranes due to increased blood flow following injury of the skin that may be caused by an allergic reaction, underlying skin condition, or trauma. The inspection of skin integrity is also considered during the performance of a skin examination. Abnormal findings would include skin breakdown, pressure ulcers related to poor vasculature and/or in pressure point areas, and chronic skin conditions such as atopic dermatitis.

LESIONS

The inspection and observation of abnormal lesions may be indicative of local or systemic diseases. Primary lesions are those that arise from direct consequence of the disease process. Secondary lesions are those lesions that are characteristically brought about by modification of the primary lesion either by the individual with the lesion or through the natural evolution of the lesion. In the observation of a primary or secondary lesion, documentation of the lesion must include its location, distribution, size, color, and configuration. Skin cancer lesions can be either primary or secondary lesions and are classified as squamous cell carcinoma, basal cell carcinoma, or malignant melanoma. The mnemonic for malignant melanoma, ABCDE, should be utilized during the encounter of an abnormal lesion during the process of inspection (Figure 5.19). The ABCDEs of melanoma represent the following:

A: Asymmetry

B: Borders—Irregular

C: Color variations

D: Diameter >6 mm

E: Evolution

The recognition of an abnormal mole with the use of ABCDE melanoma mnemonic can considerably alter one's life expectancy with early detection and primary prevention (Figure 5.20). Vascular lesions can also signify an abnormality that is associated with bleeding, circulatory conditions, aging, and hepatic disease, among many other diseases. Examples of vascular lesions that are considered an abnormal finding include petechia, ecchymosis, and hematoma.

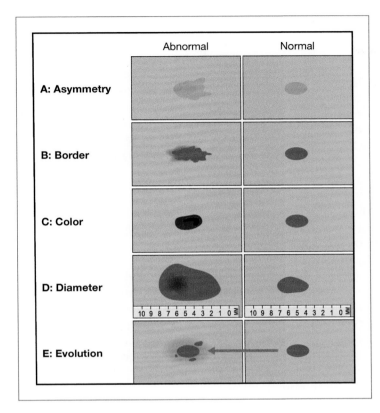

FIGURE 5.19 ABCDEs of melanoma. This figure represents the acronym used to classify characteristics of a melanoma during skin examination. Asymmetry (**A**) defines a lesion that is irregular and not symmetric; border (**B**) of a cancerous lesion may be scalloped or notched and not well defined as seen in a benign lesion; color (**C**) that is very dark or the presence of more than one color (e.g., blue, black, brown, tan) can be a warning sign of melanoma; diameter (**D**) of a concerning mole is often >6 mm; evolution (**E**) or change in a lesion, such as bleeding, pruritus, or pain, may signal warning signs of melanoma.

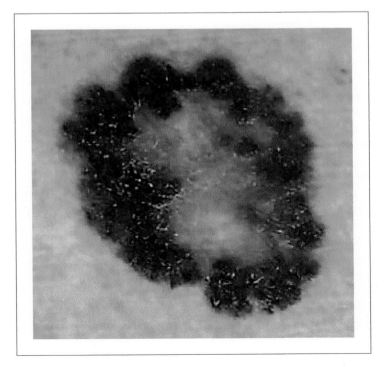

FIGURE 5.20 Malignant melanoma. This figure demonstrates all of the characteristics that classify a melanoma, such as asymmetry, irregular borders, mixed color, larger than 6 mm, and significant change.

PALPATION OF THE SKIN

The skin examination should include the palpation of the skin with particular detail to any abnormalities that warrant further evaluation. The normal skin finding is typically smooth and even, whereas, in those with abnormal skin, the skin on palpation may be rough, dry, and flaky. This skin abnormality is often found in patients with a medical history of hypothyroidism. Very thin skin may signify arterial insufficiency or systemic steroid use. Skin surfaces may alternate between moist to dry depending on environmental factors, temperature, or anatomical locations. However, increased moisture or diaphoresis (profuse sweating) may be present in conditions such as fever or hyperthyroidism. Decreased moisture occurs with dehydration or hypothyroidism. Clammy cold skin occurs during periods of shock or low blood pressure. Cool skin may accompany arterial insufficiency whereas, very warm skin may signal a febrile state.

INSPECTION OF THE HAIR

Inspection of the hair and scalp during the skin examination is important in the event of hair disease that may represent a manifestation of an underlying condition. Excessive generalized hair loss, known as telogen effluvium, may occur with infection, hormonal disorders, thyroid or liver disease, drug toxicity, hepatic or renal failure, or be stress induced. Significant hair loss may be attributed to chemotherapy or radiation treatments. Self-induced plucking or breaking of the hair is called trichotillomania. Trichotillomania is associated with psychological stress or a personality disorder. Round or oval patches of hair loss commonly represent alopecia areata, a nonscarring alopecia that is postulated to be a hair-specific autoimmune disease (Figure 5.21). Nutritional deficiencies may cause patchy gray hair in some patients. Severe malnutrition in African American

children may cause a copper-red hair color. Patchy hair loss may result from infections of the scalp, discoid systemic lupus erythematosus, and some types of chemotherapy. In contrast to hair loss, hypertrichosis represents the growth of an excessive amount of hair. Hirsutism is defined by the presence, in women, of terminal hairs in a male pattern (Figure 5.22). Hirsutism is related to an increase in androgen levels or the end-organ response to androgens.

PALPATION OF THE HAIR

The palpation of the scalp and hair will identify any abnormalities such as tumors, cysts, hair loss, and infection. The palpation of excessive scaliness may indicate dermatitis, psoriasis, or infection (Figure 5.23). Raised lesions may indicate infections, tumor growths, or cysts. Nonmelanoma skin tumors such as basal cell carcinoma and squamous cell carcinoma are often found in the male or female patient suffering from alopecia, as a result of excessive sun exposure or sunburns to the scalp. Pilar cysts are firm benign tumors that are commonly found on the scalp. Pilar cysts, also known as trichilemmal cysts, may be solitary, but more frequently are multiple. Dull, dry hair may be seen in hypothyroidism or malnutrition.

INSPECTION OF THE NAILS

The inspection of the nails should include the observation for abnormal findings. Dirty, dystrophic, or jagged fingernails may be indicative of poor hygiene. Pale or cyanotic nails may represent hypoxia or anemia. Beau's lines are transverse depressions in the nail plate that are often found to be parallel to the shape of the lunula (Figure 5.24). Beau's lines often occur after an acute illness or trauma to the nail (manicuring) and eventually

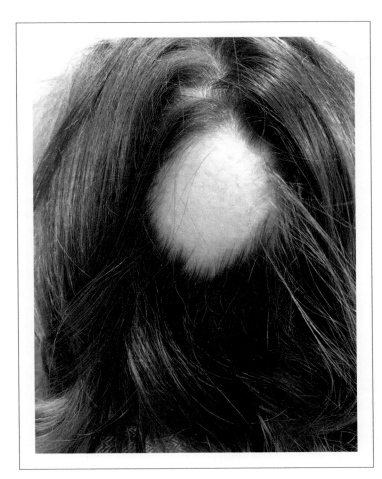

FIGURE 5.21 Alopecia areata. Alopecia areata can be diagnosed clinically by the presence of round or oval patches of hair loss with exclamation point hairs found at the periphery. Alopecia areata is a nonscarring autoimmune disease of the hair follicle. In the majority of cases, one or two small patches of alopecia are identified in the scalp, eyebrows, or body hair. Alopecia areata is seen equally in both sexes and in patients of all ages and ethnicities.

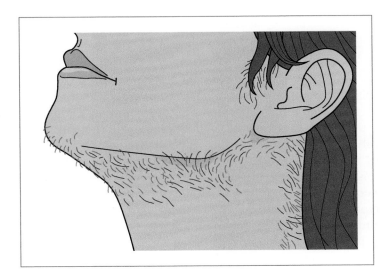

FIGURE 5.22 Hirsutism in a female. Hirsutism occurs in areas where a high level of androgen is required for hair growth, such as the chin, chest, stomach, thighs, upper lip, and upper back. Hirsutism is caused by excessive androgen-dependent male-pattern terminal hair growth in females. Hirsutism can be caused by polycystic ovary syndrome or Cushing disease.

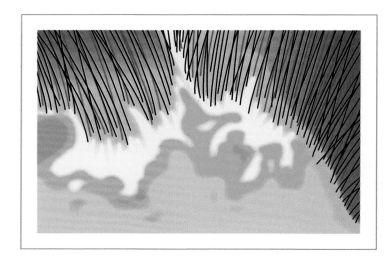

FIGURE 5.23 Psoriasis of the scalp. Psoriasis is a chronic, inflammatory disease that is characterized by sharply demarcated erythematous, silvery, scaly plaques more commonly seen on the scalp, elbows, and knees.

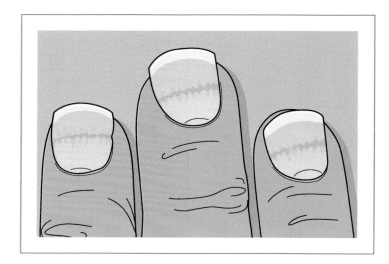

FIGURE 5.24 Beau's lines. Beau's lines are transverse depressions in the nail plate that are seen to be parallel to the shape of the lunula. Beau's lines are common and nonspecific nail changes that can be caused by trauma or local disease involving the nail fold, such as manicuring. As the nail plate grows distally, the Beau's lines will disappear.

grow out. Yellow discoloration of the nail may be seen in infections or psoriasis. Onychomycosis is a fungal infection caused by a dermatophyte fungus and, less frequently, by molds or yeast that results in a yellow thickening and discoloration of the nail (Figure 5.25). Other infections of the nail include acute paronychia, which is caused by bacteria, most commonly *Staphylococcus aureus* or *Streptococcus pyogenes*. Paronychia of the affected digit is swollen, red, and painful. Compression of the nail fold may produce pus drainage. Nail pitting involves punctate depressions of the nail surface seen in psoriasis, alopecia areata, and eczema patients. Traumatic nail abnormalities consist of hemorrhage or crust,

absence of the cuticle, inflammation of the proximal nail fold, nail plate abnormalities (e.g., longitudinal central depression), and melanonychia. Detachment of the nail plate from the nail bed is seen in idiopathic onycholysis, which is often a consequence of repetitive water immersion and exposure to irritants. The affected nail is detached from the nail bed and often displays an abnormal color due to secondary microbial contamination of the subungual space. Clubbing of the nail involves a change in the shape or structure of the nail plate, which is often related to cardio-thoracic disorders. Spooning of the nails, which represents a concave structure of the nail bed, may be present with iron deficiency anemia.

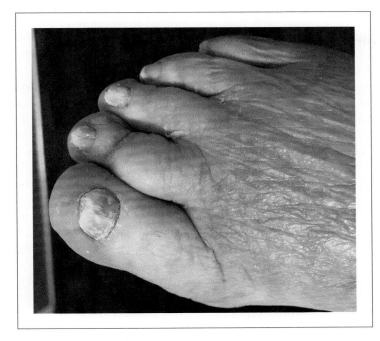

FIGURE 5.25 Onychomycosis of the toenails. The figure displays onychomycosis of the toenails that is caused by a dermatophyte fungi and, less frequently, nondermatophyte molds or yeasts. Onychomycosis is more common in men and is more commonly linked to concurrent disease of tinea pedis. It affects toenails more commonly than fingernails.

PALPATION OF THE NAILS

The palpation of the nail in an abnormal state will assist the provider in formulating a diagnosis. The palpation of a nail in a diseased state can also serve as the primary treatment. For example, the manual expression of the affected nail in acute paronychia will not only allow drainage of a pus-filled pocket that is harboring bacteria but will also aid in immediate pain relief. In addition, palpation of the nail is utilized when assessing for capillary refill (abnormal is >2 seconds), which may reveal respiratory or cardiovascular disease in the state of hypoxia.

Holistic Assessment

SPECIFIC HEALTH HISTORY

History taking is fundamental in dermatology. Its purposes are: (a) to allow the patient to verbalize the complaint and develop a rapport with the provider; (b) to determine factors that may have set off or aggravated the problem; (c) to determine the course of the disorder and whether it is acute or chronic; and (d) to determine whether there are associated systemic complaints. Prior to a diagnosis, it is important to obtain information on when, where, and how the skin condition started. Other relevant information includes what the initial lesions looked like and the course of evolution. Gather information on symptoms related to the problem, such as itching or painful areas, as well as aggravating, alleviating, or exacerbating factors. The patient's medical history is also imperative during the history-taking process, including any previous skin diseases or atopic symptoms. Family history of skin diseases is crucial in obtaining a history as skin conditions can be genetically inherited. Psoriasis and atopic eczema have a substantial hereditary component. Other than the importance of genetic syndromes, a family history may disclose that other family members have had a recent onset of eruption similar to that of the patient, indicating an infection or infestation.

SAFETY

Obtaining a social and occupational history may be a contributing or causative factor of a skin condition. Occupational exposures can induce contact dermatitis or other skin problems; therefore, it is valuable to have the patient explain what he or she does at work. Occupational contact dermatitis accounts for 90% of all cases of work-related cutaneous disorders. Work-related dermatitis consists of irritant contact dermatitis (80% of cases) and allergic contact dermatitis. In the majority of cases, both types will present as eczematous lesions on exposed parts of the body, notably the hands. Accurate diagnosis is highly dependent on meticulous history taking, thorough physical examination, careful reading of Material Safety Data Sheets, and comprehensive patch testing to confirm or rule out allergic sensitization.

DISTRESS

There is evidence linking psychological stress to exacerbation of certain skin diseases. Both the clinical and the basic science evidence, however, can be hard to interpret in light of the difficulty of defining and quantifying psychological stress as well as the questions regarding the etiologic significance of neuroimmunologic findings in skin diseases. Numerous case reports and studies have suggested that psychological stress may have a role in the onset or exacerbation of a variety of skin diseases. While stress may indeed worsen the patient's response to a skin condition, it is not a significant factor in the development of the skin disorder. The psychological burden of skin disorders has been documented in many studies to cause distress. Adults with atopic dermatitis are 2.24 times more likely to suffer moderate depression and 5.64 times more likely to be severely depressed compared to adults without the disease, as reported in a clinical research letter published in 2015 in the *Journal of Investigative Dermatology*. A 2015 article published in *Medicine* showed that, in children, there is a dose-dependent relationship between atopic dermatitis severity and psychologist distress. Adolescents with atopic dermatitis were more likely to suffer suicidal ideation than healthy teens.

NUTRITION AND EXERCISE

A growing number of studies suggest that diet influences general skin health and specific diseases, from acne and eczema to skin aging. In order to maintain healthy skin, one's diet must be rich in antioxidants, which are also anti-inflammatory. Free radical damage has been shown to be an important factor in the aging process and in the development of cancer. It is also thought to be the root cause of wrinkles and aging skin. Diet is thought to be a key method of controlling psoriasis, one of many suspected sensitivities that may keep the skin reacting. Some patients with psoriasis also show an elevated sensitivity to gluten and improve tremendously after a gluten-free diet. Exercise is also very crucial to the psoriasis patient as well as other patients with chronic skin conditions such as hidradenitis suppurativa. Exercise can assist in reducing the acute flare-ups that patients experience in these chronic conditions. Patients with psoriasis, independent of other risk factors, have higher risk for hypertension, diabetes, heart disease, and other types of inflammatory conditions.

FINANCIAL IMPLICATIONS

Costs of medications for patients with dermatological skin conditions have been on the rise. Patients with significant and imminently treatable skin disorders go without therapy for financial reasons alone. Prices of generic drugs have also skyrocketed over the past years, but they remain a bargain compared to the name-brand medications. If there is a generic equivalent, there is no reason to prescribe the branded drug, with very few exceptions. There is virtually no published data to support the notion that generic drugs do not work as well as branded medications.

SPIRITUAL CONSIDERATIONS

Integrative dermatology, also known as holistic medicine, when implemented appropriately can have life-changing therapeutic outcomes of certain dermatologic conditions. Integrative therapies could include alterations in diet, nutritional supplements, the use of botanicals and herbal medicine, as well as mind–body interventions such as hypnosis. Integrative dermatology treatments may be practical for those skin conditions that are uncontrolled to the traditional therapies and/or for those patients who prefer to limit their exposure to pharmaceuticals. Nevertheless, integrative dermatology may not replace gold standard treatment for certain diseases or conditions, for example, treatment of melanoma.

CASE STUDY

DOCUMENTATION

Chief Complaint: Changing mole of the right upper back that continues to itch

History of Present Illness: A 34-year-old female who is fair-haired and fair-skinned enjoys spending hours in the sun. Reports numerous incidences of blistering sunburns. History of atypical nevi. She reports evolutionary changes of a mole on her right upper back that has darkened, grown larger, and is constantly itchy. No symptoms of bleeding, swelling, or inflammation. She presents to the office for further evaluation and management as well as a full skin examination.

Medical History: None

Surgical History: Surgical excision of an atypical nevus of the right forearm in 2010

Medications: None

Allergies: Penicillin

Family History: Paternal grandfather: malignant melanoma; maternal grandmother: basal cell carcinoma

Social History: No alcohol or tobacco use

EXAMINATION

General: Well developed and well nourished. Awake, alert, and oriented. Appears stated health.

(*continued*)

(continued)

Integumentary: Skin is warm, dry, and intact. Light brown/tan macules of the upper chest, back, and shoulders. Medium brown soft papules of the back, abdomen, and chest. Medium brown macules of the arms, back, and chest. Well-healed surgical scar of the right forearm, no signs of lesion recurrence. Dark-brown irregular-shaped lesion with notched borders >6 mm in diameter of the right upper back. Nail beds pink with no cyanosis or clubbing.

Head: Normocephalic and atraumatic without tenderness, and no visible or palpable masses. Hair is of normal texture and evenly distributed.

Eyes: Conjunctivae are clear without exudate or hemorrhage. Sclera is nonicteric. Extraocular muscle intact. Pupils equal, round, react to light, accomodation.

Ears: External ear and ear canal are nontender without swelling. Canal clear with no discharge. Hearing intact.

Nose: Nasal mucosa is pink and moist. Nasal septum is midline. Nares are patent bilaterally.

Throat/Neck: Oral mucosa is pink and moist with good dentition. Tongue normal in appearance without lesions and with good symmetrical movement. No buccal nodules or lesions. The neck is supple without adenopathy. Trachea is midline. Thyroid gland is normal without masses.

Lymphatic: Neck, groin, and axilla without adenopathy

Cardiovascular: External chest appears normal without lifts, heaves, or thrills. Heart rate and rhythm are normal.

Respiratory: The chest wall is symmetric and without deformity. Lung sounds are clear in all lobes without rales, rhonchi, or wheezes.

Abdominal: Soft, symmetric, and nontender without distention. Bowel sounds are present and normoactive in all four quadrants.

Review of Systems: A focused review of systems was performed. New darkening mole, pruritic. No new rashes or nonhealing sores.

Diagnostic Plan: Biopsy of lesion of the right upper back to rule out malignant melanoma

Diagnosis: Malignant melanoma

ICD-10-CM Diagnosis Code: C43.9 Malignant Melanoma of the Skin, Unspecified

Differential Diagnosis: Moderate-to-severe atypical melanocytic nevus, Spitz nevus

Treatment Plan: Excision of malignant melanoma per American Academy of Dermatology (AAD) national guidelines. Melanoma skin exams per AAD guidelines.

Additional Notes: Referral to surgical oncology for sentinel lymph node biopsy to rule out metastasis dependent on stage of melanoma reported on pathology report once finalized.

Assessment of Special Populations

ELDERLY POPULATION

The elderly patient's skin becomes pale due to decreased melanin production and decreased dermal vascularity. As we age, skin lesions develop as a normal process; examples of those lesions include the following: seborrheic or senile keratoses, senile lentigines, cherry angiomas, purpura, and cutaneous tags and horns. An elderly patient's skin may feel dryer than a younger patient's skin because sebum production decreases with age. The elderly patient loses his or her skin turgor because of a decrease in elasticity and collagen fibers. Therefore, sagging or wrinkled skin appears in the face, breast, and scrotal areas. Older patients generally have thinner hair because of a decline in hair follicle productivity. Pubic, axillary, and body hair also decrease with aging. Alopecia is seen, particularly in men when compared to women. Hair loss is seen from the periphery of the scalp and moves to the center. Elderly women may have terminal hair growth on the chin owing to hormonal changes. In the elderly, patient nails may appear thickened, yellow, and brittle because of decreased circulation in the extremities.

PEDIATRIC POPULATION

Atopic dermatitis is a condition that is becoming much more prevalent in the pediatric population. Although a common condition, it is also highly personalized and may vary from case to case. The underlying causes, triggers, and symptoms should be investigated as well as familial predisposition. Profound data has linked food allergies as a prevailing cause of atopic dermatitis in the pediatric population. Treatment of atopic dermatitis in the pediatric patient differs from that in the adult patient, particularly in the use of topical steroids. Integrative dermatology should be considered either in combination or as monotherapy in these patients depending on severity of disease.

PREGNANT POPULATION

Pregnant women experience multiple skin changes, most of which are physiological in nature. Physiological skin changes in pregnancy include changes in pigmentation and alterations of the connective tissue and vascular system. Several skin eruptions seem to be specifically related to pregnancy and are best known as pregnancy specific dermatoses. The commonly encountered skin changes include pigmentation changes such as melasma, linea nigra, secondary areola, and localized or general hyperpigmentation. Vascular alterations include the development of palmar erythema, spider angiomas, and varicosities. Pregnant women may also develop striae distensae as well as hair and nail changes. Pigmentary skin changes constitute the most common cutaneous alteration seen in up to 90% of pregnant women.

PATIENTS WITH DISABILITIES

Individuals with lack of sensation and limited mobility because of disability or chronic illness are at increased risk for pressure ulcers. Therefore, the examination of the skin must include those areas of the skin prone to shear and pressure forces. These may include the previously identified pressure point areas (i.e., sacrum, hips, elbows). Different areas of the body are more likely to be subject to skin breakdown depending on the patient's continual use of a wheelchair versus lying in bed. It is important to inspect all skin areas in those with physical disabilities to assess for breakdown or friction.

Diagnostic Reasoning

Common Differential Diagnoses: Hair

Physical Finding	Diagnoses
Alopecia, nonscarring	• Alopecia areata • Androgen alopecia • Anagen effluvium • Tinea capitis • Telogen effluvium • Trichotillomania
Alopecia, scarring	• Tinea capitis with inflammation • Trauma • Neoplasm • Lichen planopilaris • Folliculitis decalvans • Discoid lupus erythematosus • Congenital • Bacterial folliculitis • Central centrifugal scarring alopecia
Hypertrichosis (excessive hair growth)	Drugs • Cyclosporine • Dilantin • Hexachlorobenzene • Minoxidil • Penicillamine Systemic Illness • Anorexia nervosa • Dermatomyositis • Hypothyroidism • Malnutrition • Porphyria

Common Differential Diagnoses: Skin	
Physical Finding	**Diagnoses**
Bullous disease, intraepidermal (fragile blisters)	• Bullous impetigo • Paraneoplastic pemphigus • Pemphigus foliaceus • Pemphigus vulgaris • Staphylococcal scalded skin syndrome
Bullous disease, subepidermal (tense blisters)	• Acute graft-versus-host reaction • Arthropod bite reaction • Bullous drug reaction • Bullous pemphigoid • Dermatitis herpetiformis • Burns • Epidermolysis bullosa • Herpes gestationis • Leukocytoclastic vasculitis • Urticaria pigmentosa • Toxic epidermal necrosis
Cutaneous color changes: blue	• Cardiovascular disease • Pulmonary disease • Raynaud's disease
Cutaneous color changes: brown	• Adrenocorticotropic hormone-producing tumor • Liver disease • Pituitary disease • Localized: Nevi, neurofibromatosis • Pituitary disease

(continued)

Common Differential Diagnoses: Skin (*continued*)	
Physical Finding	**Diagnoses**
Cutaneous color changes: red (erythema)	• Anxiety reaction • Fever • Generalized urticaria • Localized: Inflammation, infection, Raynaud's disease • Polycythemia • Viral exanthems
Cutaneous color changes: white	• Albinism • Raynaud's disease • Vitiligo
Cutaneous color changes: yellow	• Anemia • Chronic renal failure • Hepatitis, liver disease • Hypothyroidism • Increased intake of vegetables containing carotene • Localized: Resolving hematoma, infection, peripheral vascular insufficiency
Cutaneous infections	• Folliculitis • Furuncles • Herpes simplex • Impetigo • Molluscum contagiosum • Tinea cruris • Tinea pedis • Verruca vulgaris

(*continued*)

Common Differential Diagnoses: Skin (*continued*)

Physical Finding	Diagnoses
Exanthems (eruptive skin rash)	• Kawasaki syndrome • Erythema infectiosum (fifth disease) • Epstein-Barr virus • Enterovirus infections • Adenovirus • Meningococcemia • Rocky Mountain spotted fever • Roseola exanthema • Rubella • Scarlet fever • Varicella
Fever and rash	• Drug hypersensitivity: Penicillin, sulfonamides, thiazides, anticonvulsants, allopurinol • Dermatomyositis • Allergic vasculitis • Erythema marginatum • Erythema multiforme • Erythema nodosum • Herpes zoster • Other infections: Meningococcemia, scarlet fever, typhoid fever, *Pseudomonas* bacteremia, Rocky Mountain spotted fever, Lyme disease, secondary syphilis, bacterial endocarditis • Viral infection: Measles, rubella, varicella, erythema infectiosum, roseola, enterovirus infection, viral hepatitis, infectious mononucleosis, acute HIV • Pityriasis rosea • Serum sickness • Systemic lupus erythematosus

(*continued*)

Common Differential Diagnoses: Skin (*continued*)

Physical Finding	Diagnoses
Finger lesions, inflammatory	• Dyshidrotic eczema • Herpes simplex type 1 (herpetic whitlow) • Psoriatic arthritis • Paronychia • Bacterial endocarditis (Osler's nodes)
Flushing	• Agnogenic flushing • Anxiety • Carcinoid syndrome • Chronic myelogenous leukemia • Drugs: Nicotinic acid, diltiazem, nifedipine, levodopa, bromocriptine, vancomycin, amyl nitrate • Ingestion of alcoholic beverages • Ingestion of hot peppers and hot drinks • Menopause • Renal cell carcinoma • VIPoma (Verner–Morrison syndrome)
Foot dermatitis	• Dyshidrotic eczema • Neuropathic foot ulcers • Peripheral vascular insufficiency • Tinea pedis • Psoriasis • Allergic contact dermatitis • Tylosis (mechanically induced hyperkeratosis, fissuring, and dryness)
Foot lesions, ulcerating	• Cellulitis • Plantar wart • Plantar fibromatosis • Pseudoepitheliomatous hyperplasia • Squamous cell carcinoma

(continued)

Common Differential Diagnoses: Skin (*continued*)

Physical Finding	Diagnoses
Genital sores	• Condyloma acuminatum • Chancroid • Herpes genitalis • Granuloma inguinale • Neoplastic lesion • Syphilis • Trauma • Lymphogranuloma venereum
Hyperpigmentation	• Hemochromatosis • Drug induced (antimalarials) • Addison's disease • Melanoma • Malabsorption syndrome (Whipple's disease) • Pregnancy • Psoralen and ultraviolet radiation (PUVA) therapy for psoriasis or vitiligo
Hypopigmentation	• Atopic dermatitis • Idiopathic guttate hypomelanosis • Nevoid hypopigmentation • Tinea versicolor • Vitiligo • Sarcoidosis

(*continued*)

Common Differential Diagnoses: Skin (*continued*)	
Physical Finding	**Diagnoses**
Livedo reticulitis (mottled reticulated vascular pattern)	• Congenital • Antiphospholipid antibody syndrome • Drugs (quinine, quinidine, amantadine, catecholamines) • Cryoglobulinemia, cryofibrinogenemia • Emboli • Leukocytoclastic vasculitis • Pancreatitis • Systemic lupus erythematosus • Thrombocythemia or polycythemia
Nodular lesions, skin	• Lipoma • Pyogenic granuloma • Nodular melanoma • Hemangioma • Cherry angioma • Classic Kaposi's sarcoma
Nodules, painful	• Arthropod bite or sting • Angiolipoma • Dermatofibroma • Erythema nodosum • Tumor • Leiomyoma • Neuroma • Osler's node • Sweet's syndrome • Vasculitis • Panniculitis

(*continued*)

Common Differential Diagnoses: Skin (*continued*)

Physical Finding	Diagnoses
Oral mucosa, erythematous lesions	• Candidiasis • Geographic tongue • Burn from hot beverage • Erythroplakia • Pemphigus vulgaris • Viral infection • Allergy • Plasma cell gingivitis
Oral mucosa, pigmented lesions	• Addison's disease • Chloasma • Nevi • Melanoma • Drug reaction: Minocycline, quinacrine, chlorpromazine • Neurofibromatosis • Melanotic macule • Peutz–Jeghers syndrome
Oral mucosa, vesicles and ulcers	• Aphthous stomatitis • Behcets syndrome • Coxsackievirus • Drug reaction • Herpes simplex • Chron's disease • Reiter's syndrome • Erythema multiforme • Pemphigus • Pemphigoid • Systemic lupus erythematosus • Fungi (histoplasmosis) • Syphilis

(*continued*)

Common Differential Diagnoses: Skin *(continued)*	
Physical Finding	**Diagnoses**
Oral mucosa, white lesions	• Allergy • Benign intraepithelial dyskeratosis • Candidiasis • Leukoedema • Leukoplakia • Lichen planus • Squamous cell carcinoma • White, hairy leukoplakia • Pachyonychia congenita
Papulosquamous diseases	• Dermatophytosis • Lichen planus • Mycosis fungoides • Parapsoriasis • Pityriasis rosea • Pityriasis rubra pilaris • Pityriasis lichenoides • Psoriasis • Secondary syphilis • Tinea versicolor
Penile rash	• Condyloma acuminate • Herpes simplex 2 • Fordyce spots (sebaceous glands) • Balanitis • Molluscum contagiosum • Lichen nitidus • Pearly penile papules • Pediculosis pubis • Scabies

(continued)

Common Differential Diagnoses: Skin (*continued*)

Physical Finding	Diagnoses
Photodermatoses	• Chronic actinic dermatitis • Phototoxicity and photoallergy • Polymorphous light eruption • Solar urticaria
Photosensitivity	• Drug-induced (doxycycline) • Photoallergic reaction • Phototoxic reaction • Polymorphous light eruption • Systemic lupus erythematous • Solar urticaria
Pruritus	• Acquired immunodeficiency syndrome • Carcinoma: Breast, lung, gastric • Cholestatic liver disease • Chronic renal failure • Drug-induced eruption, fiberglass exposure • Dry skin (xerosis) • Endocrine disorders: Diabetes mellitus, thyroid disease, carcinoid, pregnancy • Iron deficiency • Myeloproliferative disorders: Mycosis fungoides, Hodgkin's lymphoma, multiple myeloma, polycythemia vera • Neurosis • Scabies • Sjogren's disease • Skin diseases

(*continued*)

Common Differential Diagnoses: Skin (*continued*)	
Physical Finding	**Diagnoses**
Purpura	• Disseminated intravascular coagulation • Hemolytic-uremic syndrome • Meningococcemia • Rocky Mountain spotted fever • Thrombocytopenia • Trauma • Viral infection: Echovirus, coxackivirus

Sexually transmitted diseases, anorectal region	Nonulcerative
	  • Chlamydia (Chlamydia trachomatis)
	  • Condyloma acuminatum
	  • Gonorrhea
	  • Syphilis
	Ulcerative
	  • Chancroid (*Haemophilus ducreyi*)
	  • Cytomegalovirus
	  • Early syphilis
	  • Herpes simplex virus
	  • Idiopathic (usually HIV positive)
	  • Lymphogranuloma venereum

Verrucous lesions	• Acanthosis nigricans • Deep fungal infection • Lichen simplex • Nevus sebaceous • Scabies (Norwegian, crusted) • Seborrheic keratosis • Verrucous carcinoma • Warts

(continued)

Common Differential Diagnoses: Skin (*continued*)

Physical Finding	Diagnoses
Vesiculobullous diseases	• Bullous pemphigoid
	• Dermatitis blisters
	• Diabetic blisters
	• Epidermolysis bullosa
	• Erythema multiforme
	• Herpes simplex
	• Herpes zoster
	• Impetigo
	• Mucous membrane pemphigoid
	• Pemphigus (vulgaris, foliaceus, paraneoplastic)
	• Staphylococcal scalded skin syndrome
	• Varicella
Vulvar lesions	Dark lesions
	• Lentigo
	• Melanoma
	• Nevi (mole)
	• Reactive hyperpigmentation
	• Seborrheic keratosis
	• Pubic lice
	Red lesions
	Infections
	• Behcet's syndrome
	• Candida
	• Folliculitis (*Staphylococcus aureus*)
	• Erythrasma (*Corynebacterium minutissimum*)

(*continued*)

Common Differential Diagnoses: Skin (*continued*)	
Physical Finding	**Diagnoses**
Vulvar lesions (*continued*)	• Granuloma inguinale (*Calymmatobacterium granulomatis*) • Hidradenitis suppurativa • Intertrigo • Scabies (*Sarcoptes scabiei*) • Tinea cruris *Inflammation* • Chemical irritation (lubricants, hygiene sprays, spermicide) • Irritation from semen, saliva • Mechanical trauma: Scratching • Medications *Neoplasm* • Squamous cell carcinoma, melanoma, Paget's disease, Bowen's disease • Vulvar intraepithelial neoplasia
Vulvar, ulcerative lesions	• Bartholin cyst or abscess • Basal cell carcinoma • Chancroid • Behcet's disease • Condyloma acuminatum • Crohn's disease • Granuloma inguinale • Herpes simplex • Hidradenitis suppurativa • Lymphogranuloma venereum • Molluscum contagiosum • Neurofibroma • Pemphigoid

(*continued*)

Common Differential Diagnoses: Skin (*continued*)

Physical Finding	Diagnoses
Vulvar, ulcerative lesions (*continued*)	• Pemphigus • Squamous cell carcinoma • Keratocanthoma • Primary syphilis (*Treponema pallidum*)
Vulvar, white lesions	• Lichen sclerosus • Intertrigo • Partial albinism • Radiation treatment • Vitiligo

Common Differential Diagnoses: Nails

Physical Finding	Diagnoses
Melanonychia (pigmented longitudinal band within the nail plate)	• Bowen's disease • Lichen planus • Medications (e.g., 5-fluorouracil, psoralens, doxorubicin, azidothymidine) • Addison's disease • Melanocyte hyperplasia • Nail matrix melanoma • Nail matrix nevus • Trauma • Subungual keratosis • Onychomycosis • Pregnancy

(*continued*)

Common Differential Diagnoses: Nails (*continued*)	
Physical Finding	**Diagnoses**
Nail clubbing (change in nail structure)	• Chronic obstructive pulmonary disease • Cirrhosis • Chronic bronchitis • Congenital heart disease • Endocarditis • Familial • Idiopathic • Asbestosis • Pulmonary malignancy • Inflammatory bowel disease • Trauma
Nail, horizontal white lines (Beau's lines)	• Idiopathic • Malnutrition • Pemphigus • Prolonged systemic illnesses • Raynaud's disease • Trauma
Nail onycholysis (detachment of the nail)	• Infection • Connective tissue disorder • Hyperthyroidism • Nutritional deficiencies • Psoriasis • Sarcoidosis • Trauma
Nail pitting	• Alopecia areata • Psoriasis • Reiter's syndrome • Trauma • Idiopathic

(*continued*)

Common Differential Diagnoses: Nails (*continued*)	
Physical Finding	**Diagnoses**
Nail whitening (Terry's nails)	• Hyperthyroidism • Liver disease (cirrhosis, hepatic failure) • Malnutrition • Idiopathic • Trauma
Nail yellowing	• Lymphedema • Nephrotic syndrome • Immunodeficiency • Tobacco use • Thyroiditis • Rheumatoid arthritis • Pleural effusions • Chronic infections (sinusitis, tuberculosis)

BIBLIOGRAPHY

Bolognia, J. L., Jorizzo, J. L., & Rapini, R. P. (Eds.). (2008). *Dermatology* (2nd ed.). St. Louis, MO: Mosby/Elsevier.

Cui, C.-Y., & Schlessinger, D. (2015). Eccrine sweat gland development and sweat secretion. *Experimental Dermatology, 24*(9), 644–650. doi:10.1111/exd.12773

Ferri, F. (Ed.). (2019). *Ferri's fast facts in dermatology* (2nd ed.). Philadelphia, PA: Elsevier.

Gawkrodger, D. J., & Ardern-Jones, M. R. (2017). *Dermatology: An illustrated colour text* (6th ed.). Edinburgh, Scotland Churchill Livingstone/Elsevier.

Hassan, I., Bashir, S., & Taing, S. (2015). A clinical study of the skin changes in pregnancy in kashmir valley of north India: A hospital-based study. *Indian Journal of Dermatology, 60*(1), 28–32. doi:10.4103/0019-5154.147782

Hilton, L. (2018). Psychological distress: Emotional burden of skin conditions may be rooted in physiology. *Dermatology Times, 39*(8), 1, 28–29. Retrieved from https://www.dermatologytimes.com/sites/default/files/legacy/mm/digital/media/dt0818_ezineR1.pdf

Jain, S. (2017). *Dermatology: Illustrated study guide and comprehensive board review*. Cham, Switzerland: Springer.

Kimyai-Asadi, A., & Usman, A. (2001). The role of psychological stress in skin disease. *Journal of Cutaneous Medicine and Surgery, 5*(2), 140–145. doi:10.1177/120347540100500208

Kolarsick, P. A. J., Kolarsick, M., & Goodwin, C. (2011). Anatomy and physiology of the skin. *Journal of the Dermatology Nurses' Association, 3*(4), 203–212. doi:10.1097/JDN.0b013e3182274a98

Levine, N. (2018). What can be done about high drug prices? *Dermatology Times, 39*(7), 10. Retrieved from https://www.dermatologytimes.com/drug-costs/what-can-be-done-about-high-drug-prices

Marks, J. G., Jr., & Miller, J. J. (2019). *Lookingbill and Mark's principles of dermatology* (6th ed.). Philadelphia, PA: Elsevier.

McKay, M. (1990). The dermatologic history. In H. K. Walker, W. D. Hall, & J. W. Hurst (Eds.), *Clinical methods: The history, physical, and laboratory examinations* (3rd ed., Chap. 104). Boston, MA: Butterworths. Retrieved from https://www.ncbi.nlm.nih.gov/books/NBK207

McLafferty, E., Hendry, C., & Farley, A. (2012). The integumentary system: Anatomy, physiology and function of skin. *Nursing Standard, 27*(3), 35–42. doi:10.7748/ns2012.09.27.3.35.c9299

OpenStax. (n.d.) *Anatomy and physiology* (Chapter 5). Retrieved from https://opentextbc.ca/anatomyandphysiology/chapter/5-1-layers-of-the-skin

Petrou, L. (2013). Holistic CARE. *Dermatology Times, 34*(5), 28–32.

Purves, D., Augustine, G. J., Fitzpatrick, D., Katz, L. C., LaMantia, A.-S., McNamara, J. O., & Williams, S. M. (Eds.). (2001). *Neuroscience* (2nd ed, Chapter 9). Sunderland, MA: Sinauer Associates. Retrieved from https://www.ncbi.nlm.nih.gov/books/NBK10895

Sasseville, D. (2008). Occupational contact dermatitis. *Allergy, Asthma, and Clinical Immunology, 4*(2), 59–65. doi:10.1186/1710-1492-4-2-59.

Shimizu, H. (2006). *Shimizu's textbook of dermatology.* Retrieved from https://www.derm-hokudai.jp/shimizu-dermatology/ch01/

Sodano, W. (2016). Integrative medicine approach to eczema (atopic dermatitis). *Nutritional Perspectives: Journal of the Council on Nutrition, 39*(4), 20–22.

Watkins, J. (2013). Skin rashes, part 1: Skin structure and taking a dermatological history. *Practice Nursing, 24*(1), 30–33. doi:10.12968/pnur.2013.24.1.30

Weber, J.R. & Kelley, J.H. (2018). *Health Assessment in Nursing* (6th ed.). Philadelphia, PA: Wolters Kluwer Health.

6

ADVANCED HEALTH ASSESSMENT OF THE CARDIOVASCULAR SYSTEM

Allison Rusgo

CHAPTER CONTENTS

(continued)

HOLISTIC ASSESSMENT
  Specific Health History
  Safety
  Distress
  Nutrition and Exercise
  Financial Implications
  Spiritual Considerations

CASE STUDY

ASSESSMENT OF SPECIAL POPULATIONS
  Transgender Population
  Pediatric Population
  Elderly Population
  Patients With Disabilities
  Veteran Population
  Pregnant Population

DIAGNOSTIC REASONING
  Common Differential Diagnoses: Atherosclerotic Diseases
  Common Differential Diagnoses: Heart Failure
  Common Differential Diagnoses: Arrhythmias
  Common Differential Diagnoses: Pericardial, Myocardial, and Endocardial Diseases
  Common Differential Diagnoses: Valvular Heart Diseases
  Common Differential Diagnoses: Heart Muscle Diseases
  Common Differential Diagnoses: Vasculature Diseases

Overview of Anatomy and Physiology

The cardiovascular system, composed of the heart (Figure 6.1) and great vessels, is the body's circulatory mechanism. The right side of the heart receives deoxygenated blood from the superior and inferior venae cavae (SVC and IVC), while the left side of the heart pumps oxygenated blood into the aorta for distribution to all organs and tissues. As this circulatory process is vital for survival, it is imperative that providers understand the anatomy and physiology of the cardiovascular system. This knowledge will allow clinicians to evaluate this body system thoroughly and aid in the diagnosis of patients with cardiac-related complaints.

From a surface anatomy perspective, the heart and roots of the great vessels are surrounded by the pericardial sac located in the middle of the thorax. The heart, approximately the size of a fist, is bordered laterally and posteriorly by the lungs and anteriorly by the sternum and the third through fifth ribs on the left.

PERICARDIAL AND CARDIAC MEMBRANE

The heart is encased by the pericardial sac, a double-walled membrane located posterior to the sternum and the costal cartilage between the fifth through eighth thoracic vertebrae. The pericardium composes the outer fibrous and inner serous layers. The fibrous pericardium affixes the heart to the mediastinum and protects it from a sudden overfilling of blood. The serous pericardium is further divided into parietal and visceral components. The parietal pericardium is fused to the fibrous pericardium, while the visceral pericardium forms the epicardium or outer surface of the heart. In between the visceral and parietal layers is the pericardial space, which contains a small amount of serous fluid to lubricate and protect the heart from injury (Figure 6.2).

Similar to the multilayered pericardial sac, the heart is also composed of three layers. The

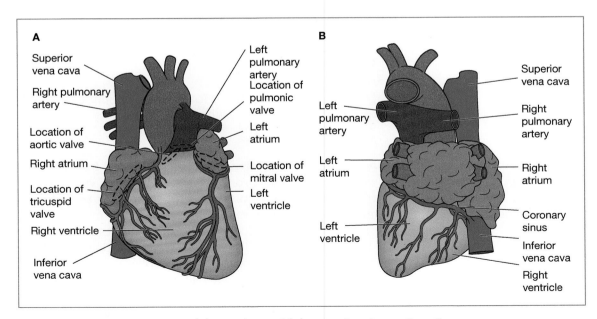

FIGURE 6.1 The heart: (**A**) anterior and (**B**) posterior views of cardiac anatomy depicting the four chambers, the valves (aortic, pulmonic, mitral, tricuspid, and pulmonic), and key vasculature including the pulmonary arteries and vena cavae (superior and inferior).

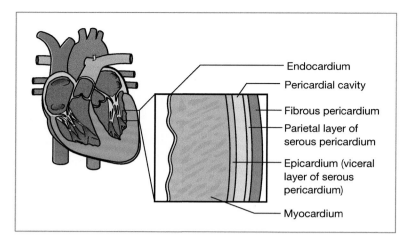

FIGURE 6.2 Pericardial anatomy: pericardial layers and cardiac wall.

Source: Reproduced from Tkacs, N., Herrmann, L., & Johnson, R. (Eds.). (in press). *Advanced physiology and pathophysiology: Essentials for clinical practice* (Figure 10.2A). New York, NY: Springer Publishing Company.

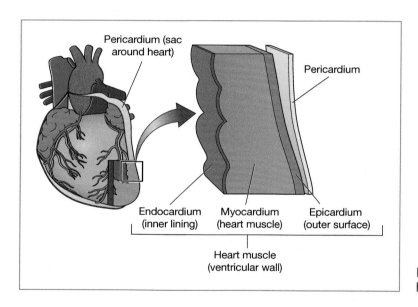

FIGURE 6.3 Anatomical layers of the heart.

epicardium is the outermost membrane formed by the visceral pericardium. The myocardium is the thick middle layer composed of cardiac muscle, and the endocardium is the innermost layer that lines the heart (Figure 6.3).

CARDIAC CHAMBERS

The heart itself contains four chambers—a right and left atria and a right and left ventricle (LV). The right atrium (RA) is located at the right heart border.

It receives deoxygenated blood from the SVC, IVC, and coronary sinus, the latter of which connects to the cardiac veins that supply the myocardium. The inferior portion of the RA is a muscular wall with individual openings for the SVC, IVC, and coronary sinus. The RA also contains a right atrioventricular (AV) opening where deoxygenated blood is pushed into the right ventricle (RV; Figure 6.4).

The RV comprises the majority of the anterior and inferior portions of the heart. The RV meets the pulmonary artery at the sternal angle, which is the *base* of the heart. The RV receives deoxygenated blood from the RA through the aforementioned right AV orifice. This area is surrounded by the tricuspid valve, which is made up of the valvular cusps, the tendinous chords, and three papillary muscles. Once the RV receives oxygen-poor blood, it is pushed through the pulmonary valve to the pulmonary artery and into the lungs where it is reoxygenated and subsequently returned to the left atrium (LA). Another important component of the RV is the right bundle branches of the AV bundle. This anatomical feature is an integral part of the heart's electrical conduction system, as it allows for organized cardiac contractions. Finally, the interventricular septum is located between the RVs and LVs. This muscular barrier separates the chambers where a significant portion encroaches into the RV due to the increased pressure from the powerful flow of blood from the LV (Figure 6.4).

The LA encompasses the majority of the heart's base. This chamber has a thicker muscular wall when compared to the RA and this helps maintain its integrity against forceful blood flow. Within the LA, two superior and two inferior pulmonary veins converge at its posterior wall and allow for the transfer of oxygenated blood from the lungs. The LA also has a left AV aperture where blood is pushed into the LV for distribution to the rest of the body (see Figure 6.4). The LV is located slightly posterior and leftward of the RV. It covers the majority of the pulmonary and diaphragmatic aspects of the heart, which equates to the organ's left lateral border. The tip of the LV also forms the *cardiac apex*, which is an important landmark in the cardiac physical examination. During the palpation portion of the exam, one can appreciate the *point of*

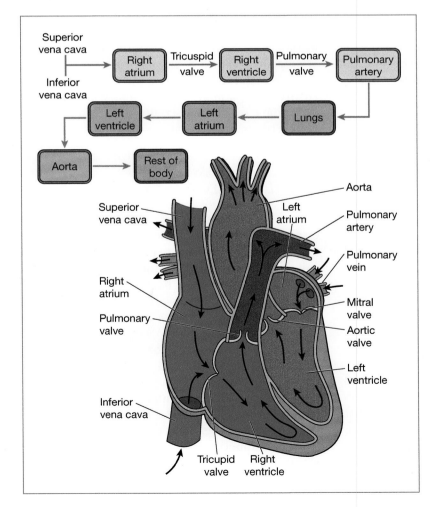

FIGURE 6.4 Cardiac circulatory pathway. Circulation of blood through the cardiopulmonary system—tracing the flow of deoxygenated blood from the vena cavae through the right side of the heart and into the lungs where it is oxygenated and returned to the left side of the heart and pumped to the aorta and the rest of the body.

maximal impulse or *PMI*, which is located at the apex. Anatomically, this pulsation is helpful when delineating the heart's left lateral border and should be located at the fifth intercostal space in the left midclavicular line. The location of the PMI is also an important factor when evaluating patients with conditions such as hypertension and congestive heart failure (CHF); this will be discussed in future sections of this chapter.

The LV needs to be stronger than the RV because it withstands a powerful contraction as oxygenated blood moves into the aorta. Therefore, its walls are significantly thicker and more muscular than the RV. An important landmark within the LV is the mitral, or bicuspid, valve, which is used to funnel blood from the LA. This valve is designed to maintain its integrity and prevent the backflow of blood into the LA despite the high-pressure environment generated by strong contractions from the LV. Also located inside the chamber is the aortic orifice, which is encased by a fibrous ring that is connected to the aortic valve. This valve allows for blood flow from the LV to the ascending aorta, which is the final destination of oxygenated blood before it is forcefully pumped into all other organs and tissues (see Figure 6.4).

CARDIAC CIRCULATION

When the atria and ventricles contract, a designated amount of blood is forcefully pumped into the pulmonary arteries and aorta; this is cardiac output (CO). CO equates to the volume of blood that is discharged from the LV in 60 seconds. It is composed of two components—heart rate and stroke volume, the latter of which is the amount of blood ejected per heartbeat. Both heart rate and stroke volume can vary based on three factors—preload, afterload, and the contractile ability of the heart.

Preload is defined as a given volume of blood that causes cardiac cells to stretch prior to contraction. This corresponds to the amount of blood that remains in the RV at the end of diastole or cardiac relaxation. Afterload is the pressure the heart has to work against in order to eject blood during its contractile phase. It can also be thought of as the amount

of pressure that the atria and ventricles have to create in order to successfully eject a sufficient amount of blood into the circulatory system and pulmonary arteries. Contractility is guided by the cardiac muscle cells' ability to work against a given volume of blood—the sarcoplasmic reticulum of the cells stretch when under pressure and their recoil allows the atria and ventricles to contract.

The concepts of preload, afterload, and cardiac contractility are especially important when evaluating patients with suspected heart failure. For example, in one type of heart failure, the aorta or ventricles dilate. When this occurs, the chambers require a greater amount of pressure, as compared to a healthy heart, to overcome the aortic pressure needed to eject an adequate amount of blood for circulation. Over time, the cardiac cells develop an inability to compensate with these higher pressures and thus circulation is compromised. Although there are various types, severity levels, and underlying etiologies for CHF, in many instances preload, afterload, and contractility are affected. Therefore, it is important for providers to understand these physiological mechanisms to ensure that patients who present with signs and symptoms of cardiac compromise can receive proper treatment and management.

CARDIAC VALVES

Cardiac circulation is guided by a series of valves that function on a pressure gradient system. These valves are very important for maintaining proper blood flow through the heart. The mitral (bicuspid) and tricuspid valves are located between the LA and LV and the RA and RV, respectively. They are also known as the AV valves. The pulmonic and the aortic valves are located between the RV and pulmonary artery and the LV and the aorta, respectively. The pulmonary and aortic valves are also known as the semilunar valves due to their half-moon appearance. As each of these valves open and close, the vibrations from the valve leaflets in conjunction with the movement from the blood itself and the individual cardiac structures generate the familiar *"lub-dub"* sounds heard during cardiac auscultation. Clinically, these normal heart sounds are defined as S1 and S2, while there are also two pathological sounds termed S3 and S4. If a provider does appreciate one of the abnormal heart sounds, this can signify diseases such as heart failure or ischemia.

CARDIAC CYCLE AND HEART SOUNDS

The cardiac cycle is another important physiological concept because it forms the basis for understanding circulatory blood flow as well as valvular and cardiac chamber function. These components are integral portions of the cardiac exam and can help providers better evaluate and treat patients with cardiac diseases. By definition, the cardiac cycle describes the period of time between the origination of one heartbeat to the next. Two important terms are systole, the period of ventricular contraction, and diastole, the period of ventricular filling and relaxation. To start the cycle, diastole begins as the aortic and pulmonic valves close. This process prevents the backflow of blood into the LV (from the aorta) and the RV (from the pulmonary artery). Also during diastole, the mitral valve is open to allow blood to move from the LA into the LV. This filling process helps the LV prepare for its contraction of blood into the aorta during systole. The tricuspid valve is also open during diastole so that blood can flow into the RV from the RA. Once the ventricles have filled sufficiently, atrial contraction occurs at the end of diastole. This creates an increased pressure gradient across the valves and systole begins. During systole, the tricuspid and mitral valve close to prevent regurgitation of blood into the LA and RA, respectively. Additionally, the aortic and pulmonic valves open so that blood can move into the ascending aorta (from the LV) and pulmonary artery (from the RV; Figure 6.5).

Focusing on the concept of heart sounds, the S1 and S2 sounds equate to the timing of systole and diastole. The "*lub*" sound occurs when blood moves from the atria to the ventricles, and the "*dub*" is appreciated during ventricular contraction. Most commonly, it is believed that the actual sound is generated by the closing of the valvular leaflets.

During diastole, the pressure in the atria is slightly higher than the ventricles and the mitral valve is open so that blood can flow from the LA to the LV. During systole, the LV contracts; this significantly elevates the pressure in the LV. Additionally, this accentuates the pressure difference between the LA and LV; thus, the mitral valve is forced closed and the S1 heart sound is generated. As the pressure in the LV continues to rise, it exceeds the pressure in the ascending aorta; thus, the aortic valve opens and blood can move from the LV into the aorta. Once the LV has discharged most of its blood, its pressure decreases below the pressure inside the aorta and the aortic valve subsequently closes. This creates the S2 heart sound. This also prompts another cycle of diastole to begin with the opening of the mitral and tricuspid valves.

As previously mentioned, there are several heart sounds that can be heard if a patient has a cardiac pathology related to valvular or chamber dysfunction. Typically, when the mitral valve opens during diastole, this is silent. However, if a patient has a stenotic or stiff valve, one might appreciate a snap-like sound as the valve leaflets "pop" open to allow blood to flow between the LA and LV. In adults, a provider might hear an S3 heart sound, which can indicate ventricular failure or myocardial ischemia. This occurs because of an abrupt deceleration of blood flow across the mitral valve. In children and older adolescents, however, the S3 sound can be a normal variant heard during cardiac auscultation. Finally, an S4 sound, also pathological in adults, occurs immediately prior to S1 and represents ventricular dysfunction, typically stiffness.

In addition to each of the heart sounds, one can also appreciate a separation, or splitting, of the S1 and S2 heart sounds (Figure 6.6). This finding can be a normal variant or indicative of a cardiac pathology. When auscultating the right side of a patient's heart, one may appreciate two discernable sounds for S2. This is defined as an A2 and P2—the former representing the aortic valve closing and the latter equating to the pulmonic valve closing. During the cardiac cycle, this phenomenon occurs because events that occur on the left side of the heart occur slightly before those on the right side of the heart. To determine the clinical value of this finding, one

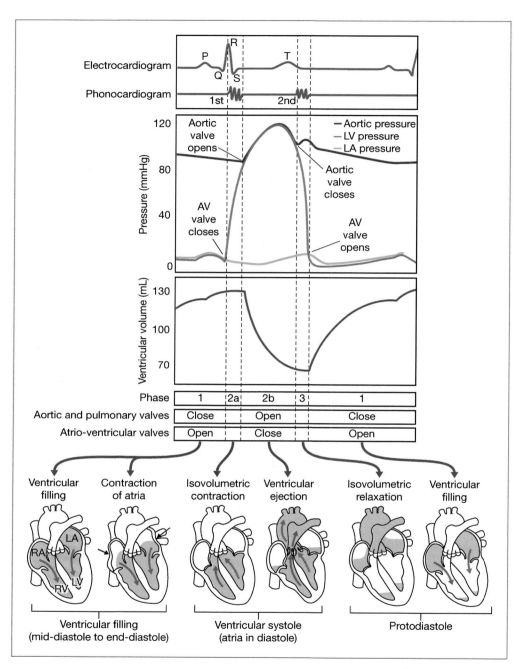

FIGURE 6.5 Elements of the cardiac cycle. The top figure is an EKG representation of the cardiac cycle in conjunction with corresponding pressures, volumes, and valvular activity during each phase. The bottom figure outlines the contraction of each chamber and direction of blood flow during each portion of the cycle.

AV, atrioventricular; LA, left atrium; LV, left ventricle.

Source: Reproduced with permission from Marieb, E. N. (2005). *Essentials of human anatomy and physiology* (8th ed., Figure 18.20).

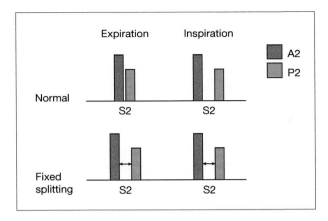

FIGURE 6.6 Splitting of the S2 heart sound during the cardiac cycle. When performing cardiac auscultation, one may appreciate a split or two discernable sounds for S2 defined as A2 and P2. This finding can be physiological or pathological; thus, it requires further investigation. The splitting of S2 into A2 and P2 can be a normal variant during inspiration; however, if it is also appreciated during expiration, it can signify cardiac abnormalities such as valvular disease or septal irregularities.

should coordinate the auscultation with a patient's respiratory cycle. During inspiration, the time required to fill the right side of the heart is slightly increased. This process delays the closing of the pulmonic valve (as compared to the aortic valve); therefore, each valve closure's sound is appreciated separately. When a provider is investigating heart splitting, it is best heard between the second and third intercostal spaces near the sternum, where A2 is slightly louder than P2 due to the increased pressure within the aorta. An S2 split (into A2 and P2 components) can occur physiologically during inspiration; however, if it persists during exhalation, it is defined as a fixed split. This finding is pathological and requires further evaluation for underlying valvular diseases or other structural abnormalities, particularly within the septal walls. There are also additional variants such as a wide S2 split or a paradoxical split, which signal the presence of cardiac pathology.

The S1 heart sound can also be split; however, it does not vary with respiration. The S1 is broken down into the closure of the mitral valve and the tricuspid valve, respectively. The mitral aspect is significantly louder than the tricuspid sound because pressures are higher on the left side of the heart. One can appreciate the mitral component of S1 at the cardiac apex. This is the location of the LV, which contains the mitral valve. The sound of the tricuspid valve closing can be heard best along the left sternal border near the RV.

CARDIAC MURMURS

In conjunction with the four heart sounds, heart murmurs are also distinct sounds that one might appreciate during a cardiac assessment. The majority of heart murmurs are indicative of valvular pathology and can affect any of the AV or semilunar valves; however, some murmurs can be normal variants in childhood/adolescents.

Patients with valvular heart disease can present with a variety of chief complaints (CCs); thus, it is imperative that providers understand murmur physiology and develop a keen ability to recognize the sounds during a cardiac physical exam. In general, heart murmurs are generated by turbulent blood flow. As blood is forced from one chamber to the next, if a specific valve is not functioning properly, the smooth movement of blood is disrupted; this creates an abnormal vibratory sound at a given precordial location, which corresponds to the affected valve. The two primary types of valvular disease are stenosis and regurgitation. These findings can occur because of various underlying disease etiologies or secondary to normal aging. When a valve narrows, blood is forced through a smaller than usual aperture and this creates the characteristic murmur of stenosis. On the contrary, if a valve has weak walls that become "floppy," it is unable to close properly. As blood flows across this defective valve, its once impermeable seal becomes penetrable and blood flows backward;

this disrupts proper circulation and generates the murmur of regurgitation.

Anatomically, it is important to remember where each of the heart valves is located on the precordium. This will increase the likelihood of not only appreciating a heart murmur but also understanding which valve is the culprit. Murmurs of the aortic valve are best heard near the cardiac apex at the right second intercostal space; this corresponds to its location between the LV and the ascending aorta. Mitral stenosis and regurgitation are also usually heard near the cardiac apex since this valve is located between the LA and ventricle. Murmurs that affect the tricuspid valve are usually the loudest near the lower aspect of the left sternal border, which corresponds to its location between the RA and RV. Finally, abnormalities associated with the pulmonary valve are best heard near the left second intercostal spaces, which correspond to its location near the RV and pulmonary artery.

Given this anatomical information, it is apparent that the locations of some murmurs can overlap. To help differentiate, one can note characteristics such as timing during the cardiac cycle, sound radiation, and pitch (Table 6.1). This information will increase a provider's diagnostic accuracy when evaluating a patient with suspected valvular heart disease.

TABLE 6.1
Detailed Characteristics of Heart Murmurs

Type of Murmur	Precordial Location	Timing in Cardiac Cycle	Radiation	Pitch	Sound Quality	Special Maneuvers
Aortic stenosis	Right second and third intercostal spaces	Mid-systolic	Toward carotid arteries	Medium; crescendo–decrescendo	Harsh	Best heard with patient sitting and leaning forward
Mitral stenosis	Apex	Diastole	None	Low; decrescendo	Rumbling	Use bell of stethoscope at PMI; best heard with patient in left lateral decubitus position
Aortic regurgitation	Left second to fourth intercostal spaces	Diastole	Toward apex	High	Blowing	Best heard with patient sitting and leaning forward with breath held following exhalation

(continued)

TABLE 6.1
Detailed Characteristics of Heart Murmurs (*continued*)

Type of Murmur	Precordial Location	Timing in Cardiac Cycle	Radiation	Pitch	Sound Quality	Special Maneuvers
Mitral regurgitation	Apex	Holosystolic	Toward left axilla	Medium/high	Harsh	Murmur should not vary with respiration
Tricuspid regurgitation	Lower left sternal border	Holosystolic	Toward xiphoid process	Medium	Blowing	Murmur will increase with inspiration
Pulmonic stenosis	Left second and third intercostal spaces	Mid-systolic	May radiate to left shoulder	Medium; crescendo–decrescendo	Harsh	None

PMI, point of maximal impulse.

CARDIAC CONDUCTION

To fulfill its role as the circulatory hub for the body, the heart maintains a coordinated electrical system that allows for synchronous cardiac muscle contraction and relaxation.

The main components of cardiac conduction are the sinoatrial (SA) node, AV node, the bundle of His, the left and right bundle branches, and the Purkinje fibers. These components create a unified pathway for cardiac electrical impulses to travel.

An action potential occurs when there is a change in voltage across a cellular membrane. As charged particles travel between the inside and outside of a cell, the membrane potential changes. When this occurs, a cardiac impulse can be generated and move through the cell membrane to cause contraction. Action potentials from the heart differ slightly from those created by other cells because they have automaticity. This means that the specialized cells at the SA node can create their own action potentials without relying on nervous system activity. The main ions that are involved are sodium (Na), potassium (K), and calcium (Ca) in conjunction with various membrane transport proteins, which move the charged particles against the electrochemical gradient. As the ions travel between the inside and outside of the cardiac cells, the voltage across the membranes alternates between (+) and (−); this allows the cardiac chambers to depolarize or repolarize based on the given voltage potential. On a macrolevel, this electrochemical process sets the heart's rate and allows it to rhythmically contract and relax. It also helps to create the cardiac cycle that is depicted graphically via EKGs to show the heart's underlying cardiac activity.

In terms of the anatomical components of cardiac conduction, the SA node is a 13.5-mm structure within the RA near the superior vena cava. It is the pacemaker of the heart because it is composed of a group of specialized cardiac cells that can generate impulses that travel to all other cardiac tissues. In a well-functioning heart, the SA node creates approximately 60 to 90 impulses per minute, which match one's normal resting heart rate. This unique electrical property ensures that the SA node is the only designated area for the initiation of cardiac impulses. The SA node is innervated by sympathetic nerves and branches from the vagus nerve, and its surrounding tissues function via calcium channel activation. These properties allow impulses from the SA node to travel in a slow and decremental fashion. The node is also directly connected to the cardiac cells of the right atrial wall; this allows impulses to travel between the SA node and the next point in the cardiac circuit.

Once a beat is generated by the SA node, it moves slowly to the atrial tissues and then is funneled more quickly to the AV node, which is approximately 5 mm. This small structure is composed of a group of specialized cardiac cells located between the atrial and ventricular septa. Primarily, it serves as a transition zone where each impulse is temporarily held before moving toward the ventricles. This slight delay at the AV node is representative of the time needed to stimulate the atria for contraction. The next portion of the conduction system is the bundle of His, which is a collection of myocardial cells surrounded by a fibrous outer sheath. Anatomically, this structure is very important because it is the only direct connection for impulses to travel between the atria and the ventricles. The bundle of His then bifurcates into left and right bundle branches, which wind through the interventricular septum independently. At this juncture, the left bundle travels toward the apex of the LV, while the right bundle branch moves toward the apex of the RV. Finally, the two bundle branches coalesce into the Purkinje fibers, which disperse into the subendocardium of the myocardium. Once an electrical impulse travels through the bundle branches to the Purkinje fibers, the ventricles contract and one beat of the cardiac cycle is complete (Figure 6.7).

Conceptually, one can understand the heart's electrical conduction system; however, it cannot be seen during a physical exam. Therefore, one way to evaluate a patient with a suspected conduction abnormality is an electrocardiogram (EKG). This diagnostic test is useful because its individual waveforms represent the electrical impulses of the heart, specifically, and its contraction and relaxation phases. The main components of an EKG are the P-wave, QRS complex, and T-wave. The cardiac cycle, and thus the EKG, begins with the P-wave, which is atrial activation or depolarization. The QRS complex represents ventricular depolarization and the T-wave equates to ventricular relaxation or repolarization. Specific heart sounds and timing of the cycle can also be applied to the EKG's waveforms. For example, S1 can be mapped to the QRS complex because it corresponds to ventricular contraction when the mitral valve closes and the aortic valve opens during systole. Additionally, S2 represents the beginning of diastole with the closing of the aortic valve and the opening of the mitral and tricuspid valves. Finally, the ventricles relax; this is represented by the EKG's T-wave.

BLOOD PRESSURE

An additional component of the cardiac physical exam is the evaluation of blood pressure (BP). While this information is technically documented as a vital sign, it is something to be mindful of during a cardiac exam because BP has a direct correlation with cardiovascular health. As blood circulates during the cardiac cycle and moves into the arterial system, a pulse is created. The force that is generated during this process is essentially a measure of one's BP. During cardiac contraction or systole, the pressure reaches its highest level and then falls to its nadir during diastole or relaxation. The pressure at these two extremes is the two numbers that comprise a patient's systolic and diastolic BPs that are measured with a sphygmomanometer (BP cuff). The difference between the systolic and diastolic BP is defined as pulse pressure and it can be narrowed or widened in various cardiac conditions. There are also several factors that affect BP such as left ventricular stroke volume, vascular

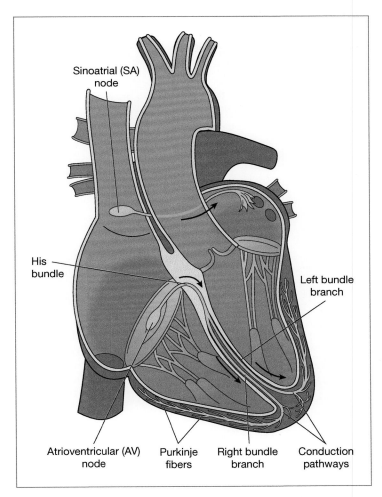

Sinoatrial (SA)
node

His
bundle

Left bundle
branch

Atrioventricular (AV)
node

Purkinje
fibers

Right bundle
branch

Conduction
pathways

FIGURE 6.7 Electrophysiological pathway of cardiac conduction. Tracing an impulse from the SA node to the AV node through the bundle of His where it bifurcates into the left and right bundle branch blocks and terminates at the Purkinje fibers to allow the ventricles to contract and complete one beat of the cardiac cycle.

stiffness, volume of blood in the arterial system, and integrity of the aorta.

Although BP is helpful in the evaluation of cardiac abnormalities, it cannot be used to directly assess pressures within the heart. One noninvasive method to assess a patient's overall volume status is to examine the jugular venous system. The jugular veins can help provide an estimation of the pressures within the RA, pericardium, and RV (specifically right ventricular end-diastolic pressure). Additionally, it can help determine the integrity of the tricuspid and pulmonary valves because the right internal jugular (IJ) is connected to the RA.

During a cardiac physical exam, one should evaluate the jugular veins (Figure 6.8). As the pressures fluctuate in the RA during contraction and relaxation, the same will occur in the jugular system and pulsations can be appreciated via inspection. Jugular venous pressure (JVP) will increase when there is an excess of fluid in the cardiovascular system. This often occurs in patients who are suffering from exacerbations of congestive failure. The JVP can also fall in settings of hypotension and acute blood loss. The procedure for properly examining and measuring the JVP will be reviewed later in this chapter when reviewing the steps of the cardiac physical examination.

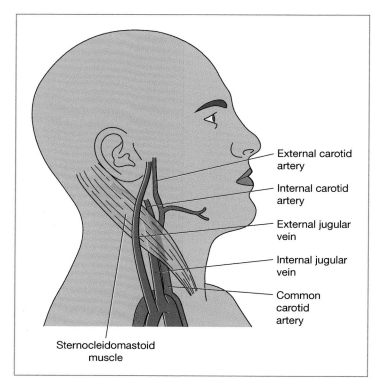

External carotid
artery

Internal carotid
artery

External jugular
vein

Internal jugular
vein

Common
carotid
artery

Sternocleidomastoid
muscle

FIGURE 6.8 Basic anatomy of jugular venous system: external and internal jugular veins, the carotid artery vasculature, and the sternocleidomastoid muscle.

Screening Health Assessment and Normal Findings

BLOOD PRESSURE EVALUATION

An assessment of the cardiovascular system will consist of inspection, palpation, and auscultation of the precordial area in addition to the evaluation of the jugular veins and systemic BP. Using a manual sphygmomanometer and a stethoscope, a provider will begin by checking a patient's BP. In order to obtain the most accurate BP reading, it is important to have a patient remain seated in a quiet room with his or her feet firmly on the floor for at least 5 minutes prior to obtaining the measurement. In addition, providers should ensure that patients have not utilized tobacco products or consumed caffeine for a minimum of 30 minutes prior to a BP evaluation, as these substances can result in falsely elevated readings. As sphygmomanometers come

in multiple sizes, providers should select a cuff that is the right size for their patient. Using a cuff that is too large can result in a BP reading that is too low and a cuff that is too tight can cause an inaccurately high BP measurement. In adults, a properly fitting BP cuff should encircle 80% of the upper arm closest to the brachial artery and the width should be 40% at this same point. The tubing between the device and the cuff should be a standard 27.5 inches (70 cm) long.

PATIENT POSITIONING

Patient positioning is also crucial during this portion of the exam (Figure 6.9). The American Heart Association (AHA) BP guidelines state that patients should be seated with their backs

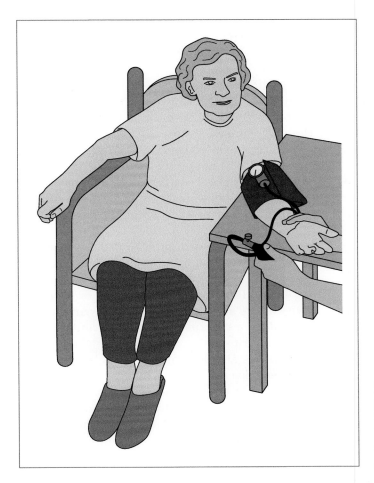

FIGURE 6.9 Patient positioning for blood pressure evaluation. When taking a patient's blood pressure, the individual's arm should be exposed, and he or she should be seated with the feet firmly on the floor and arm at approximately heart level.

supported, feet flat on the floor, legs uncrossed, and relevant arm exposed. It is important that patients do not roll-up their sleeves because this can create a tourniquet-like effect above the cuff, leading to an inaccurate BP reading. Research has also shown that if a patient is sitting in a backless chair, diastolic pressure can be falsely elevated; while crossed legs can increase systolic pressure. Ideally, the mid-point of the cuff on the arm should be at the level of the RA, which is close to the sternum. This position can be achieved by having the patient rest his or her arm on a small table or pillow. If the arm is placed below heart level, the BP could be falsely elevated, and if the arm is too high, the value obtained could be lower than the patient's actual BP.

PROCESS

Step 1: Wrap the bladder of the BP cuff around the patient's upper arm, approximately 2 to 3 cm above the antecubital fossa, which is the location of the brachial artery. One can also palpate the brachial pulse; this would be the proper location to place the cuff.

Step 2: Place the pads of the index and middle fingers on the patient's radial pulse and slowly inflate the cuff using the other hand. Once the provider can no longer feel the patient's pulse, the number reached on the BP cuff should be noted. This is because AHA guidelines recommend inflating the cuff 30 mmHg above this value to achieve the most accurate BP reading. Once the baseline value is obtained, the cuff should be deflated. The patient can rest for a moment, and the provider can prepare to obtain the actual reading.

Step 3: Place the diaphragm of the stethoscope at the brachial artery and inflate the cuff to 30 mmHg above the value that was just obtained. Next, the provider should slowly deflate the cuff at approximately 2 to 3 mmHg per second. If the cuff is deflated too quickly, the diastolic pressure will be falsely elevated and the systolic pressure will be lower than it should be. As the cuff is deflated, one should listen for the first two consecutive heartbeats or Korotkoff sounds—the number on the BP monitor at this point marks the patient's systolic pressure. Then, continue to deflate the cuff slowly and listen for the pulse to disappear—the number on the BP device at this point denotes the patient's diastolic pressure.

During a physical examination, the AHA recommends obtaining two BP readings with a 1-minute interval in between. Several studies have shown that the average of the systolic and diastolic values, respectively, is the most accurate determination of a patient's BP because the initial reading is often abnormally elevated due to a variety of factors. It is also noted that additional readings should be done if the difference between the first two measurements (systolic and diastolic, individually) is greater than 5 mmHg.

When conducting an exam on a new patient, AHA guidelines state that BP should be taken in each arm. This is a recommendation because significant differences in these readings can signal anatomical abnormalities such as coarctation of the aorta or an upper-extremity arterial occlusion.

Mastering the ability to obtain accurate BP is essential because this vital sign provides clues about structural abnormalities, cardiac dysfunction, and determines whether a patient has hypertension (elevated BP). This is especially important because chronic untreated hypertension can result in cardiac damage and affect other organ systems such as the eyes, the lungs, the vascular system, and the kidneys.

INSPECTION OF THE PRECORDIUM

This portion of the exam should be conducted with the patient supine, head angled to 30 degrees, and the provider standing on the patient's right side. The only equipment necessary for this exam is a penlight to enhance visibility. (Throughout the cardiac exam, it is important for providers to maintain patient modesty with gowns and sheets and explain to patients that certain portions of their precordium will need to be exposed during the exam.)

When looking at the anterior chest, one should note any obvious congenital deformities such as pectus excavatum or carinatum (Figures 6.10 and 6.11). Pectus excavatum results in a concavity at the sternum, while pectus carinatum is marked by a protrusion at the sternum and its associated ribs.

Providers should look for the location of the apical impulse or PMI. This impulse equates to the pulse of the LV as it contracts against the chest wall. The ability to see the pulsations will depend on a patient's body habitus, as it may be difficult to appreciate in obese patients. If needed, one can shine a tangential light across the patient's chest to increase the likelihood of its visualization. Additionally, one can ask the patient to turn on his or her left side, into the left lateral decubitus position; this moves the LV closer to the chest wall and makes the PMI easier to recognize. The expected position for the PMI is at the cardiac apex—fifth intercostal space in the midclavicular line (Figure 6.12). If displaced, most commonly the PMI shifts laterally toward the left axilla. The most common etiology for this abnormality is left ventricular dilation due to increased pressures within the cardiac system. Patients with laterally displaced PMIs often have long-standing hypertension, which can progress to concomitant heart failure.

With the patient repositioned supine, providers should examine the anterior precordium for any lifts or heaves, both of which are abnormal findings. In patients with an enlarged LV or RV, one may appreciate a heaving motion of the left side of the

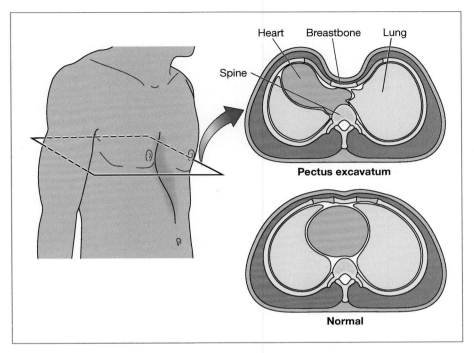

FIGURE 6.10 Pectus excavatum deformity and its effect on cardiopulmonary anatomy.

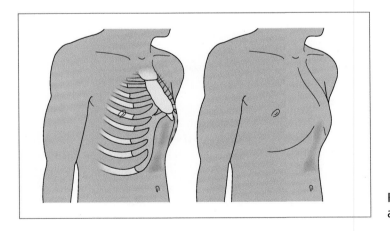

FIGURE 6.11 Pectus carinatum deformity and its effect on cardiopulmonary anatomy.

chest with each pulsation. In a setting of right-sided pressure or volume overload, the area around the sternum will appear to elevate or lift slightly from the rest of the chest wall with each heartbeat. Both of these findings show that a patient's heart is under stress due to increased pressures and/or volumes.

PALPATION OF THE PRECORDIUM

For this portion of the examination, the patient should remain supine and head angled at 30 degrees with the provider on the patient's right side. The

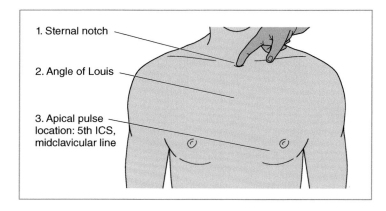

FIGURE 6.12 Location of PMI. To accurately locate the anatomical position of the PMI, one should begin at the sternal notch, then gradually move downward to appreciate the angle of Louis, and then proceed to the left side of the chest at the fifth intercostal space midclavicular line where the apical impulse can be felt.

ICS, intercostal space; PMI, point of maximal impulse.

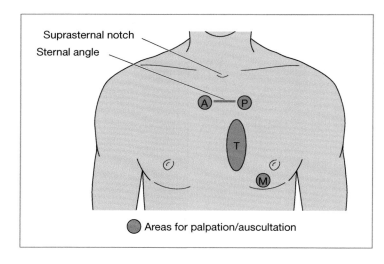

FIGURE 6.13 Key anatomic locations/landmarks that should be used during the cardiac examination:

   A: Aortic—palpate for thrills, auscultate for aortic valve murmurs

   P: Pulmonic—palpate for thrills, auscultate for pulmonic valve murmurs

   T: Tricuspid—inspect for right ventricular lifts/heaves, palpate for thrills, auscultate for tricuspid valve murmurs

   M: Mitral—palpate for thrills and PMI, auscultate PMI and for mitral valve murmurs

PMI, point of maximal impulse.

only equipment needed to complete this exam is a ruler to measure the PMI and a stethoscope to appreciate its duration. As previously mentioned, patient modesty should be respected and only the area being examined should be exposed. In addition, when examining a female with large breasts, the provider should explain to the patient that he or she is going to gently lift the patient's left breast with the back of his or her (provider's) left hand, or one can ask the patient to perform this maneuver. The goal of this exam is to palpate the precordial area, specifically the second right and left interspaces, down the sternal border, and the apex for lifts, heaves, thrills, and the PMI (Figure 6.13).

To palpate for a lift or heave, one should place the palm of his or her hand flat against a patient's anterior precordium (Figure 6.14). With each cardiac impulse, if the provider's palm slightly elevates from the chest wall, this indicates either a lift or heave due to an enlarged cardiac chamber.

The presence of a cardiac thrill is directly associated with murmurs, specifically those that are more severe. When palpating for a thrill, one will use the ball of his or her hand pressed firmly against the patient's anterior chest. If a thrill is present, it will feel like a vibration or hum secondary to turbulent blood flow from incompetent valves. It is important to palpate for thrills at the right and left second interspaces, down the sternum, and at the apex, concentrating on areas where valves are located.

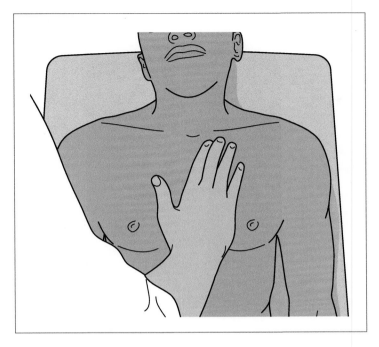

FIGURE 6.14 Proper technique for precordial palpation for a lift or heave, which can indicate ventricular hypertrophy.

APPRECIATING POINT OF MAXIMAL IMPULSE

For this exam, patients can remain supine; however, it may be advantageous to ask patients to move into the left lateral decubitus position because the apical impulse is easier to feel when patients are on their left side. To feel for the pulse, one should place the tip of his or her index or middle finger against the patient's chest at the fourth or fifth intercostal space in the midclavicular line (Figure 6.15). To further accentuate the impulse, one can ask patients to inhale, exhale, and hold their breath for several seconds to enhance the sound. If one still cannot locate the impulse, it will be important to note this finding and shift his or her fingers slightly laterally and downward, toward the left axilla; this is the most common location for PMI displacement due to left ventricular volume overload. Once the PMI is detected, its location, diameter force, and amplitude should be noted.

In a healthy patient, the PMI should be located at the midclavicular line between the fourth and fifth intercostal space. It should measure 2 cm in diameter, and its amplitude should be brisk and feel like a light tapping motion against the provider's fingertip.

The examination of the PMI is important because there are many pathologies that alter its normal position, size, or force. Although abnormalities of the PMI are somewhat nonspecific, if something is noted to be amiss, it should prompt further investigation. For example, an apical impulse that lasts longer than expected is defined as sustained and can occur with aortic stenosis (AS) or chronic hypertension. If one measures an enlarged (<3–4 cm) and diffuse PMI, this can indicate heart failure due to left ventricular enlargement from pressure and volume overload. If the PMI's amplitude feels hyperkinetic, this can be a normal variant in young adults (especially after physical activity); however, it is usually pathological in adult/elderly patients secondary to the heart working in overdrive. This hyperkinesis can occur in high-metabolic states such as severe blood loss anemia and hyperthyroidism or secondary to cardiac etiologies, including hypertension and AS (due to increased LV pressure) or aortic regurgitation because of LV volume overload.

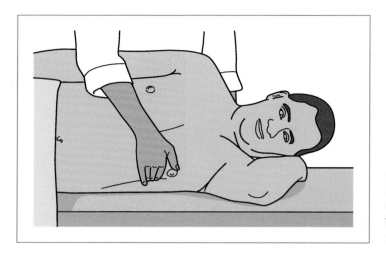

FIGURE 6.15 Location of PMI. The PMI can be felt at the fourth or fifth intercostal space of the midclavicular line with the patient in the left lateral decubitus position.

PMI, point of maximal impulse.

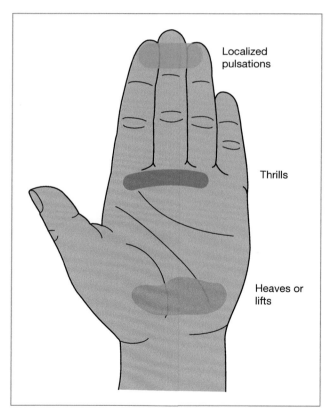

Localized pulsations

Thrills

Heaves or lifts

FIGURE 6.16 Precordial palpation techniques. During the palpation portion of the cardiac exam, one will use his or her fingertips to feel pulses (such as the PMI), the base of the fingers to detect thrills (caused by valvular dysfunction), and the base of the hand to detect lifts or heaves (concerning for ventricular hypertrophy in diseases such as heart failure).

PMI, point of maximal impulse.

DURATION OF THE APICAL BEAT

To determine the duration of the apical beat, the provider should place his or her stethoscope at the patient's cardiac apex, while the fingertip remains on the patient's PMI (Figure 6.16). The goal is to correlate the pulsation of the apical impulse with the start of systole (via cardiac auscultation of S1 and S2 sounds). In a properly functioning cardiovascular system, the apical pulsation should last for approximately two-thirds of systole and cease prior to the S2 beat. Pathologically, if the impulse is sustained, this can indicate left ventricular dysfunction. If it occurs in conjunction with lateral displacement, one should consider an etiology such as left ventricular volume overload while an elevated amplitude is usually due to chronic hypertension.

AUSCULTATION OF THE PRECORDIUM

The final step in the cardiovascular examination is auscultation. The majority of this evaluation can occur with the patient supine (head angled at 30 degrees); however, if any murmurs are suspected, one can use special maneuvers for additional confirmation. These techniques will be reviewed in the following section. The only instrument necessary for this examination is a stethoscope.

There are many types of stethoscopes that are available—for example, ones designed for infants, those that record heart sounds for playback, and others with tunable diaphragms. As a student, it will be helpful to use a simple stethoscope with a diaphragm and bell to build a solid foundation of basic auscultation skills (Figure 6.17).

The diaphragm of the stethoscope is best for listening to high-pitched sounds such as S1, S2, and regurgitation murmurs (aortic and mitral). The bell of the stethoscope is better at accentuating the low-pitched sounds of S3, S4, and mitral stenosis. When using the bell, it is best to apply light pressure against the chest. If one presses it too firmly, the bell's function becomes negated and it will act more like a diaphragm and detect high-pitched sounds. In some instances, however, this can be helpful. For example, if a provider thinks he or she hears a pathological S3 or S4 heart sound with the bell (using light pressure) and then applies more pressure and the sounds disappear, this could help confirm the suspicion.

During auscultation, the provider listens to each landmark, first with the diaphragm and then the bell. To begin, listen at the right second interspace, move to the left second interspace, then down the left sternal border (second to fifth interspaces), and then finish at the apex (see Figure 6.13). At each precordial location, the goal is to identify the S1 and S2 sounds. With practice, one will be able to discern how these sounds differ in intensity at each landmark. For example, at the base, S2 should sound louder than S1, while the reverse occurs at the apex. Physiologically, this occurs because the S1 sound equates to the closure of the mitral and tricuspid valves. S1's intensity is primarily driven by the anterior leaflet of the mitral valve and left ventricular action; therefore, it follows suit that S1 will be loudest at the apex, which is the location of the LV. To help discern S1/S2, systole (interval

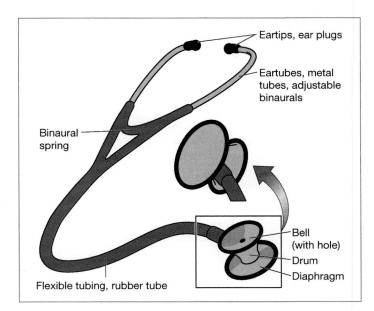

FIGURE 6.17 Components of a stethoscope. It is important to be familiar with the components of a stethoscope including the eartips, eartubes, rubber tubing, and most importantly the diaphragm and bell, which have unique acoustic properties for identifying physiological and pathological heart sounds. The diaphragm is best for detecting high-pitched sounds (S1 and S2) and regurgitation murmurs, while the bell is helpful when listening for lower-pitched sounds (S3 and S4) and mitral stenosis murmurs.

between S1 and S2), and diastole (interval between S2 and S1) at each precordial location, one can apply light pressure to the patient's right carotid artery, noting that S1 occurs right before the upstroke and S2 immediately after it.

During auscultation, the provider should listen for any obvious splitting of the S1 and S2 heart sounds. This is best heard at the left second and third interspaces. For this skill, one should coordinate his or her listening with the patient's respirations—initially listening as the patient breathes normally and then instructing the patient to breathe deeper. Physiologically, one should appreciate an S2 split (into A2 and P2) only during inspiration, but if it is fixed with respiration, this can indicate a pulmonic or aortic valve pathology. If the split is heard during expiration, as opposed to inspiration, this can also equate to a valvular abnormality.

With respect to the pathological S3 sound, it is best heard during diastole (at the rapid ventricular filling phase) with the bell. It can be appreciated on the left or right side of the precordium and indicates heart failure. On the left side, the sound is best heard at the apex. Studies have also confirmed that in patients with chronic heart failure, this left-sided sound is directly correlated with a high occurrence of cardiac morbidity and mortality. On the right side, S3 is best heard at the lower left sternal border and can be enhanced during inspiration. It may also be helpful to have patients in the left lateral decubitus position to accentuate this sound.

The S4 heart sound occurs in diastole during atrial filling and left ventricular expansion. It is also best heard with the bell in the same location as S3 also enhanced with patients in the left lateral decubitus position. Acutely, an S4 can occur in conjunction with myocardial infarctions/ischemia; chronically, it can indicate left ventricular dysfunction. One should also be aware that S3 and S4 sounds can be normal variants in children and young adults, especially those who are very physically active, but in adults, these sounds are pathological.

CARDIAC MURMURS

During cardiac auscultation, it is paramount to listen for any cardiac murmurs. Although it can be challenging to discern faint murmurs, one can become

proficient with dedicated practice. When decoding murmurs, one should listen for the following characteristics—location, timing, radiation, intensity, and shape of the sound (see Table 6.1). With respect to timing, this refers to whether the sound is heard during systole or diastole, and it can be helpful to remember that systole corresponds to the carotid upstroke. Additionally, diastolic murmurs are almost always pathological, whereas those in systole can be normal variants or signify valvular disease.

Murmurs that occur in systole can be mid-, late-, or holosystolic (pansystolic). Those that occur in mid-systole begin after S1, cease prior to S2, and correspond to blood flow across the aortic and pulmonary valves. Late-systolic murmurs commence in mid-systole and last up to the S2 heart sound. The most commonly heard late systolic murmur is that of mitral valve prolapse (MVP) where an opening "snap" or "click" sound is usually heard immediately prior to the murmur, as the valve pops open. Additionally, the murmur of mitral regurgitation is characterized as late systolic. Pansystolic murmurs begin in S1 and stop prior to S2. They differ from mid-systolic murmurs in that there is not an audible gap between the murmur stopping and the second heart sound starting. These murmurs typically occur because of retrograde flow across the mitral and tricuspid valves.

Diastolic murmurs can be defined as early-, mid-, or late-diastolic. An early-diastolic murmur is one that begins right after S2 and ceases prior to the subsequent S1 sound. Typically, these murmurs occur because of backflow in the aortic or pulmonic valves. A mid-diastolic murmur commences after S2 (following a short gap) and becomes inaudible by the start of the next S1. Murmurs that occur in late diastole begin after S2 (following a considerable silent gap) and continue right until the start of S1. Both mid- and late-diastolic murmurs refer to pathology within the mitral or tricuspid valves.

One can think of a murmur's shape as the type of sound that is generated. For example, the systolic murmur of AS is characterized by a crescendo–decrescendo sound, meaning that, initially, it will grow in loudness and then fade to silence. This is in contrast to a mitral regurgitation murmur, which is holosystolic and maintains the same level of sound throughout S1 and S2. In conjunction with a murmur's shape, one can also become skilled at noting its quality and pitch, as certain murmurs have distinct sounds. For example, aortic regurgitation creates a high-pitched blowing-like sound, whereas mitral stenosis sounds like a low-pitched rumble. Another important clue when trying to discern a specific cardiac murmur is if the sound radiates to another location on the precordium. This information is used in conjunction with noting the murmur's primary location where it is loudest on the chest. This radiation phenomenon occurs because of the reverberation of sound (from the blood flow) through the bones of the thorax. The

two most common points of radiation are the carotids in AS and the axilla with mitral regurgitation.

During auscultation, positioning is also important because the sounds of certain murmurs can be enhanced when a patient is not supine. For example, the diastolic murmur of mitral stenosis can be accentuated if a patient is lying in the left lateral decubitus position while the provider listens with the bell of the stethoscope over the PMI (Figure 6.18). This technique brings the LV closer to the surface of the

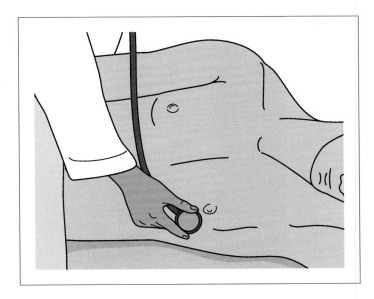

FIGURE 6.18 Technique for appreciating a murmur of mitral stenosis with patient in the LLD position. Provider listens over the mitral valve area near the PMI with the bell of the stethoscope.

LLD, left lateral decubitus; PMI, point of maximal impulse.

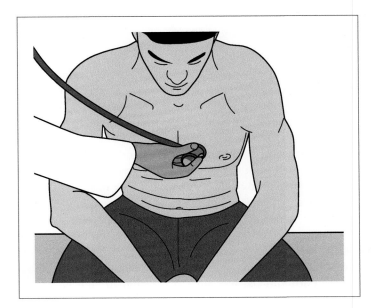

FIGURE 6.19 Patient positioning to accentuate murmur of aortic regurgitation. Patient should be sitting up and instructed to inhale and then simultaneously lean forward, exhale completely, and hold his or her breath. At this point, the provider should listen at the aortic, pulmonic, and tricuspid landmarks with the diaphragm of the stethoscope.

TABLE 6.2 Levine Scale of Cardiac Murmurs	
Murmur Grade	**Description**
Grade 1	Quite faint; may require special maneuvers for accentuation and usually requires listening for at least several seconds
Grade 2	Quiet, but easily and immediately heard when stethoscope applied to precordium
Grade 3	Moderately loud
Grade 4	Loud; (+) palpable thrill
Grade 5	Very loud; (+) palpable thrill and may be heard without stethoscope firmly applied to precordium
Grade 6	Very loud; (+) palpable thrill and may be heard without use of stethoscope

chest wall to make the murmur more audible. With aortic regurgitation, it is helpful to have the patient sit up, inhale deeply, subsequently exhale, and then lean forward while the provider listens with the diaphragm of the stethoscope down the left sternal border (Figure 6.19).

Finally, one should note how loud a murmur is because this correlates with its severity. To minimize subjectivity, the Levine scale was created. This tool is a six-level standardized grading system to help determine murmur intensity. Table 6.2 outlines the six gradations of severity.

Focused Health Assessment and Abnormal Findings

When a patient presents to a provider with a focused CC in the cardiovascular system, the following health assessment techniques with their rationales would be performed.

JUGULAR VENOUS PRESSURE EVALUATION

If a provider is concerned about a patient's overall volume status, one can perform a JVP measurement. This skill is somewhat complex; however, it can be very helpful in determining whether a patient is fluid overloaded and placing excess strain on his or her

heart. The goal of this technique is to gain information regarding central venous and right atrial pressures. The first step is to locate the IJ vein, which is one of the anatomical landmarks. It is preferred to use the IJ instead of the EJ (external jugular vein) because the IJ does not contain any valves and it is more closely aligned with the SVC and RA. Traditionally, the JVP is measured as the vertical distance between the top of the pulsation at the IJ and the sternal angle (angle of Louis) where the manubrium meets the sternum. To perform this assessment, the provider must find the highest point of pulsation within the IJ, which is the oscillation point. This exam is usually conducted with the patient supine and his or her head elevated to 30 degrees; however, depending on current volume status, the provider may be unable to locate the oscillation point at this angle. Therefore, one can adjust a patient's head to either 60 or 90 degrees to obtain the measurement.

Current research also shows that the area between the angle of Louis and the RA can vary based on a patient's body habitus and the angulation of his or her head during the exam (30, 45, or 60 degrees). Since this distance is not standardized, there is concern for an underestimation of central venous pressure. To account for this difference, a mathematical adjustment is used when calculating the actual JVP height.

Another option is to use the clavicle as the second reference point because its distance from the RA is approximately 10 cm and a JVP >8.0 cm is considered abnormal. Therefore, if the provider appreciates any venous pulsations above the clavicular line, the JVP height would be significantly greater than the accepted threshold of 8.0 cm. For

documentation purposes, note that although one is measuring the JVP in centimeters of water, this value should be converted to mmHg because it is the most accurate way to assess hemodynamics (1.36 cm H_2O = 1.0 mmHg).

To perform this examination, the only necessary equipment is a ruler (centimeter). In terms of positioning, the required angle of the patient's head will depend on his or her volume status and the provider's ability to locate the JVP's oscillation point. Once the patient is adequately positioned, there are several steps to follow. First, place a pillow behind the patient's head to relax the sternocleidomastoid muscles (SCMs) and turn the patient's head away from the side that is being assessed. If necessary, use a penlight to visualize the IJ vein and then inspect for pulsations immediately posterior to the SCM. To obtain the height of the JVP, locate the oscillation point in the IJ and align the bottom of the ruler with the patient's sternal angle (Figure 6.20). Next, note

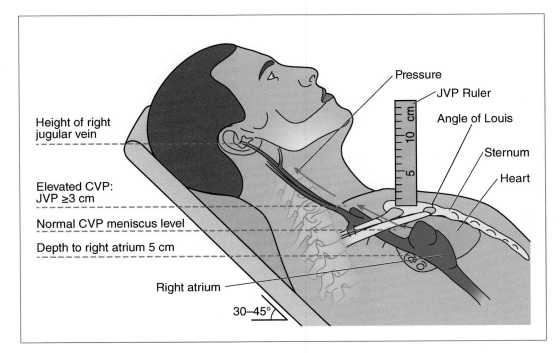

FIGURE 6.20 Measurement of JVP. To obtain a patient's JVP, locate the oscillation point in the IJ and align the bottom of a ruler with the sternal angle. Then, note the vertical distance of the pulsation above the sternal angle—a value greater than 3 cm is an indication of elevated CVP. Additionally, add 5 cm to that value to account for the extra distance between the sternal angle and the RA. This result is the best estimation of JVP.

CVP, central venous pressure; IJ, internal jugular; JVP, jugular venous pressure; RA, right atrium.

the vertical distance of the pulsation above the sternal angle; if it is greater than approximately 3 cm, this is an indication of elevated central venous pressure. Additionally, once this value (in cm) is determined, add 5 cm to account for the extra distance between the sternal angle to the RA; this value is the best estimation of a patient's JVP.

One common pitfall during this examination is unknowingly focusing on the pulsations in the carotid artery as opposed to those from the IJ. To avoid this mistake, remember that the carotid pulse is palpable, whereas impulses from the IJ are not. In addition, the JVP will vary with respiration and patient positioning; however, the carotid pulse will not change as patients breathe or move from supine to sitting to standing. Another difference between the two pulsations is that if one applies light pressure on the veins above the sternal end of the clavicle, the JVP will be obliterated while the carotid pulse will remain palpable.

Clinically, this information is helpful in the evaluation of patients with specific cardiac pathologies. For example, JVP can be low if patients are hypovolemic, which can occur because of acute blood loss or sepsis (systemic infections). JVP can be increased in heart failure (due to fluid overload), tricuspid stenosis, and constrictive pericarditis, the latter of which occurs when the

pericardium is too stiff for proper cardiac contraction and relaxation; this results in increased cardiac pressures. An elevated JVP is also indicative of an increase in left end-diastolic pressure and a decrease in ejection fraction (EF). EF is the percentage of blood discharged from the LV with each contraction and serves as a good estimation of overall cardiac function. This is because a low EF signals that the heart is unable to work hard enough to provide an adequate amount of circulating blood volume for the body's needs.

When examining the oscillations in the IJ vein there are four discernable phases that directly correspond to the pressure variations of the RA during the cardiac cycle. These are termed as the *a-wave, x-descent, v-wave,* and *y-descent* (Figure 6.21). Beginning with systole, just prior to the generation of the S1 heart sound, there is a presystolic a-wave. This waveform in the IJ correlates to the increased pressure in the RA immediately prior to contraction. The x-descent consists of the time between the RA relaxing, the RV contracting (still in systole), and ends immediately prior to the production of the S2 heart sound. The next portion of the IJ oscillation is the v-wave. In the cardiac cycle, this is marked by the closing of the tricuspid valve and subsequent elevation in pressure of the RA as it fills with blood. The final phase of the oscillation is the y-descent that corresponds

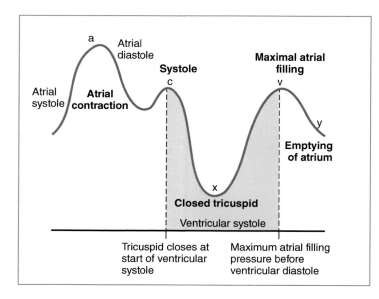

FIGURE 6.21 JVP waveforms. Within the internal jugular vein there are four phases corresponding to the variations in pressures within the RA during the cardiac cycle. In systole, prior to S1, there is a presystolic a-wave that corresponds to the increase in RA pressure prior to cardiac contraction. The x-descent is time between the RA relaxing and the right ventricle contracting, ending just prior to S2. The v-wave denotes the closure of the tricuspid valve where the RA fills with blood and its pressure begins to rise. The final phase is the y-descent (in diastole) where the tricuspid valve opens, blood moves into the right ventricle, and the pressure in the right atrium decreases.

JVP, jugular venous pressure; RA, right atrium.

to diastole as the tricuspid valve opens, blood moves into the RV, and pressure in the RA decreases.

One can also inspect the height and the timing of the jugular venous pulsations because these abnormalities can indicate cardiac pathologies such as arrhythmias or valvular disease. To appreciate the timing, one can visualize the IJ pulsations while auscultating the precordium for the S1 and S2 heart sounds. In a normally functioning heart, the a-wave comes immediately prior to S1, the v-wave occurs with S2, and the y-descent follows soon after. If one cannot appreciate an a-wave, meaning its amplitude is undetectable, one possibility is the conduction disorder, atrial fibrillation. If an elevated a-wave is detected, this can signal tricuspid stenosis marked by significant resistance to atrial contraction. If the v-wave is observed to have an increased height, one possible etiology is tricuspid regurgitation because this portion of the oscillation occurs during diastole when the tricuspid valve would normally close and allow for the pressure to build within the RA as it fills with blood.

INSPECTION AND PALPATION OF THE CAROTID ARTERIES

For patients with pre-existing cerebrovascular disease (or at high-risk for developing it) or who present with complaints related to the cerebrovascular system, the next step in the cardiovascular examination is to evaluate the carotid arteries (see Figure 6.8). This consists of inspecting for symmetry, timing, amplitude, and duration, as well as auscultating for bruits (sound created by turbulent blood flow). Physiologically, the carotid pulse will vary depending on stroke volume, EF, and the integrity of the vascular system. This examination can also be challenging in patients with peripheral vascular or arterial disease as well as those with conduction disorders such as atrial fibrillation; however, it can be very useful in detecting pathologies relating to valvular disease and heart failure.

To begin, a patient should be supine with his or her head angled at 30 degrees. In this position, one can appreciate the carotid pulse medial to the SCM muscles near the cricoid cartilage. After inspecting

this area for the pulse, providers should palpate it using the pad of their index or middle fingers in the lower aspect of the neck. It is important to never palpate both carotid pulses simultaneously or use force during this exam because those techniques can induce carotid hypersensitivity and syncope, especially in elderly patients. Once a strong impulse has been located, one should assess its amplitude, contour, and timing.

The height of the pulsation should correspond to a patient's pulse pressure, and its contour refers to the characteristics of its waveforms. With practice, one can become proficient at denoting the speeds of the upstroke and downstroke as well as the timing of the plateau period. In a healthy heart, the upstroke is quick, the plateau is smooth, and the downstroke is slightly less rapid than the upstroke. With respect to timing, it can be helpful to simultaneously auscultate the heart during this exam because the carotid pulse waveforms correspond to the cardiac cycle. For example, the carotid upstroke follows S1 (and precedes S2) and the plateau occurs during the middle of systole.

The inspection and palpation of the carotid arteries are important because there are various pathologies that can be detected during this portion of the examination. For example, if one notes a weak carotid pulse, this could signal a myocardial infarction, sepsis, or cardiogenic shock. In patients with severe aortic regurgitation, one might appreciate a sharp rise and rapid fall of the carotid upstroke (termed Corrigan's or water hammer pulse), or recognize a pulse called bisferiens where two systolic peaks occur due to the aortic valve's inability to open and close properly. It is also common to palpate a bounding pulse in patients with aortic regurgitation. With respect to AS, the valve's stiffness causes a delayed carotid upstroke (*tardus*) in combination with a weak impulse on palpation (*parvus*).

Another pulse-related abnormality is *pulsus alternans*. This finding is particularly concerning because it corresponds to severe left ventricular dysfunction. It occurs when the rhythm of the pulse is steady; however, the force of the impulses will alternate (*alternans*) between strong-and weak-feeling beats. One can also confirm his or her suspicions by using the sphygmomanometer to check the patient's BP while listening for specific sounds. To perform this technique, raise the pressure of the BP monitor to the patient's known systolic BP and then listen to the Korotkoff sounds. Initially, the sound of each beat will be fairly loud; however, as the pressure is lowered, one should appreciate soft and loud beats in an alternating fashion or a sudden doubling of the pulse.

One can also use the BP cuff and stethoscope to assess for a *paradoxical pulse*. This is defined as a greater than 10 mmHg drop in a patient's systolic BP during inspiration. This finding can indicate cardiac and respiratory diseases such as severe chronic obstructive pulmonary disease (COPD), pericardial tamponade, pulmonary emboli, or a tension pneumothorax. To perform this test, inflate the BP cuff to the level of the patient's systolic pressure. As the cuff is slowly deflated, the provider should listen for the first Korotkoff sound that appears and disappears during inspiration. The pressure value at this point should be noted. Then, as the cuff is consistently deflated, listen for the first Korotkoff sound that no longer

disappears as the patient inspires. This value should also be noted. In a patient with a well-functioning cardiovascular and respiratory system, this difference between those two values should be no more than 4 mmHg, while anything greater than 10 mmHg equates to an abnormal finding that requires further investigation.

AUSCULTATION OF THE CAROTID ARTERIES

The final portion of the carotid pulse exam focuses on auscultation, specifically listening at the carotid arteries for sounds of turbulent blood flow. This finding can occur in conditions such as arterial stenosis (secondary to atherosclerosis; Figure 6.22), external carotid artery disease, thoracic outlet syndrome, complications from hyperthyroidism, and tortuously shaped arterial walls. Additionally, the

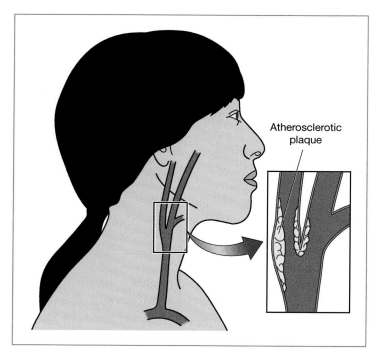

Atherosclerotic plaque

FIGURE 6.22 Carotid artery atherosclerosis. As plaque accumulates within the carotid arteries, they become stiff and narrow. When this occurs, one can appreciate a bruit, which is the sound generated by turbulent blood flow through a stenotic area.

murmur of AS radiates to the carotids; it is important to differentiate between a carotid bruit and a transmitted murmur from an incompetent valve. Because the differential diagnoses associated with carotid bruits are so broad and somewhat nonspecific, the U.S. Preventive Services Task Force (USPSTF) recommends against routine carotid artery auscultation. This exam should only be used in elderly patients or those who are at high-risk for cerebrovascular disease.

To conduct the exam, the only necessary equipment is a stethoscope. First, the provider should instruct the patient to take a deep breath in and hold it; this ensures that carotid bruits are not confused with respiration sounds. Next, place the diaphragm of the stethoscope (best used for detecting lower-pitched bruit-type sounds) over the carotid artery right below the angle of the mandible (Figure 6.23). Anatomically, this positioning is important because it marks the bifurcation of the common carotid artery in the internal and external carotid arteries. It is the best location to hear a carotid bruit without mistaking it for a radiated sound from the heart. The provider should listen for approximately 15 to 20 seconds before assessing the opposite carotid artery.

SPECIAL MANEUVERS FOR AUSCULTATION OF THE CAROTID ARTERIES

If a provider suspects a murmur after performing basic precordial auscultation, there are various techniques that can be used to determine whether a murmur is present and, if so, which one. The majority of these maneuvers require patients to change positions; therefore, they should only be used if patients are clinically and hemodynamically stable. The principal techniques require that the patient transition between standing and squatting and perform a Valsalva maneuver (such as bearing down as if having a bowel movement).

Physiologically, these movements are beneficial in differentiating between AS, MVP, and a genetic condition termed hypertrophic obstructive cardiomyopathy (HOCM). Anatomically, HOCM results in a thickened myocardium at the interventricular septum and a left ventricular

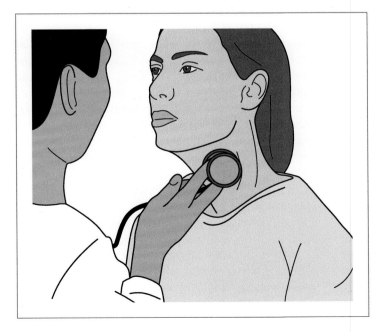

FIGURE 6.23 Technique for auscultation of carotid bruits. The patient should be instructed to hold his or her breath while the provider places the diaphragm of the stethoscope over the carotid artery directly below the angle of the mandible. The process is then repeated on the opposite side.

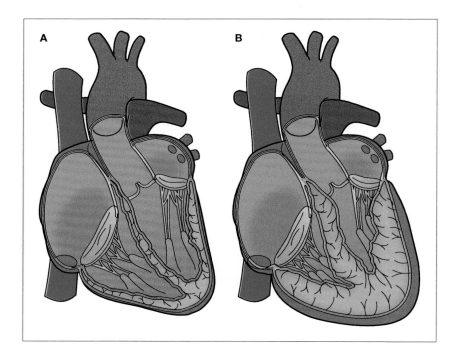

FIGURE 6.24 Anatomical representation of HOCM. (**A**) Normal heart. (**B**) Heart with HOCM. Anatomically, HOCM results in a thickened myocardium at the interventricular septum and a left ventricular outflow tract obstruction, thus affecting the heart's contractile ability.

HOCM, hypertrophic obstructive cardiomyopathy.

outflow tract obstruction, thus affecting the heart's contractile ability (Figure 6.24). Clinically, this condition can result in heart failure, dangerous arrhythmias, mitral regurgitation, and sudden cardiac death (SCD); therefore, if the provider notes an HOCM-type murmur, further investigation should be conducted immediately. The murmur of HOCM is very similar to that of AS because it is mid-systolic, high-pitched, and crescendo–decrescendo; however, unlike AS, it is nonradiating and best heard at the lower left sternal border and apex. To further differentiate a HOCM murmur from AS, the provider should instruct a patient to perform a Valsalva maneuver. This technique enhances the murmur of HOCM because it increases intrathoracic pressure, decreases left ventricular filling (i.e., preload), and increases left ventricular contractility. Physiologically, this creates more strain on the heart, especially at the intraventricular septum, and worsens the left ventricular outflow obstruction; therefore, the murmur intensifies. If patients with AS perform the identical technique, the decrease in blood volume pushed into the aorta leads to a quieter sounding murmur (Figure 6.25).

Another skill is dynamic auscultation, where a patient is asked to stand and then squat while the provider listens to the heart at each position (Figure 6.26). When a patient stands, venous return to the heart, peripheral vascular resistance, and arterial BP decrease; therefore, left ventricular blood volume also declines. This process accentuates HOCM's LV outflow tract obstruction and enhances its murmur. In AS, standing equates to a lower volume of blood moving into the aorta; therefore, its murmur sounds quieter. When a patient squats, there is an increase in arterial pressure, peripheral vascular resistance, venous blood return to the heart, and LV volume. Physiologically, this minimizes the LV outflow tract obstruction and decreases the murmur of HOCM; however, more blood flow is also ejected into the aorta; thus, the AS murmur is enhanced.

Both of these maneuvers can also be used when trying to identify the murmur of MVP. When auscultating, one will appreciate that squatting decreases the duration of the MVP's "click" while standing and Valsalva techniques will generate a more pronounced sound that lasts longer within systole.

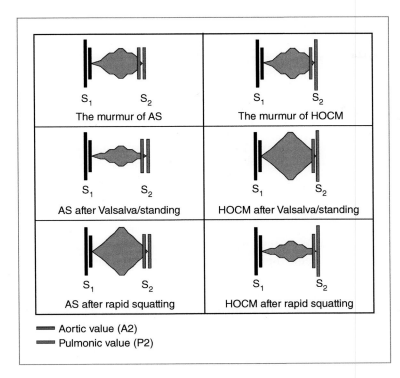

Aortic value (A2)
Pulmonic value (P2)

FIGURE 6.25 Comparing AS and HOCM murmurs. The murmurs of HOCM and AS are similar; however, HOCM's murmur is nonradiating and best heard at the lower left sternal border and apex. Additionally, if a patient performs a Valsalva maneuver, the murmur of HOCM becomes louder (due to increased intrathoracic pressure and a worsening of the left ventricular outflow obstruction), while the murmur of AS softens because there is a decrease in blood volume flowing to the aorta.

AS, aortic stenosis; HOCM, hypertrophic obstructive cardiomyopathy.

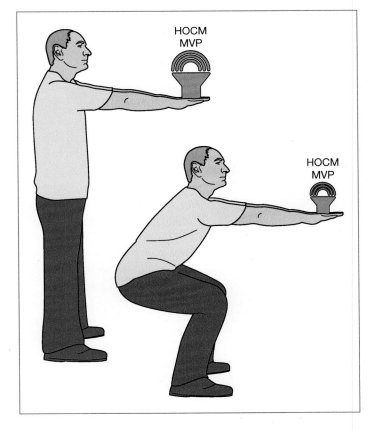

FIGURE 6.26 Detecting HOCM from MVP murmurs using dynamic auscultation. During dynamic auscultation, a patient stands and then squats while the provider auscultates the precordium. While standing, venous return to the heart, peripheral vascular resistance, and arterial blood pressure decrease. This process accentuates HOCM's LV outflow tract obstruction and enhances the murmur. This technique can also be used to identify the murmur of MVP—squatting decreases the duration of the MVP's "click" while standing and Valsalva motions generate a louder sound that lasts longer during systole.

HOCM, hypertrophic obstructive cardiomyopathy; LV, left ventricle; MVP, mitral valve prolapse.

Holistic Assessment

SPECIFIC HEALTH HISTORY

When a patient presents with a cardiovascular complaint, it is imperative to gain a comprehensive understanding of his or her primary symptom. This also includes a detailed history of the present illness (HPI) and review of systems (ROS). When assessing the characteristics of the main symptom, the provider should focus on onset and duration to determine whether the problem is acute or chronic, as well as identify aggravating or alleviating factors and associated symptoms, especially those related to the pulmonary, peripheral vascular, and neurological systems.

As with all other body system evaluations, one should inquire about past medical history (PMH), family history (FH), and social history (SH). For a cardiovascular patient's PMH, important information to document is a history of valvular disease, arrhythmias, hyperlipidemia, hypertension, CHF, coronary artery disease (previous myocardial infarctions), diabetes mellitus (DM) II, chronic kidney disease, and cerebrovascular disease. In addition, the provider should acquire the results of any recent diagnostics, such as stress tests, heart catheterizations, echocardiograms, and EKGs. This information is important because it can help risk-stratify patients, especially in emergent situations, and provide clues for potential differential diagnoses. In SH, the provider should learn about a patient's diet, activity level, and use of tobacco or other substances. In terms of substances, remember that cocaine can cause acute infarctions or arrhythmias, intravenous drug users are at risk of cardiac infections (particularly endocarditis), and excess alcohol can result in dilated cardiomyopathy (a type of heart failure). The provider should also obtain a detailed FH for all patients with cardiovascular complaints and note if any first- or second-degree relatives died from SCD at a young age.

SAFETY

Identifying patients at risk for cardiac decompensation is an important aspect of the comprehensive cardiovascular health assessment. The goal is to help these individuals avoid morbidity or mortality from conditions such as myocardial infarctions, CHF, valvular pathologies, hypertension, and arrhythmias. To do this, the provider should educate the patient (and their support system) about their respective diagnoses and the signs and symptoms of cardiac emergencies. The provider should also confirm that patients are safe in their current living situations and have adequate community resources and social support. The patient should also be well-connected with their primary care provider and cardiologist because these clinicians coordinate follow-up appointments, arrange diagnostic testing, and manage medications.

DISTRESS

It is important to identify and understand the effect that a given cardiovascular disease (CVD) is having on a patient's life. For example, is this someone who was previously very active and independent, but suddenly limited by his or her condition? The provider should aim to provide the patient with resources to manage their CVD while maximizing his or her activity level (as much as possible); for example, finding ways that the patient can continue hobbies and interests that are important to them while maintaining cardiovascular stability.

NUTRITION AND EXERCISE

For the patient with CVD, proper diet and exercise are paramount to survival. CVD consists of hypertension, coronary artery disease, heart failure, and stroke, and it is the leading cause of death in the United States. Therefore, the provider and patient need to focus on prevention strategies, such as those relating to lifestyle and behavior. The providers should educate the patient about disease-specific dietary guidelines and refer them to a nutritionist for additional monitoring. Although there are many cardiovascular diets, one of the most popular is the Dietary Approaches to Stop Hypertension (DASH) regiment that was created by the National Heart, Lung, and Blood Institute (NHLBI), which is a branch of the National Institute of Health (NIH). The initial version of this diet was designed and studied in the late 1990s where researchers determined that it reduced systolic BP by 11 mmHg and diastolic BP by 6 mmHg in patients with hypertension. Individuals on this diet eat a high volume of fruits, vegetables, whole grains, fish, and poultry, while limiting red meat, sugars, and other fats. After the first DASH study, additional trials were done that focused on sodium use. This research determined that when a salt restriction (1500 mg/d) is combined with pre-existing DASH guidelines, patients have an even greater reduction of systolic and diastolic BP. It should also be noted that for patients with CHF, sodium restrictions are equally as important because salt has a direct effect on volume status and overall cardiac function. In addition, heart failure patients may benefit from individualized fluid restriction plans to help prevent water retention and CHF exacerbations.

Although less disease specific, the AHA provides dietary guidelines for maintaining good cardiovascular health. For example, it recommends that individuals consume a diet rich in fruit, vegetables, whole grains, low-fat dairy, legumes, and skinless poultry and fish, while limiting alcohol, red meat, sugars, sodium, and trans-fats.

In regard to exercise, the provider should consider a patient's baseline activity level in conjunction with his or her cardiovascular status before recommending physical activity guidelines. For patients without any significant cardiovascular limitations, the AHA recommends 40 minutes of moderate-to-intense aerobic exercise three to four times per week to lower overall BP and cholesterol. However, for patients with severe valvular disease, chronic CHF, or other physically limiting comorbidities, this regiment may be implausible. Therefore, the provider needs to consider the whole patient before providing specific activity guidelines.

In addition, certain patients may qualify for guided cardiac rehabilitation programs to improve their overall cardiac status. These customized outpatient initiatives are typically prescribed for patients who are recovering from cardiac surgery, experienced a recent myocardial infarction, or were diagnosed with cardiac conditions that limit their ability to perform unsupervised physical activity. During cardiac rehabilitation, patients are engaged in a multifaceted program for several months where they focus on physical and emotional well-being and lifestyle changes. Trained cardiac rehabilitation providers help patients regain their strength, learn about their cardiovascular status, and reduce the risk of further cardiac damage. It is important for the provider to be aware of these programs because they can be very beneficial for patients who require additional outpatient resources to improve their cardiovascular health.

FINANCIAL IMPLICATIONS

Ask the patient if there are any financial implications because of his or her cardiovascular condition. Inquire about the patient's occupation/employment status and, for a patient who is working, determine whether his or her job is high-stress or requires intense physical activity. These questions are important when evaluating a patient's cardiovascular health in conjunction with his or her ability and need to return to work.

SPIRITUAL CONSIDERATIONS

Identify areas where the patient has turned for help in the past, including his or her faith and other means of support. Ask the patient how he or she addresses challenging situations and what methods he or she uses for self-care. Additionally, if there is a possibility that a patient may need an invasive procedure, the provider should ask that individual if he or she is a practicing Jehovah's Witness and, if so, determine the patient's wishes regarding the use of blood products.

CASE STUDY

DOCUMENTATION

Chief Complaint: Chest pain

History of Present Illness: Onset was sudden and acute after completing 2 hours of strenuous yard work. Pain is aggravated by physical activity and improved with rest and one dose of 325 mg oral aspirin. The discomfort is described as a pressure-like sensation located in the left chest area without radiation. Rates the severity as a 6/10 with activity and lessened to a 1/10 with rest and one dose of oral aspirin. States that when the pain occurred, it was constant and lasted for approximately 15 minutes. Also denies any previous occurrences of chest pain.

REVIEW OF SYSTEMS

Constitutional: No complaints of fever, chills, malaise, diaphoresis, or changes in weight

Integumentary: Denies rashes, lesions, peripheral edema

Gastrointestinal: Denies abdominal pain, nausea, vomiting, reflux, change in bowel habits

Neurological: Denies numbness, tingling, paresthesias, weakness, dizziness, lightheadedness, near-syncope/syncope

Respiratory: Denies cough, pleuritic chest pain, shortness of breath, dyspnea on exertion, orthopnea, or paroxysmal nocturnal dyspnea

PHYSICAL EXAMINATION

General: Well-developed, well-nourished male; neatly groomed, speech is clear and goal-directed, answers questions appropriately and appears in no acute distress

Integumentary: Olive complexion, warm, smooth, moist with rapid turgor. Villous hair evenly distributed to fingers and toes. Nails curved; nail beds pink with capillary refill <1 second. No erythema, edema, ecchymosis, cyanosis, jaundice, ulcers, or clubbing noted

Cardiovascular: Rate and rhythm: Regular at 68 minutes. Precordium: Flat without lifts, heaves, or visible pulsations. PMI: Palpable 9 cm lateral to the MSL in the left, fifth ICS; approximately 1 cm diameter; strong, and lasting approximately two-thirds of systole. S1> > S2 at apex. No murmurs, gallops, rubs, or fixed splitting of heart sounds. Carotid upstrokes: Strong bilaterally and synchronous with S1, no carotid bruits

(continued)

(continued)

Respiratory: Bony thorax: Symmetrical on quiet and deep respirations. Respirations: Unlabored, regular rhythm at 16 minutes. Chest wall: Nontender. Respiratory excursion equal bilaterally. Breath sounds: Vesicular in distal airways; bronchovesicular over larger airways. No wheezes, rales, or rhonchi

Gastrointestinal: Normal active bowel sounds × four quadrants. Slightly obese abdomen. Umbilicus: Midline. No visible peristalsis, scars, striae, bulging flanks, venous patterns, diastasis recti. Mixed tympany and dullness. Abdomen is soft, nontender, and nondistended without masses, rebound tenderness, tenderness, guarding, or fluid wave

Neurological: Alert and oriented to person, place, time, and purpose. Cranial nerves I to XII intact; no focal neurological deficits

Diagnosis: Unspecified Chest Pain

ICD-10-CM Diagnosis Code: R07.9 Chest Pain, Unspecified

Assessment of Special Populations

TRANSGENDER POPULATION

When caring for the transgender population, providers need to be sensitive to their individual needs. During the encounter, providers need to be *gender affirming*, meaning that correct pronouns are used throughout the visit. In addition, providers should talk with patients about their preferred use of terminology for certain body parts. These techniques help build a trusting patient–provider relationship and create an environment where patients are comfortable asking questions and sharing concerns. Providers must also ensure patient modesty and only expose body areas that are being examined. Some transgender patients may also use torso binders and be apprehensive to remove them. Care should be taken to explain to patients why it is important to expose their precordial area and that sheets and gowns will be provided; however, patients should never be forced to do anything that makes them feel uncomfortable. Providers should be hypervigilant of patient comfort and any anxieties that patients may have about physical touch during examinations.

In terms of cardiovascular-based patient education for this population, providers need to consider personal and family cardiovascular history in conjunction with any current use of testosterone or estrogen supplementation. Many studies show that the cardiovascular risk in transgender men using testosterone therapy is not statistically different than that of cisgendered women. There is some research that found increased morbidity and mortality from heart attacks and strokes among transgender women; however, the majority of this work did not control for factors such as tobacco use, obesity, and comorbid DM II, which are integral variables when measuring cardiovascular health. It has also been noted that among transgender women, tobacco use, sedentary lifestyles, obesity, hyperlipidemia, and DM II are very common; therefore, healthy lifestyle choices should be emphasized. Additionally, for transgender women with underlying cardiovascular risk factors who are using estrogen therapy, the transdermal route is preferred because it carries a lower risk of thromboembolic diseases and hyperlipidemia.

When evaluating any patient's overall cardio-vascular health, many providers employ mathematical tools to determine their risk of suffering from a heart attack or stroke within a 10-year period. The most commonly used is the Atherosclerotic Cadiovascular Disease (ASCVD) Risk Estimator Plus based on AHA and American College of Cardiology guidelines (https://tools.acc.org/ASCVD-Risk-Estimator-Plus/#!/calculate/estimate). This tool takes sex into account; therefore, providers should be mindful when using this calculator for transgender patients. According to current research, whether a provider uses natal sex or affirmed gender should be patient-specific. This is particularly focused on whether a patient is using hormones and, if so, what age that began and the duration of their use.

PEDIATRIC POPULATION

The infant and pediatric patient will have unique findings during the cardiovascular examination. It is important to obtain a detailed history of the infant from the parents and learn about any pregnancy-related complications. If there is a concern for cardiac disease, constitutional symptoms such as poor feeding, irritability, failure to thrive, and weakness must be noted. During the complete physical exam, providers should look for evidence of tachypnea, clubbing, and hepatomegaly because these findings can be indicative of cardiac pathologies. For example, the triad of tachycardia, tachypnea, and hepatomegaly are common in infants with CHF.

VITAL SIGNS

With respect to vital signs, it can be difficult to obtain an accurate BP on infants and children. Typically, it is not performed until age 3; however, this information is necessary for premature infants or those with certain congenital/genetic diseases. If a BP cuff cannot be used, there is a special Doppler, which notes arterial blood flow, converts it to a systolic pressure, and then displays this value as a digital number on the device. In a healthy child, systolic pressure increases as the child grows. For example, at birth, systolic pressure is approximately 70 mmHg and then it progresses to 85 mmHg at 1 month and 90 mmHg by 6 months of age. If there is a concern for consistently elevated BP in infants, possible differential diagnoses are renal artery stenosis, congenital kidney disease, or coarctation of the aorta; these conditions require prompt referral to specialists for further evaluation and treatment.

Infants' heart rates are also much faster than those of older children or adults. The average pulse from birth to 1 month is 140 beats/min and it decreases to 115 beats/min between 6 months and 1 year of age. As the infant grows, the rate decreases until it reaches that of a healthy adult. A pulse rate of greater than 180 beats/min could indicate paroxysmal supraventricular tachycardia, while bradycardia can result from conditions such as hypoxia, congenital neurological diseases, or heart block. To obtain the pulse, use the femoral or brachial areas because it can be challenging to record an accurate radial pulse in an infant. Additionally, all newborns should have a femoral pulse evaluation because decreased or absent femoral pulses could indicate aortic coarctation.

CENTRAL CYANOSIS

Another unique component of the infant cardiovascular exam is examining for central cyanosis. This finding is always abnormal, and without any respiratory symptoms, it suggests a congenital cardiac abnormality. Physiologically, central cyanosis occurs because of right to left shunting of blood. The underlying etiology depends on the age at presentation. At birth, consider transposition of the great arteries (TGA), tetralogy of Fallot (TOF), and pulmonary valve atresia. Within a few days of birth, another possible etiology is hypoplastic left heart syndrome; as the infant grows, other pulmonary vascular diseases with right to left shunting can manifest.

There are varying degrees of central cyanosis and mild cases may be difficult to detect. In addition to examining the perioral region, one should focus on the mucous membranes of the mouth and eyes. A light-pink appearance of these areas is normal, while a deeper red hue denotes an emergent decrease in oxygen saturation (Figure 6.27).

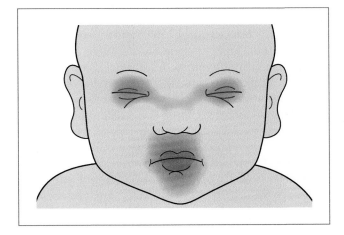

FIGURE 6.27 Central cyanosis in the infant. When an infant presents with concern for central cyanosis, the exam should focus on the perioral and conjunctival mucous membranes. In healthy babies, these areas are light pink; however, as depicted in the figure, when they become a darker reddish-blue, this indicates an urgent decrease in oxygen saturation.

PALPATION OF THE PRECORDIUM

During palpation of the precordial area, it is difficult to locate the PMI in infants. Starting in young childhood, it will be palpable in the fourth intercostal space at the midclavicular line because the heart is positioned more horizontally in kids. If a heave is detected at the left sternal border, this is concerning for right ventricular overload/strain while a similar motion at the apex could signify left ventricular dysfunction. If one sees and feels increased cardiac pulsations, this means that the heart is functioning in overdrive due to metabolic etiologies or ineffective cardiac contractility. When palpating for thrills in infants and children, the location of the vibration on the precordium will help diagnose the specific valvular abnormality. For example, if the vibration is felt near the right sternal border and carotids, one should consider AS, while an abnormality near the lower left sternal border can indicate a ventricular septal defect.

AUSCULTATION

Auscultation is the final step in the pediatric cardiovascular examination and there are dedicated stethoscopes that one can use for infants (bell size: ¾ inch) and pediatric patients (bell size: 1 inch). The provider will listen in the same precordial spaces as adults. Similar to adults, the goal is to appreciate the S1 and S2 heart sounds. This

can be difficult in infants and young children, but with practice one can improve his or her skills. In this patient population, one should be able to hear the S1 and S2 sounds independently, but during expiration, the two sounds will blend into one. It is also important to note the splitting of the S2 heart sound. In infants, this helps rule out the majority of life-threatening congenital cardiac diseases and is best accomplished when the patient is sleeping. If one detects a very loud P2 component, this is concerning for pulmonary hypertension, while a persistent splitting of S2 (one that does not vary with respiration) could equate to an atrial septal defect, right ventricular volume overload, or pulmonary vein abnormalities.

When auscultating, it is common for young children to have a sinus dysrhythmia where the heart rate increases on inspiration and decreases on expiration. This is considered a normal variant in childhood (not infancy) and can be confirmed by coordinating the rhythm with the patient's breathing. Some neonates and infants also have atrial or ventricular skipped beats. If they are physiological, they can be eliminated by increasing the patient's heart rate via stimulation such as crying or physical activity. The most common arrhythmia in infants and children is paroxysmal atrial tachycardia (PAT). Patients with PAT can be asymptomatic or in distress because of tachycardia and tachypnea. It is more common for infants and younger children with PAT to be very ill, whereas older children can compensate better. Typically, patients experiencing PAT will have a heart rate of 240 beats per minute; as the child ages, the episodes can vary in duration and frequency. Infants and children can also have other cardiac arrhythmias secondary to structural or conduction-related heart disease; however, providers should be mindful of other etiologies such as infections, metabolic diseases, endocrine abnormalities, or toxic ingestions.

The most challenging portion of the cardiac physical exam in the pediatric patient is detecting heart murmurs and determining which are physiological versus pathological. Similar to evaluations for adults, one will classify murmurs by their location, timing, duration, and sound quality. The vast majority of children will have at least one benign murmur that will dissipate before adulthood; these patients will not have any other concerning noncardiac signs or symptoms. For patients with murmurs secondary to severe structural heart disease, it is common to appreciate failure to thrive, poor feeding, weakness, or obvious genetic defects.

Two very common benign murmurs that occur between birth and 1 year of age are a peripheral pulmonary flow murmur and a closing ductus murmur. A closing ductus murmur is a soft, crescendo–decrescendo, holosystolic sound best detected in the upper left sternal border. The peripheral pulmonary flow manifests in newborns and disappears by age 1.

It occurs because of the improper growth of the pulmonary artery while in utero and is defined as soft, holosystolic, and best heard at the upper left sternal border with radiation to the axillae. If a pulmonary flow murmur is detected in a newborn in conjunction with other associated symptoms, one should be concerned for diseases such as congenital rubella.

There are two main categories of pathological pediatric murmurs—obstructive and left-to-right shunts. Obstructive murmurs occur when blood tries to flow through underdeveloped valves or those that are too small. They are appreciated immediately after birth because they are not related to the decrease in pulmonary vascular resistance that happens during the first moments of life. Murmurs that occur because of left-to-right shunts are directly related to the immediate decrease in pulmonary vascular resistance; therefore, some of these murmurs are undetectable until several weeks after birth and others may not be diagnosed until a child is at least 1-year-old. High-pressured shunts such as ventricular septal defect and patent ductus arteriosus can be heard within a week after birth while low-pressured shunts as atrial septal defects can take at least a year to manifest. Table 6.3 provides additional information regarding the most common pathological murmurs related to structural heart disease in infants and children.

TABLE 6.3
Congenital Structural Cardiac Abnormalities and Corresponding Murmurs

Murmur	Mechanism	Details	Other Physical Examination Findings
Pulmonic stenosis	Valve leaflet fusion restricting blood flow	Location: Upper left sternal border Radiation: May radiate to the lung fields Quality: Loud ejection click in early systole	P2 heart sound becomes soft in severe stenosis Newborn growth is unaffected Typically, characterized as an acyanotic abnormality, but if severe, it can result in central cyanosis and respiratory failure

TABLE 6.3
Congenital Structural Cardiac Abnormalities and Corresponding Murmurs (*continued*)

Murmur	Mechanism	Details	Other Physical Examination Findings
Patent ductus arteriosus	Ductus arteriosus fails to close at birth; results in continuous blood flow from aorta to pulmonary artery	Location: Upper left sternal border Radiation: To the back Quality: Harsh machinery-like sound throughout systole and diastole	Defined as an acyanotic abnormality Can be diagnosed at birth (if premature) if bounding pulses, murmur, and dynamic precordial activity Diagnosed later in infancy (if full-term) when pulmonary vascular resistance decreases Large defect can result in heart failure by 1–2 months of age
Aortic stenosis	Congenital bicuspid valve or structural damage from rheumatic fever	Location: Upper right sternal border Radiation: Toward carotids Quality: Harsh systolic ejection sound	Defined as an acyanotic abnormality Heart failure and diminished pulses if severe disease Mild cases may remain undetected until adulthood
Tetralogy of Fallot	Combination of: 1. Ventricular septal defect 2. Right ventricular outflow obstruction 3. Rotation of the aorta 4. Right to left shunt at the ventricular septum	Location: Upper left sternal border Radiation: Left sternal border Quality: Systolic ejection sound	Will have central cyanosis that worsens with activity Can have cyanotic episodes resulting in altered mental status Persistent cyanosis can result in polycythemia and failure to thrive
Atrial septal defect	Defect in atrial septum results in left-to-right shunt	Location: Upper left sternal border Radiation: Posteriorly Quality: Soft systolic ejection sound	Will hear widely fixed split of S2 heart sound Often not heard until after 1 month of age Can note weight loss as defect worsens in size

(*continued*)

TABLE 6.3
Congenital Structural Cardiac Abnormalities and Corresponding Murmurs (*continued*)

Murmur	Mechanism	Details	Other Physical Examination Findings
Transposition of great arteries	Life-threatening abnormality: 1. Aorta connects to the right ventricle 2. Pulmonary artery connects to the left ventricle	No characteristic murmur	More common in male newborns (ratio of 3:1) Very prominent central cyanosis Will show signs of severe heart failure Will note tachypnea secondary to elevated pulmonary blood flow and metabolic acidosis Chest x-ray will show cardiomegaly and narrow mediastinum
Ventricular septal defect	Occurs as blood travels through defect in the septum from left ventricle (high-pressure) to right ventricle (low-pressure); results in murmur secondary to turbulent blood flow	Location: Lower left sternal border Radiation: None Quality: Harsh holosystolic sound that can mask S1 and S2	Defined as an acyanotic abnormality Will present with a murmur shortly after birth but remain asymptomatic until 1 month of age In small shunts, no growth disturbance; large defects can cause growth retardation due to heart failure

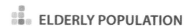

ELDERLY POPULATION

When examining the elderly population, providers should be mindful of age-related changes within the heart and all body systems. It is important to be cognizant of elderly patients' physical limitations and provide assistance during exams to minimize fall risk. Elderly patients have a higher likelihood of developing cerebrovascular disease due to atherosclerotic accumulation. Therefore, providers should conduct routine carotid artery evaluations in this population using techniques that do not induce carotid

hypersensitivity or syncope. Also, if a murmur is detected during the exam and a provider wants to investigate it further via dynamic auscultation, one should ensure that the patient is physically able to perform these maneuvers, as some could pose a fall risk. The remaining steps of the cardiac evaluation for this population should remain the same.

From a patient history and education perspective, there are also several things to consider in the elderly population. Many cardiovascular medications, especially those for BP, have side effects such as dizziness, bradycardia, and hypotension. All of these can be very dangerous for older patients.

It is the responsibility of the primary care provider, cardiologist, and pharmacist to collaborate and ensure that geriatric patients do not have issues of polypharmacy and using the lowest dose and least amount of medications to control their CVDs. Elderly patients should also be educated on healthy lifestyle guidelines and the importance of certain screening tests. One example is a one-time abdominal aortic aneurysm (AAA) ultrasound to evaluate for the presence of an AAA. Currently, this is recommended by the USPSTF in males age 65 years old to 75 years old who have ever smoked. Ba sed on the results of this initial scan, further follow-up and diagnostics may also be required.

PATIENTS WITH DISABILITIES

During the cardiovascular evaluation of a patient with a disability, providers should learn about their patient's abilities and baseline level of function, including the use of any assistive devices and the amount of support that a patient has at home. This information will help guide discussions about patient education and determine the level of assistance that a patient might need during the physical examination in terms of positioning, transferring, and performing certain maneuvers. If necessary, providers can modify the cardiovascular physical examination according to a patient's physical limitations, thus limiting the risk of falls or other injuries during an encounter. The most important aspect of CVD in individuals with disabilities is the recognition that patients with disabilities have the same risk factors for cardiovascular disorders as other patients and that CVD is the leading cause of mortality. Therefore, the same attention should be given to cardiovascular assessment in this population as with other patient populations.

With respect to physical activity guidelines to help patients maintain their cardiovascular health, it will be important to consider a patient's baseline level of function. It may also be helpful to refer patients with certain physical disabilities to physical therapists or specialized athletic trainers who have experience with creating safe physical activity plans for this population.

When referring a patient with a disability for further testing (e.g., imaging studies), it is important to refer the patient to a facility or site that can accommodate patients with various disabling conditions. It is also important to discuss transportation issues if a patient with a disability requires transport to another facility or site for such testing.

VETERAN POPULATION

When conducting a cardiovascular-focused patient encounter with a veteran, it is appropriate to learn about his or her military experience in conjunction with all other aspects of the veteran's history. One should inquire about any previous traumatic injuries (especially those affecting the cardiothoracic system), CVDs, and any invasive cardiac procedures and note where/how those conditions were managed. This aspect is important because veterans may have been treated by multiple providers nationally and internationally based on where they were stationed during their military service, and it is helpful to maintain complete patient records.

The cardiovascular physical exam for veterans should be the same used for any other patient based on age and cardiovascular history/risk factors. In addition, providers should consider any previous exposures or hazards in this population and how these factors could lead to an increased risk of developing CVD. Although not directly related to the cardiovascular exam, providers should assess overall mental health. When talking with veterans, it is important to discuss issues of chronic pain, substance abuse, and degree of family/friend support while ensuring that they are receiving available resources through Veterans Affairs (VA) – sponsored organizations.

PREGNANT POPULATION

Pregnant patients will require routine cardiovascular assessments during pregnancy. If any abnormalities are noted or if patients have complex pre-existing cardiac diseases, they are often referred to maternal-fetal medicine providers and cardiologists who specialize in treating this patient population.

When conducting physical examinations for pregnant females, the providers should be mindful of patients' physical limitations. It is especially important to note BP because persistent hypertension in pregnancy can be dangerous and requires immediate attention. During the precordial evaluation, providers might appreciate that the apical impulse (or PMI) has shifted slightly upward and to the left near the fourth intercostal space due to the increase in uterine size. When performing auscultation for a patient in the later stages of pregnancy (or while breastfeeding), it is possible to detect a venous hum or *mammary souffle*, which is a sound produced secondary to increased blood flow throughout the circulatory system. This sound is best heard at the second or third intercostal space at the sternal border and occurs during both systole and diastole. If a provider hears an S3 heart sound in patients during their third trimester of pregnancy, this is a normal variant; however, if any murmurs are detected, providers should promptly refer patients for further evaluation, especially if there is a concern for AS or pulmonary hypertension. These two findings can be dangerous for the mother and fetus. Finally, one should evaluate all pregnant patients (especially those in the third trimester) for any signs or symptoms of heart failure because there is a risk of peripartum cardiomyopathy in this population.

Diagnostic Reasoning

Common Differential Diagnoses: Atherosclerotic Diseases	
Diagnosis	**Key History and Physical Examination Differentiators**
Myocardial infarction	Males >45 years old, females >55 years old; family history of CAD in first-degree relatives; PMH of DM II, HTN, obesity, and HLD increases risk; intense crushing chest pain with radiation to jaw/left arm (usually >30 minutes); associated dyspnea, diaphoresis, nausea, syncope; can have SCD (usually due to ventricular fibrillation)
Prinzmetal angina	Occurs secondary to cardiac vasospasm—can occur in patients with or without atherosclerosis; angina at rest; during cardiac catheterization, administration of IV ergonovine will reproduce the vasospasm
Stable angina	Males >45 years old, females >55 years old; family history of CAD in first-degree relatives; chest pain or pressure <10 minutes secondary to activity and relieved with rest, ASA, or nitroglycerine
Unstable angina	Males >45 years old, females >55 years old; family history of CAD in first-degree relatives; chest pain at rest or unrelieved by rest or nitroglycerine; any change in stable angina symptoms or initial presentation of angina

ASA, acetylsalicylic acid (aspirin); CAD, coronary artery disease; DM, diabetes mellitus; HLD, hypersensitivity lung disease; HTN, hypertension; IV, intravenous; PMH, past medical history; SCD, sudden cardiac death.

Common Differential Diagnoses: Heart Failure

Diagnosis	Key History and Physical Examination Differentiators
Congestive heart failure	Occurs when the heart cannot meet the body's metabolic or circulatory demands; can have preserved (diastolic) or decreased (systolic) ejection fraction; can also be characterized as left-sided or right-sided
Left-sided congestive heart failure	Signs and symptoms: Dyspnea, orthopnea, paroxysmal nocturnal dyspnea, confusion (due to decreased cerebrovascular perfusion), nonproductive nocturnal cough; laterally displaced PMI, S3/S4 heart sounds, rales at lung bases (due to fluid/congestion backing up into the pulmonary system)
Right-sided congestive heart failure	Signs and symptoms: Peripheral edema, increased JVD and hepatojugular reflux, ascites, and right-sided ventricular heave

JVD, jugular vein distention; PMI, point of maximal impulse.

Common Differential Diagnoses: Arrhythmias

Diagnosis	Key History or Physical Examination Differentiators
Atrial fibrillation	Tachycardic irregular ventricular heart rate (75–175 bpm); can occur alone or due to other etiologies (e.g., MI, sepsis, malignancy, aortic stenosis, post-op stress, pulmonary embolism, obstructive sleep apnea); symptoms include fatigue, palpitations, DOE, dizziness, syncope, chest pain
Paroxysmal supra-ventricular tachycardia	Most common cause of supraventricular tachycardia (150–250 bmp); can occur secondary to ischemic heart disease, excessive alcohol or caffeine, or digoxin toxicity; symptoms include fatigue, dizziness, palpitations, chest discomfort
Sick sinus syndrome	Occurs secondary to dysfunction of the heart's SA node and characterized by persistent and spontaneous sinus bradycardia; symptoms include dizziness, syncope, confusion, lightheadedness
Sinus bradycardia	Normal sinus rhythm with rate <45 bpm; can occur secondary to ischemia, increased vagal tone, or antiarrhythmic medications (can be normal variant in athletes); can be asymptomatic or occur with fatigue, decreased activity tolerance, angina, or syncope

(continued)

Common Differential Diagnoses: Arrhythmias (continued)	
Diagnosis	**Key History or Physical Examination Differentiators**
Ventricular fibrillation	Multiple foci in ventricles fire rapidly to create quivering (instead of contraction); fatal if untreated; most common cause is ischemic heart disease; patient will be unconscious (no pulse or blood pressure)
Ventricular tachycardia	Rapid regular rhythm of more than three sequential premature ventricular complexes (100–250 bmp); can be sustained (<30 seconds) or nonsustained; if sustained, can be life-threatening and progress to ventricular fibrillation; patients can be stable or unstable and pulseless; most common cause is MI; symptoms include palpitations, angina, syncope, sudden cardiac death

bpm, beats per minute; DOE, dyspnea on exertion; MI, myocardial infarction; SA, sinoatrial.

Common Differential Diagnoses: Pericardial, Myocardial, and Endocardial Diseases	
Diagnosis	**Key History and Physical Examination Differentiators**
Acute cardiac tamponade	Rapidly accumulating amount of fluid within the pericardium; the effusion impairs the ventricle's diastolic filling and results in decreased stroke volume and cardiac output; can occur because of penetrating trauma, pericarditis, postmyocardial infarction with wall rupture, or iatrogenically (e.g., central line placement, pacemaker insertion); elevated JVP with distended neck veins, muffled heart sounds, narrowed pulse pressure, and pulsus paradoxus (from BP measurements); can also have hypotension, tachypnea, and tachycardia (secondary to imminent cardiogenic shock)
Acute infectious endocarditis	Infection of the endocardium involving the valvular cusps; most often caused by *Staphylococcus aureus* or *Streptococcus viridans*; can affect native or prosthetic valves; intravenous drug use increases risk of tricuspid valve endocarditis; associated with fever of unknown origin, malaise, new heart murmur
Acute pericarditis	Inflammation of the heart's pericardium; can be idiopathic or secondary to underlying causes; common etiologies include viral (HIV, Coxsackie virus, hepatitis A or B), postmyocardial infarction, malignancy, collagen vascular diseases, amyloidosis, or as a result of medications (e.g., hydralazine or procainamide); symptoms include pleuritic chest pain that is aggravated by lying supine and relieved by sitting up/leaning; can appreciate fever and pericardial friction rub (high-pitched sandpaper-like sound best heard with patient sitting up/leaning forward after exhalation)
Myocarditis	Inflammation of the myocardium secondary to various etiologies, including viral (e.g., Coxsackie B), bacterial (e.g., Lyme, Group A streptococcus), medication-related (e.g., sulfonamides), or idiopathic; can be asymptomatic but often with fever and chest pain; can result in sudden cardiac death

BP, blood pressure; JVP, jugular venous pressure.

Common Differential Diagnoses: Valvular Heart Diseases

Diagnosis	Key History or Physical Examination Differentiators
Aortic regurgitation	Occurs secondary to backflow of the blood from the aorta into the left ventricle; results in increase of left ventricular diastolic volume; can be acute (e.g., infectious endocarditis) or chronic (e.g., HTN, rheumatic fever, bicuspid aortic valve); symptoms include orthopnea, PND, palpitations, angina; signs include wide pulse pressure (BP), lateral and downward shifted PMI, diastolic decrescendo murmur at left sternal border
Aortic stenosis	Stiffened aortic valve that results in left ventricular hypertrophy/dysfunction and decreased cardiac output; initially, can be asymptomatic but progresses to angina, syncope, and heart failure; harsh systolic crescendo–decrescendo murmur at right second intercostal space that radiates to carotids, sustained PMI, parvus et tardus of carotid pulse
Mitral regurgitation	Can be acute or chronic secondary to elevation of left atrial pressures; acute etiologies include infectious endocarditis or papillary muscle rupture from an MI; chronic causes are rheumatic fever and cardiomyopathy; symptoms include PND, orthopnea, palpitations, dyspnea on exertion; laterally displaced PMI, S3 sound, holosystolic murmur at apex which radiates to clavicles
Mitral stenosis	Stiffened mitral valve that results in elevated left atrial and pulmonary venous pressures; can eventually cause right ventricular failure; majority of cases are secondary to rheumatic heart disease; symptoms include orthopnea, PND, angina, hemoptysis, dyspnea on exertion, palpitations; low-pitched diastolic rumble murmur that is preceded by an opening "snap" and followed by a prominent S1
Mitral valve prolapse	Abnormality of the mitral valve leaflets; results in prolapse of the valve into the left atrium during systole; commonly seen in conjunction with connective tissue diseases (e.g., Ehlers–Danlos and Marfan's syndromes); often asymptomatic but palpitations and chest pain can occur; mid-systolic click with mid-systolic murmur where squatting decreases the murmur and standing/Valsalva increases the murmur
Tricuspid regurgitation	Failure of the tricuspid valve to close; results in backflow of blood into the right atrium and subsequent right ventricular failure; most common underlying etiologies are left ventricular failure, inferior wall MI, and tricuspid endocarditis; symptoms are similar to right-sided heart failure; blowing holosystolic murmur at lower left sternal border, S3 heart sound, and, often, atrial fibrillation

BP, blood pressure HTN, hypertension; MI, myocardial infarction; PMI, point of maximal impulse; PND, paroxysmal nocturnal dyspnea.

Common Differential Diagnoses: Heart Muscle Diseases

Diagnosis	Key History or Physical Examination Differentiators
Dilated cardiomyopathy	Most common type of cardiomyopathy secondary to a variety of etiologies (e.g., ischemia, infection, alcohol abuse, collagen vascular disease, thyroid disease) and results in left ventricular dysfunction; symptoms of congestive heart failure; S3/S4 heart sounds and mitral/tricuspid murmurs
Hypertrophic obstructive cardiomyopathy	Autosomal dominant genetic disorder that results in a hypertrophic left ventricle with subsequent diastolic dysfunction and outflow obstruction; symptoms are chest pain, syncope, dyspnea on exertion, palpitations, **sudden cardiac death**; on exam can appreciate sustained PMI, loud S4, systolic ejection murmur that increases with standing/Valsalva and decreases with squatting, bisferiens carotid pulse; important to screen young athletes for this anomaly
Restrictive cardiomyopathy	Impaired diastolic ventricular filling secondary to infiltration of the myocardium; can result in long-term systolic heart failure; can be idiopathic as a result of other etiologies (e.g., amyloidosis, sarcoidosis, scleroderma); symptoms include dyspnea on exertion and decreased exercise tolerance; physical exam findings of right-sided heart failure

PMI, point of maximal impulse.

Common Differential Diagnoses: Vasculature Diseases

Diagnosis	Key History or Physical Examination Differentiators
Abdominal aortic aneurysm	Abnormal dilatation of the abdominal aorta; more common in males >50 years old with tobacco use history; can occur secondary to atherosclerosis, HTN, connective tissue diseases, and vasculitis; usually asymptomatic, impending rupture, sudden severe low back/abdominal pain; signs of rupture include Grey Turner sign (ecchymosis on flanks), hemodynamic instability, Cullen's sign (ecchymosis around umbilicus)
Acute aortic dissection	Separation of the layers within the aortic walls; occurs secondary to long-standing HTN, trauma, and connective tissue disorders; symptoms include severe tearing, interscapular pain, diaphoresis, chest pain, inability to get comfortable during exam; asymmetric BP between extremities, murmur of regurgitation
Peripheral vascular disease	Chronic occlusive atherosclerotic disease of the lower extremities; typically occurs in conjunction with HTN, CAD, CHF, DM II, tobacco use; symptoms include intermittent claudication that progresses to pain at rest; decreased/absent lower extremity pulses, decreased distribution of lower extremity hair, shiny appearance to skin, thickened toenails, ischemic ulcers

BP, blood pressure; CAD, coronary artery disease; CHF, congestive heart failure; DM, diabetes mellitus; HTN, hypertension.

BIBLIOGRAPHY

Agabegi, S. S., & Agabegi, E. D. (2008). *Step-up to medicine* (2nd ed., pp. 1–61). Philadelphia, PA: Wolters Kluwer.

American Heart Association. (n.d.). *The American Heart Association diet and lifestyle recommendations*. Retrieved from https://www.heart.org/en/healthy-living/healthy-eating/eat-smart/nutrition-basics/aha-diet-and-lifestyle-recommendations#.W1oFWNVKjIU

Armstrong, C. (2018). High blood pressure: ACC/AHA releases updated guideline. *American Family Physician, 97*(6), 413–415. Retrieved from https://www.aafp.org/afp/2018/0315/p413.html

Bickley, L. S., Szilagyi, P. G., & Hoffman, R. M. (Eds.). (2017). *Bates' guide to physical examination and history taking* (12th ed.). Philadelphia, PA: Wolters Kluwer.

Deutsch, M. B. (Ed.). (2016). *Guidelines for the primary and gender-affirming care of transgender and gender nonbinary people* (2nd ed.). San Francisco: University of California San Francisco. Retrieved from www.transhealth.ucsf.edu/guidelines

Ho, S. Y., & Becker, A. E. (2011). Anatomy of electrophysiology. In V. Fuster, R. A. Walsh, & R. A. Harrington (Eds.), *Hurst's the heart* (13th ed., pp. 911–924). New York, NY: McGraw-Hill.

Lewington, S., Clarke, R., Qzilbash, N., Peto, R., & Collins, R. (2002, December 14). Age-specific relevance of usual blood pressure to vascular mortality: A meta-analysis of individual data for one million adults in 61 prospective studies. *Lancet, 360*(9349), 1903–1913. doi:10.1016/S0140-6736(02)11911-8

Moore, K. L., Agur, A. M. R., & Dalley, A. F., II. (2011). *Essential clinical anatomy* (4th ed., pp. 80–115). Philadelphia, PA: Wolters Kluwer.

O'Gara, P. T., & Loscalzo, J. (2015). Physical examination of the cardiovascular system. In D. L. Kasper, A. S. Fauci, S. L. Hauser, D. L. Longo, J. L. Jameson, & J. Loscalzo (Eds.), *Harrison's principles of internal medicine* (19th ed, Chapter 267). New York, NY: McGraw-Hill.

Sacks, F., Svetkey, L., Vollmer, W., Appel, L., Bray, G., Harsha, D., … Cutler, J. A.(2001). Effects on blood pressure of reduced dietary sodium and the Dietary Approaches to Stop Hypertension (DASH) diet. *New England Journal of Medicine, 344*(1), 3–10. doi:10.1056/NEJM200101043440101

Tkacs, N., Hermann, L., & Johnson, R. (in press). *Advanced physiology and pathophysiology: Essentials for clinical practice*. New York, NY: Springer Publishing Company.

U.S. Department of Agriculture and U.S. Department of Health and Human Services. (2010). *Dietary guidelines for Americans, 2010* (7th ed.). Washington, DC: U.S. Government Printing Office.

U.S. Preventive Services Task Force. (2014). Screening for asymptomatic carotid artery stenosis: U.S. Preventative Services Task Force recommendation statement. *Annals of Internal Medicine, 161*, 356–362. doi:10.7326/M14-1333

U.S. Preventive Services Task Force. (2014, June). *Abdominal aortic aneurysm: Screening*. Retrieved from https://www.uspreventiveservicestaskforce.org/Page/Document/UpdateSummaryFinal/abdominal-aortic-aneurysm-screening?ds=1&s=AbdominalAortic Aneurysm

7

ADVANCED HEALTH ASSESSMENT OF THE RESPIRATORY SYSTEM

Dale Robertson

CHAPTER CONTENTS

(continued)

Overview of Anatomy and Physiology

The human respiratory system, also called the ventilator system, consists of biological organs primarily responsible for gas exchange. The primary function of the major organs is to provide oxygen to body tissues for cellular respiration, removal of carbon dioxide, and to help maintain acid–base balance. The respiratory system also consists of nonvital functions such as cough, odor sensation, assistance of speech, and other nonvital functions. The respiratory system consists of the paranasal sinuses, nose, pharynx, larynx, trachea, main bronchi, right/left lungs, and diaphragm (Figure 7.1).

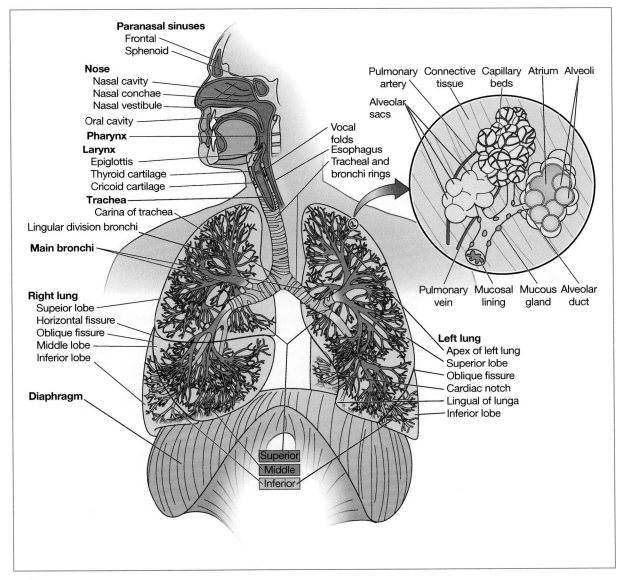

FIGURE 7.1 Respiratory system. The respiratory system consists of the paranasal sinuses, nose, pharynx, larynx, trachea, main bronchi, right/left lungs, and diaphragm.

PARANASAL SINUSES

The paranasal sinuses consist of the frontal sinuses, sphenoid sinuses, ethmoid sinuses, and maxillary sinuses (Figure 7.2). The *frontal sinuses* are the most superior in location and are triangularly shaped. They drain into the frontonasal duct and ultimately into the hiatus semilunaris. *Sphenoid sinuses* are also superiorly located, but are positioned more posteriorly. They are related to the cranial cavity and drain onto the nasal cavity. *Ethmoid sinuses* consist of the anterior (hiatus sublunary), middle (ethmoid hulla), and posterior (superior meatus), which all empty into the nasal cavity in different locations. Finally, the *maxillary sinuses* are inferiorly located and are the largest of the sinuses. They drain into the hiatus semilunaris.

NOSE

The nose is a protrusion from the face that is made up of cartilage and bone (Figure 7.3). The nose also contains nostrils which are separated by the nasal septum. The main function of the nose is to allow the passage of air to and from the lungs. Another major function of the nose is to work with the olfactory system to allow the sensation of smell. The nose contains specialized sensory cells (olfactory sensory neurons) that connect to the brain. An additional function of the nose is to warm the inhaled air entering the lungs to make it more humid. The nose also has hairs to help prevent large particles from entering the lungs. Nasal passages allow air to flow through the nose. The nasal passages also contain mucous membranes that contain many hair-like cells that move mucus toward the throat.

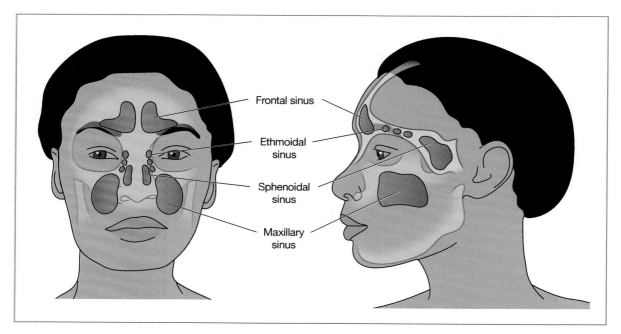

FIGURE 7.2 Paranasal sinuses. The paranasal sinuses consist of the frontal sinuses, sphenoid sinuses, ethmoid sinuses, and maxillary sinuses.

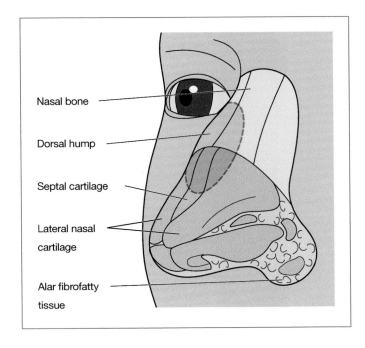

Nasal bone

Dorsal hump

Septal cartilage

Lateral nasal
cartilage

Alar fibrofatty
tissue

FIGURE 7.3 The nose. The nose is composed of cartilage and bone.

PHARYNX

The pharynx, also called the throat, is a fibromuscular tube that extends from the base of the skull to the lower border of the cricoid cartilage (Figure 7.4). Portions of the pharynx lay posteriorly to the nasal cavity, orally to the nasal cavity, and toward the larynx. These create the nasal pharynx, oral pharynx, and the laryngeal pharynx. Functions of the larynx include assisting in respiration and digestion. The pharynx assists the respiratory system by allowing air to pass into and out of the areas entering and exiting the lungs. The pharynx assists the digestive system by using its muscular walls to assist in the process of swallowing.

LARYNX

The larynx is a cartilaginous structure located below the pharynx at the area where the pharynx splits into the trachea and esophagus (Figure 7.5). Several pieces of cartilage make up the larynx; three large pieces of cartilage called *thyroid cartilage*

(anterior) make up the largest piece of the larynx and consist of the laryngeal prominence ("Adam's apple"). The *epiglottis* (superior) is a flexible piece of elastic cartilage that covers the opening of the trachea and is attached to the thyroid. The true vocal cords are vestibular folds that make up the *glottis*. The false vocal cords, called the vestibular folds, are made up of a paired section of folded mucous membranes. White membranous folds attached by muscle to the thyroid and arytenoid cartilages or the larynx on their outer edges are true vocal cords. Sound is produced by the oscillation of free inner edges of the true vocal cords. The deeper voice in males is attributed to the larger size of the folds. The act of swallowing consists of a concert of actions involving the pharynx, larynx, epiglottis, and trachea. This action involves the upward lifting of the pharynx and larynx, which in turn allows expansion of the larynx and closing of the trachea. The *cricoid cartilage* (inferior) helps to regulate the volume of air entering and leaving the lungs. The vocal folds are also located in this area and are essential for phonation. The main difference in the pharynx and larynx is that the pharynx is part of the alimentary canal and the larynx is the upper portion of the trachea. The laryngopharynx, as it extends, is lined with stratified squamous epithelium that

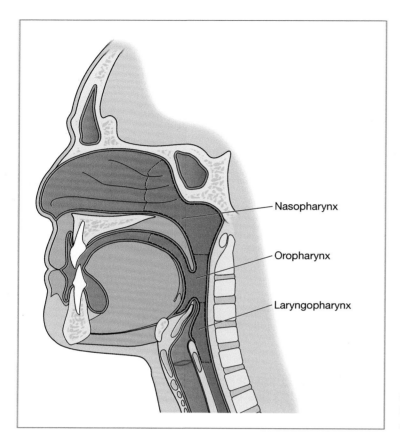

FIGURE 7.4 The pharynx. Portions of the pharynx lay posteriorly to the nasal cavity, orally to the nasal cavity, and toward the larynx. These create the nasal pharynx, oral pharynx, and the laryngeal pharynx.

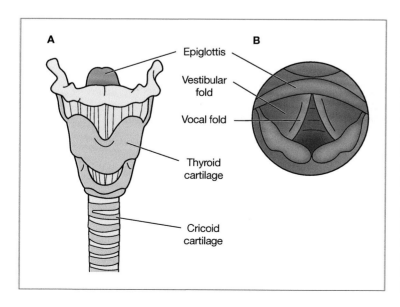

FIGURE 7.5 The larynx. (**A**) Anterior view. (**B**) Endoscopic view. Thyroid cartilage (anterior) makes up the largest piece of the larynx and consists of the laryngeal prominence ("Adam's apple"). Epiglottis (superior) is a flexible piece of elastic cartilage that covers the opening of the trachea and is attached to the thyroid. The false vocal cord, called the vestibular fold, is made up of a paired section of folded mucous membranes. The cricoid cartilage (inferior) helps to regulate the volume of air entering and leaving the lungs. The vocal folds are also located in this area and are essential for phonation.

transitions into pseudostratified ciliated columnar epithelium goblet cells. This epithelium functions similarly to the epithelium of the nasal cavity and nasopharynx, as its specialized cells produce mucus in an effort to trap foreign objects and debris entering the trachea. Functioning cilia moves the mucus upward toward the laryngopharynx, where it can be delivered to the stomach via the route of the esophagus.

TRACHEA

The trachea, sometimes referred to as the windpipe, is a large membranous tube reinforced by rings of cartilage, extending from the larynx to the bronchial tubes and conveying air to and from the lungs (Figure 7.6). Formed by 16 to 20 stacked, C-shaped pieces of hyaline cartilages that are connected by dense connective tissue, the trachea is located inferior to the thyroid cartilage and superior to the division of the left and right main bronchus. The trachea divides into the left and right main bronchus, which is known as the tracheal bifurcation, at the level of the sternal angle and of the fifth thoracic vertebra. The primary function of the trachea is to provide a passage for air to travel to and from the lungs for respiration and to allow gas exchange. The trachea also functions to expel foreign substances via its mucous lining and the ciliary goblet cells that trap foreign substances and activate coughing. The trachea also helps with thermoregulation by heating cold air before it enters the lungs in cold environments and its process of evaporating water to carry heat away from the lungs in overly warm environments.

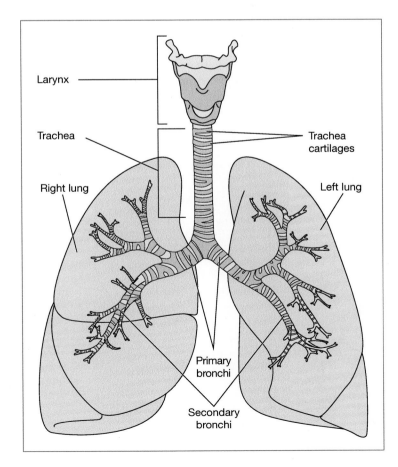

FIGURE 7.6 The trachea. The trachea is located inferior to the thyroid cartilage and superior to the division of the left and right main bronchus. The trachea divides into the left and right main bronchus, which is known as the tracheal bifurcation, at the level of the sternal angle and of the fifth thoracic vertebra.

MAIN BRONCHI AND BRONCHIAL TREE

The left main bronchus divides into two secondary bronchi or lobar bronchi (Figure 7.7) to deliver air to the two lobes of the left lung—the superior and the inferior lobe.

Extending from the trachea to the level of the carina are the right and left bronchi, which are also lined with pseudostratified ciliated columnar epithelium. These bronchi also contain goblet cells to help facilitate the removal of foreign bodies. Cough is induced by sensations to specialized nervous tissue located at the carina. This reaction to foreign bodies helps to prevent aspiration and/or the entrance of foreign materials into the lungs. Collapse is prevented by the presence of cartilaginous rings that help to support the bronchi. The bronchi continues into the branching bronchial tree. The bronchial tree is a passageway for air movement and the trapping of debris and pathogens. Tertiary bronchi extend into bronchioles and bronchioles branch into tiny terminal bronchioles. More than 1,000 terminal bronchioles per lung extend to alveoli, which is where gas exchange occurs.

RESPIRATORY ZONE

The *respiratory zone* is the area that is directly responsible for gas exchange (Figure 7.8). It is the area where the *terminal bronchioles* join respiratory bronchioles, which extend to alveolar ducts. *Alveolar ducts* open directly into a cluster of alveoli, where gas exchange actually occurs.

ALVEOLI

Alveoli are composed of alveoli ducts, alveolus, and an alveolar sac. The alveolar duct is a tubular structure, composed of smooth muscle and connective tissue. The alveolar duct opens into a cluster of alveolus which are grape-like sacs that make up the alveolar sac. The alveolar sac contains many individual alveoli that are responsible for gas exchange. The alveolus has elastic walls that allow the alveolus to expand during air intake. This expansion increases the surface area available for gas exchange. Equal distribution of air to all alveoli is accomplished by the distribution of air

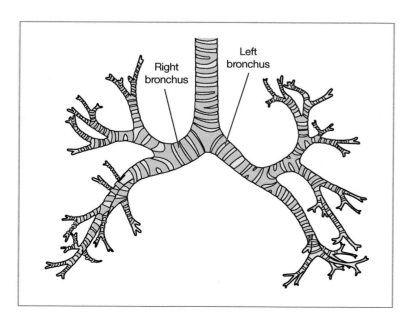

FIGURE 7.7 Lobar bronchi.

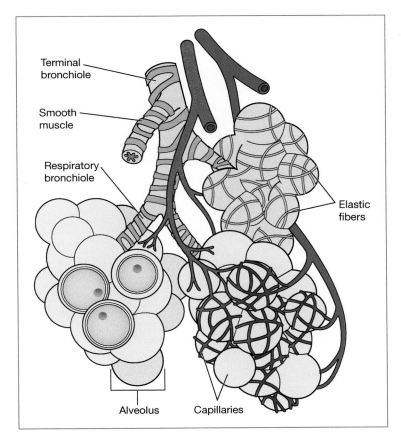

FIGURE 7.8 Respiratory zone. The respiratory zone is the area where the terminal bronchioles join respiratory bronchioles, which extend to alveolar ducts. Alveolar ducts open directly into a cluster of alveoli, where gas exchange actually occurs.

through alveolar neighboring connected alveolar pores. The alveolar wall is made up of three major types of cells: type I alveolar cells, type II alveolar cells, and alveolar macrophages. About 97% of the alveolar surface area is made up of a type I alveolar cell, which is squamous epithelial. They are about 25 nm thick and are highly permeable to gases. Scattered among these cells are type II pulmonary surfactant secreting alveolar cells (Figure 7.9). Surfactant is composed of phospholipids and proteins that reduce the surface tension of the alveoli and help to prevent collapse. Also, traveling unsystematically are alveolar macrophages. Alveolar macrophage is a phagocytic cell of the immune system that removes debris and pathogens that have reached the alveoli. Gas exchange is easily accomplished by the ease of air movement across the extremely thin endothelial membrane of capillaries that border the simple squamous epithelium formed by type I alveolar cells. The respiratory membrane is about 0.5 mm thick and is a combination of the alveoli and capillary membrane. Simple diffusion is accomplished by the respiratory membrane that permits the movement across, and allows the exchange of, CO_2 and oxygen via transport to and from the blood (Figure 7.10).

THE PLEURAE

The pulmonary pleurae or serous membranes are the two pleurae of the invaginated sac surrounding each lung and attaching them to the thoracic cavity. The parietal pleura lines the pleural cavity along the inner rib cage and the upper surface of the diaphragm. The pleural space is the space

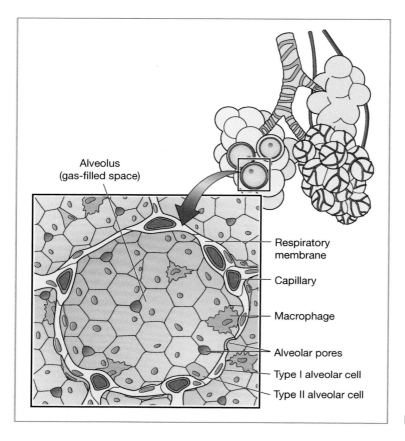

FIGURE 7.9 Type II alveolar cell.

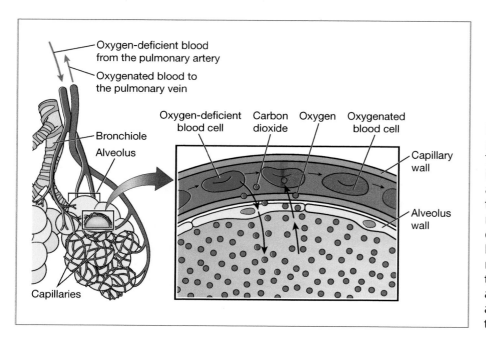

FIGURE 7.10 The respiratory membrane. The respiratory membrane is about 0.5 mm thick and is a combination of the alveoli and capillary membrane. Simple diffusion is accomplished by the respiratory membrane that permits the movement across, and allows the exchange of, CO_2 and oxygen via transport to and from the blood.

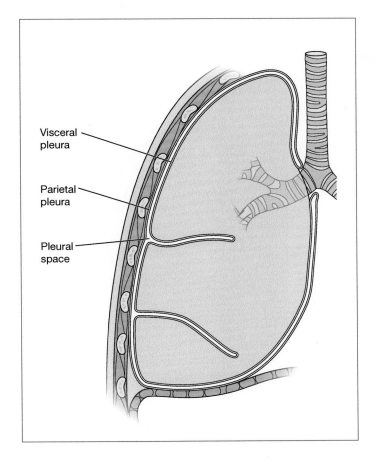

Visceral
pleura

Parietal
pleura

Pleural
space

FIGURE 7.11 Pulmonary pleurae. The parietal pleura lines the pleural cavity along the inner rib cage and the upper surface of the diaphragm. The pleural space is the space between the visceral and parietal pleura and contains pleural fluid.

between the visceral and parietal pleura and contains pleural fluid (Figure 7.11). Pleural fluid keeps the lungs in contact with the thoracic area via surface tension; this also allows the lungs to expand and contract during respiration.

RESPIRATIONS

The act of inhalation is principally facilitated by the diaphragm and is initiated by respiratory centers in the brain. The diaphragm contracts and descends during inspiration and relaxes and ascends during exhalation (Figure 7.12). The scalenes of the rib cage and the parasternal intercostal muscles also help with thoracic expansion during inhalation. Inhalation is the time during the respiratory cycle where a decrease intrathoracic pressure results in the filling of the lungs with air. This time and action also facilitates the diffusion of oxygen into the pulmonary capillaries and the exchange of carbon dioxide and oxygen via blood and adjacent alveoli. Expiration, unlike inspiration, is a passive process and usually does not require effort.

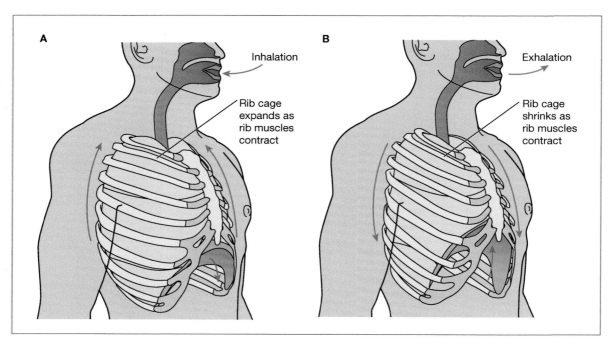

FIGURE 7.12 Inhalation and exhalation. (**A**) During inhalation, the diaphragm contracts and descends. (**B**) During exhalation, the diaphragm relaxes and ascends.

Screening Health Assessment and Normal Findings

INSPECTION OF THE ENTIRE CHEST

Inspection of the chest should be performed where the chest and key anatomical landmarks can be adequately visualized and inspected. Inspection of the entire chest should also include a midline, anterior, posterior, and bilateral axillary view. Males should be asked to remove their shirts and females should be encouraged to wear a sports bra, to allow a better view of the chest and all viewable anatomic features.

Skin should also be inspected for cyanosis or pallor.

To perform a complete physical exam, the examiner needs to be able to identify the structures and landmarks of the chest wall (Figure 7.13). Upon completion of this section, the examiner should also

be able to easily identify and locate the anatomical areas described as:

- Supraclavicular: Above the clavicles
- Intralocular: Below the clavicles
- Interscapular: Between the scapulae
- Infrascapular: Below the scapulae
- Apex of lungs: Top of lungs
- Base of lungs: Bottom of lungs
- Upper, middle, and lower lungs

The patient will need to be sitting upright with chest and abdomen exposed to allow an adequate visual and physical inspection of the anterior/posterior/lateral neck, chest, and upper abdomen. The examiner will need to be able to distinguish,

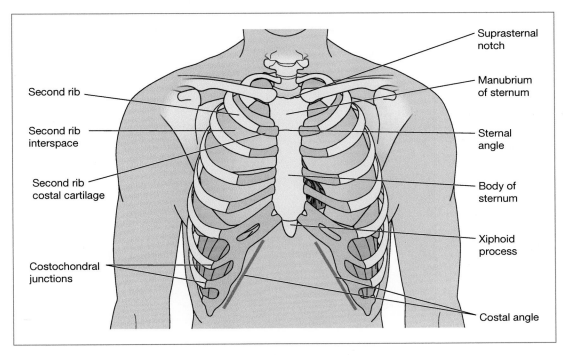

FIGURE 7.13 Structures and landmarks of the chest wall.

locate, and evaluate areas in relation to the vertical axis and circumference of the chest and neck areas.

First, locate findings in the thorax and become comfortable with numbering the ribs and intercostal spaces (Figure 7.14). Start by locating the second rib; this is done by first placing your finger in the depression of the suprasternal notch. The manubrium is about 2 inches inferior to the suprasternal notch; it is the horizontal bony ridge where the manubrium joins the sternum. This area is also called the sternal angle or the angle of Louis. The second rib is located directly, laterally adjacent to this area. To locate this rib, it is a good idea to palpate to the sternal angle and continue to remain in contact with the chest as you slide your fingers to the left or right and make contact with the second rib. Once the second rib is located, you can then use your index and middle fingers to rotate down as you maintain contact with the chest while counting the intercostal spaces. Be aware that ribs after number 8 are close and it may be difficult to determine intercostal spaces after that point.

When counting intercostal spaces on someone with moderate- to large-sized breast tissue, the breast tissue should be displaced laterally to allow a more medial palpation of ribs and intercostal spaces. The first seven ribs articulate with the sternum via costal cartilages and the eighth, ninth, and tenth ribs articulate with the costal cartilages of the seventh, eighth, and ninth ribs that are directly above them.

Palpation of the 11th and 12th ribs can be done by palpating laterally for the cartilaginous tip of the 11th rib and palpating posteriorly for the 12th rib. Locating ribs and counting intercostal spaces from the posterior of the chest is done by first identifying the 12th rib via palpation and then counting upward from the 12th rib in a reverse numerical order, via palpation of ribs and intercostal spaces.

Some other useful landmarks are the inferior tip of the scapula, which is generally located at the seventh rib or intercostal space, and the spinous process, which is observed when the neck is flexed forward (Figure 7.15). It is usually at C7 and has

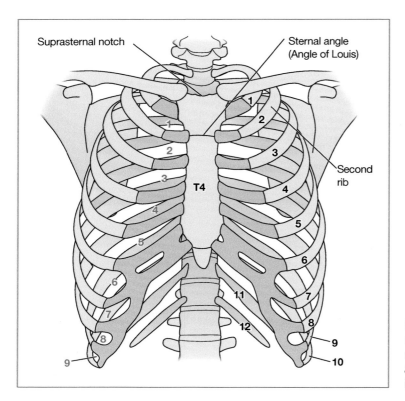

FIGURE 7.14 Numbering of ribs (black numbers) and intercostal spaces (blue numbers). Note that ribs after number 8 are close; it may be difficult to ascertain intercostal spaces after that point.

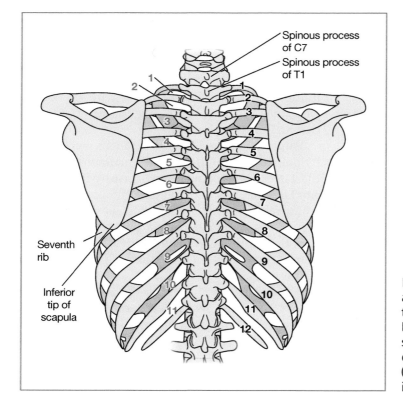

FIGURE 7.15 Inferior tip of the scapula and the spinous process. The inferior tip of the scapula, which is generally located at the seventh rib or intercostal space, and the spinous process, which is observed when the neck is flexed forward. (Black numbers: ribs; blue numbers: intercostal spaces.)

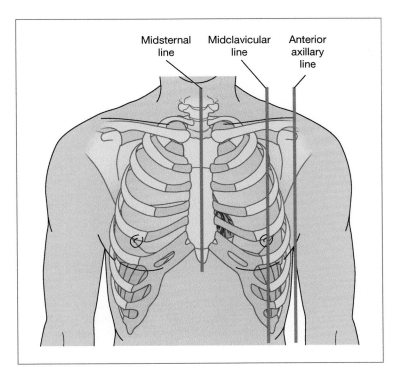

Midsternal line   Midclavicular line   Anterior axillary line

FIGURE 7.16 Midsternal, midclavicular, and anterior axillary lines. When observing an exposed chest, it is useful to visualize it in divisions, separated by vertical lines.

the greatest amount of protuberance of any vertebral process. When encountering a flexed spine, it is a useful landmark to use when counting from C7 inferiorly.

When observing an exposed chest, try to visualize it in divisions, separated by vertical lines. When viewing the anterior chest, be able to easily locate the midsternal, midclavicular, and anterior axillary lines (Figure 7.16). The midsternal line is usually easily located at the mid upper chest area and generally extends from the suprasternal notch to the zyphoid process. The midclavicular line is an imaginary vertical line located at the midclavicular point when assessing it on a horizontal plane.

When observing the anterior of an exposed chest, the examiner should be able to easily locate the vertebral line and the scapular line. The vertebral line is an imaginary line that overlies the vertebral process. The scapular line, also known as the linea scapularis, is an imaginary line that passes through the inferior angle of the scapula (Figure 7.17).

INSPECTION OF THE LUNGS

When visualizing the lungs and associated anatomical landmarks, try to visualize them in their locations to include their divisions and fissures. The tops of the lungs are identified as the apex of the lungs and the bottoms are identified as the bases. The right lung consists of the right upper lobe (RUL), right middle lobe (RML), and right lower lobe (RLL). These lobes are divided by the horizontal (minor) fissure and oblique fissures. The left lung has two lobes, the left upper lobe (LUL) and the left lower lobe (LLL), that are only divided by an oblique (major) fissure (Figure 7.18). The anterior apex of each lung extends about 1 to 1.5 inches above the inner third area of the associated clavicle. The lungs extends inferiorly to cross the sixth rib at the midclavicular line anteriorly and at the eighth rib at the midaxillary line posteriorly. The lungs expand and move inferiorly during inspiration, while also facilitating movement of the diaphragm.

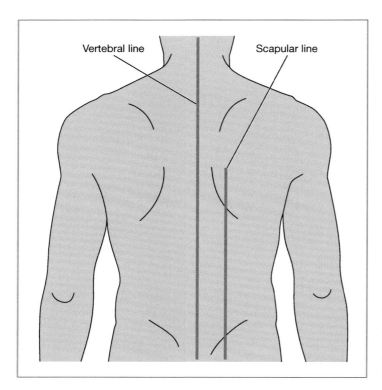

FIGURE 7.17 Vertebral and scapular lines. The vertebral line is an imaginary line that overlies the vertebral process. The scapular line, also known as the linea scapularis, is an imaginary line that passes through the inferior angle of the scapula.

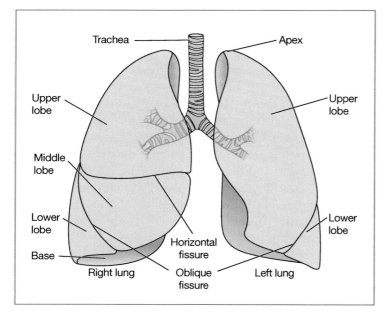

FIGURE 7.18 Right and left lungs. The right lung consists of the RUL, RML, and RLL. These lobes are divided by the horizontal (minor) fissure and oblique fissures. The left lung has two lobes, the LUL and the LLL, that are divided by the oblique (major) fissure.

RLL, right lower lobe; RML, right middle lobe; RUL, right upper lobe.

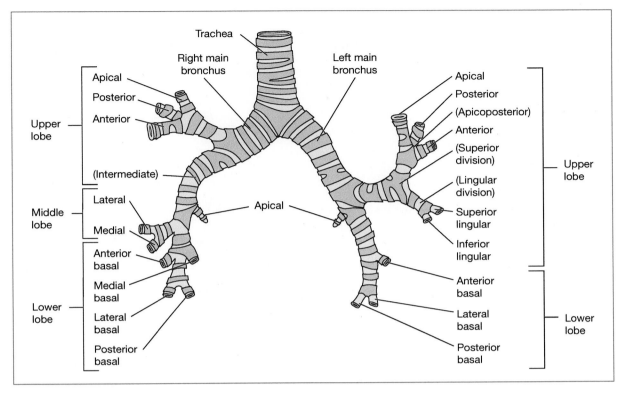

FIGURE 7.19 Tracheobronchial tree.

Each lung is responsible for gas exchange. The lungs receive deoxygenated blood from the heart via the pulmonary arteries and returns oxygenated blood to the heart via the pulmonary vein after gas exchange has occurred.

EVALUATING SOUNDS OF THE TRACHEOBRONCHIAL TREE

When listening to breath sounds, note that sounds over the trachea are harsher in quality. This is due to the cartilaginous density of the trachea as opposed to the softer less-dense tissues of the lower bronchi and surrounding tissues. The level of T4 and the sternal angle is where the trachea bifurcates into the right and left lungs. The right mainstem bronchus enters the hilum directly. It is also shorter, wider, and more vertically situated than the left. The left main bronchus, on the other hand, is below the

aortic arch, anterior to the esophagus, anterior to the aorta where it enters the hilum of the lung, and it extends below and laterally, in reference to the aortic arch. The two main bronchi extend into lobar, segmental bronchi, and bronchioles (Figure 7.19). The area of gas exchange and the end of branching is at the pulmonary alveoli (see Figures 7.8, 7.9, and 7.10).

INSPECTION OF THE POSTERIOR CHEST

Inspect the shape and configuration of the chest by evaluating the spinal processes. The spinal processes should be in a straight vertical line. The bilateral thorax and scapulas should be evaluated and assessed for symmetry.

An anterior view of the chest should be done to assess the transverse diameter. Next, a lateral/

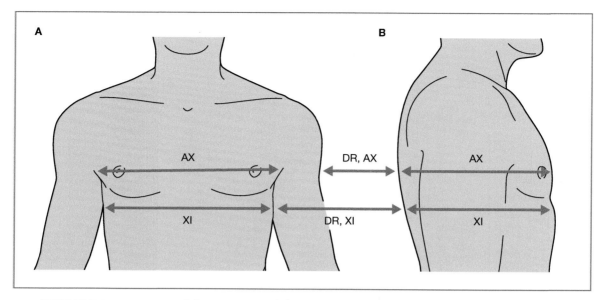

FIGURE 7.20 Transverse (**A**) and sagittal (**B**) diameters of the chest. The figure shows the points at which axillary and xiphoid measurements were taken on front- and right-side views. A comparison of the anteroposterior diameter of the chest in relation to the transverse view should have a ratio of 1:2 to 5:7.

AX, axillary; DR, diameter ratio; XI, xiphoid.

axillary view of the chest should be done to assess for anteroposterior (sagittal) diameter. A comparison of the anteroposterior diameter of the chest in relation to the transverse view should have a ratio of 1:2 to 5:7 (Figure 7.20).

Evaluation of the muscles of the neck, to include the trapezius, should be done while the patient is sitting in a relaxed position with his or her arms at the sides. The evaluation is to assess the muscles for normal development in relation to age, occupation, and exercise regimen.

PALPATION OF POSTERIOR CHEST

Chest symmetry should be confirmed by placing the palms of your hands on the posterolateral chest walls at the level of T9 or T10. With your thumbs and fingers facing upward, you should slide your hands medially to pinch up a small fold of skin between your thumbs. Ask the patient to take a deep breath and watch your thumbs move apart, as you assess them for symmetrical division.

TACTILE FREMITUS

The assessment of palpable vibration of the chest wall is termed tactile fremitus. Firmly place the palms of both hands on the patient's chest and ask the patient to repeat the words "ninety-nine." Vibrations should be assessed while moving hands from bilateral lung apices to bases assessing for unilateral vibrations. Normal fremitus is mostly felt at the scapulae and proximal to the sternum, where the major bronchi are most proximal to the chest wall. Decreased fremitus is mostly assessed as you move down the lung anatomy, progressing away from the lung apices and toward the lung bases.

CHEST WALL

Palpate the entire chest wall, using your fingers while assessing for any palpable abnormalities, tenderness, skin temperature, and moisture.

PERCUSSION OF POSTERIOR CHEST

Percussion on lungs should be performed by hyperextending the middle finger of your left hand (pleximeter finger) and pressing it firmly in the selected lung interspace. While avoiding surface contact with any other surface, strike the pleximeter finger with the right middle finger. Percussion should be in the interspaces and should start in the apical areas and progress to the bases of the lungs. A comparison should be made of the bilateral lung area and all percussion should avoid ribs or scapulae.

Resonance should be assessed and noted on all examinations.

Diaphragmatic excursion (i.e., movement of the diaphragm) should be monitored to assess for bilateral symmetry on movement. Percussion bilaterally should be done to measure the diaphragm location on inspiration and expiration to assess position.

AUSCULTATION OF POSTERIOR CHEST

With the patient sitting upright in a relaxed position, ask him or her to take a deep breath, while breathing through the nose and mouth. Listen to the following areas on the posterior: Apices at C7 to the bases, close to T10, and laterally from the axillae down to the seventh/eighth rib.

NORMAL BREATH SOUNDS

The three types of normal breath sounds are bronchial (tracheal/tubular), broncho vesicular, and vesicular. Note: If adventitious sounds (Table 7.1) are heard on initial attempt at auscultation, ask the patient to cough, and then listen again.

- Bronchial sounds: High-pitched; loud amplitude; harsh, hollow, and tubular quality sound that is heard mostly during inspiration at the trachea and larynx
- Broncho vesicular: Moderate-pitched; moderate amplitude; mixed quality sound that is heard equally on inspiration and expiration over major bronchi
- Vesicular: Low-pitched; soft amplitude; rustling/wind-like quality sound heard mostly on inspiration over peripheral lung areas

TABLE 7.1
Adventitious Breath Sounds

Sound	Characteristics
Coarse crackle or rale	Discontinuous, interrupted, explosive sounds; loud, low-pitched
Fine crackle or rale	Discontinuous, interrupted, explosive sounds; less loud than coarse crackle and of shorter duration; high-pitched
Wheeze (sibilant)	Long, continuous sounds; hissing; high-pitched
Rhonchus (sonorous)	Long, continuous sounds; snoring; low-pitched

INSPECTION OF THE ANTERIOR CHEST

Careful inspection of the anterior chest should also be done. (See also "Inspection of the Entire Chest" in this section.) When inspecting the anterior chest, the examiner should also note the facial expression of the patient, as well as the patient's level of consciousness and skin color. Cyanosis should also be evaluated by checking lips and nail beds.

PERCUSSION OF ANTERIOR CHEST

Percussion of the anterior chest should start at the apices and progress toward the bases while comparing bilateral findings. When assessing

lung sounds of the anterior chest in comparison to the posterior chest, it should be noted that there is suspected dullness at the cardiac and liver borders. Also note that there are suspected tympani (drum-like sound) over the gastric areas. (See "Percussion of Posterior Chest" section.)

AUSCULTATION OF ANTERIOR CHEST

Anterior chest auscultation should start at the apical supraclavicular areas and migrate down toward the bases. The migration should also be comparing lung sounds bilaterally. Normal lung sounds should be vesicular and heard over the majority of the anterior lung fields. (See "Auscultation of Posterior Chest" section.)

Focused Health Assessment and Abnormal Findings

CHEST INSPECTION

The normal chest has a lateral diameter that is greater than the anterolateral diameter. Figure 7.21 illustrates common deformities of the chest:

- Pigeon chest (pectus carinatum): Identified by the breastbone pushing outward instead of being flush against chest (Figure 7.21A).
- Funnel chest (pectus excavatum): Identified by an anteriorly displaced sternum and an increased anteroposterior diameter. This condition can also result in limited chest expansion (Figure 7.21B).
- Barrel chest: Identified by an increased anterior-posterior (AP) diameter and commonly associated with chronic obstructive pulmonary disease and aging (Figure 7.21C).

- Kyphosis: An exaggerated forward rounding of the spine that can occur at any age is identified as kyphosis. Severe kyphosis can resolve in limited lung expansion (Figure 7.21D).
- Scoliosis: Sideways curvature of the spine usually occurring in proximity to the start of puberty. Signs include uneven shoulders, uneven waist, or uneven hips. Can result in limited lung expansion (Figure 7.21E).

Other common abnormal findings to search for during inspection of the chest are:

- Hypertrophy of neck muscles, which may suggest excessive use (Figure 7.22).
- Patient in the tripod position is a sign of difficulty breathing (Figure 7.23).
- Clubbing of fingers is associated with chronic obstructive pulmonary diseases (Figure 7.24).

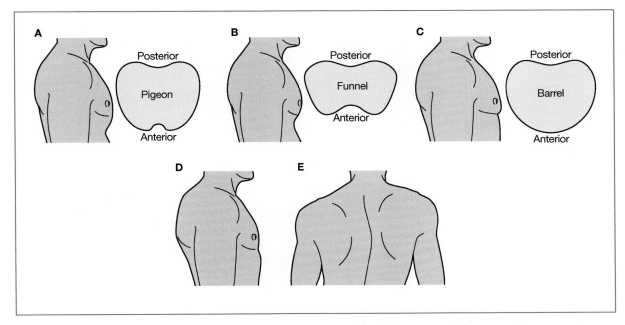

FIGURE 7.21 Common deformities of the chest. (**A**) Pigeon chest. (**B**) Funnel chest. (**C**) Barrel chest. (**D**) Kyphosis. (**E**) Scoliosis.

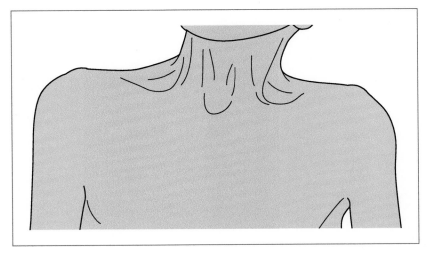

FIGURE 7.22 Hypertrophy of neck muscles.

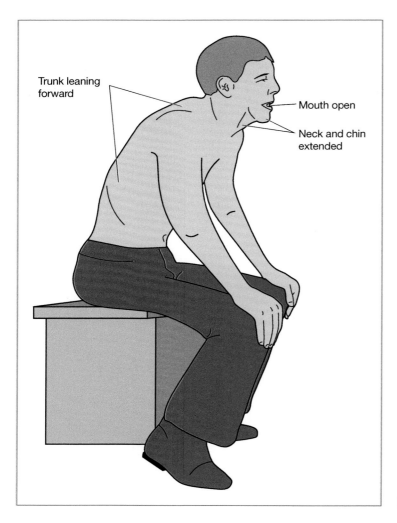

Trunk leaning forward

Mouth open

Neck and chin extended

FIGURE 7.23 Patient in tripod position.

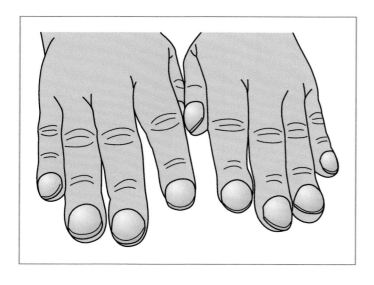

FIGURE 7.24 Clubbing of fingers.

CHEST PALPATION

Common abnormal findings to search for during palpation of the chest are as follows. *Note*: Pulmonary disease may conceal dullness that is usually palpated over the heart.

- Increased fremitus is associated with consolidation that is secondary to increased fluid.

- Unequal expansion of the chest is associated with atelectasis, pneumonia, fractured ribs, thoracic trauma, or pneumothorax.

- Pain associated with palpation of certain areas which is associated with localized musculoskeletal disorders and/or disorders of the pleura.

CHEST PERCUSSION

Some common abnormal findings to search for during percussion of the chest are:

- Dullness to percussion is associated with an increase in secretions, pleural fluid, pus, pneumonia, fibrous tissue, or tumor. Very large effusions can be detected when dullness is palpated posteriorly in supine patients. RML pneumonia is usually detected by palpated dullness behind the right breast.

- Hyperresonance is associated with air trapping. General hyperresonance is associated with chronic obstructive disease or asthma, and unilateral hyperresonance is associated with a large pneumothorax or an air-filled bulla.

CHEST AUSCULTATION

Some common abnormal findings to search for during auscultation of the chest are:

- Decreased or absent breath sounds are encountered when there is some type of obstruction or secretions blocking air movement within the bronchial tree. Other types of obstruction can be plugs, foreign body, tumor, effusion, or pleural thickening.

- Adventitious breath sounds: An increase in breath sounds over peripheral lung areas can be a result of lung disorders such as pneumonia or lung disorders that result in denser lung areas. Crackles are associated with pneumonia, interstitial lung disease, pulmonary fibrosis, atelectasis, heart failure, bronchitis, and/or bronchiectasis. Wheezes are commonly associated with asthma and emphysema (see Table 7.1).

SPECIAL TESTS

Special tests to assess suspected consolidation are as follows:

- Bronchophony (Bronchiloquy): Used to assess the abnormal transmission of sound through secretions or consolidation. The patient is asked to repeat the words "ninety-nine," while auscultating a suspected area of consolidation. Any area of increased sound transmission suggests consolidation.

- Egophony: Used to assess areas of suspected consolidation. While auscultating an area of suspected consolidation, ask the patient to say "E." If the auscultated area transmits the sound to be heard as "A," this would represent an area of suggested consolidation.

- Whispered pectoriloquy: Used to assess areas of suspected consolidation. While auscultating an area of suspected consolidation, ask the patient to whisper the numbers 1, 2, and 3. Any areas of increased sound transmission suggest consolidation.

Holistic Assessment

SPECIFIC HEALTH HISTORY

When a patient presents with a respiratory complaint, it is very important to elicit a thorough and accurate chief complaint, complete recent and chronic respiratory history, review of systems, and a complete acute and chronic social history. Some common respiratory complaints are as follows and all should raise concern and elicit a thorough history and physical exam:

- Chest pain: Usually associated with heart disease or structures of the thorax and lungs

- Shortness of breath (dyspnea): Usually associated with cardiac and pulmonary disease

- Wheezing: Usually associated with asthma and/or emphysema

- Cough: Can be of minor significance or have major implications or concerns

- Blood-streaked sputum: Can be of minor or major significance. Source can have multiple etiologies

- Daytime sleepiness or snoring and disordered sleep: Usually associated with sleep apnea

FINANCIAL IMPLICATIONS

Ask the patient if there are any financial or work-related considerations that may have contributed to or exacerbated his or her medical condition. Also, inquire about the patient's ability to work and whether he or she can work at the same level as prior to the medical condition.

SPIRITUAL CONSIDERATIONS

Identify areas where the patient has turned for help in the past, including his or her faith and support circles. Ask the patient about his or her habits for coping with difficult times, and if the patient has provisions for self-care.

CASE STUDY

DOCUMENTATION

Chief complaint: 35-year-old male with periodic productive cough with blood-streaked sputum

History of the present illness: Has had a periodic cough for about 1 year that has slowly progressed in frequency to be routine throughout the day. Over the last month, cough has progressed to have periodic blood-streaked sputum. Amount of sputum is very small and streaky in appearance. Cough is not associated with any activity and is not better or worse at any times of the day or night. Cough is also not made better or worse with any activities or interventions by the patient. Denies any current upper respiratory signs or symptoms, but admits to having recurrent upper respiratory infections (URIs) over the last year or so. Does not take any medications at this time and denies fatigue.

(continued)

(continued)

Review of systems: Denies: Chest pain, shortness of breath, fever, chills, nausea, vomiting, gastrointestinal/genitourinary, or other upper respiratory concerns

Primary medical history: None

Social history: Has chronic history of smoking. Has smoked about one pack of cigarettes a day for the last 20 years. Drinks occasionally, about one glass of wine every other day. Does not exercise. Lives at home with his wife and has been working as a bus driver for 15 years.

Family history: Father is a chronic cigarette smoker and has chronic obstructive pulmonary disease; mother has type 2 diabetes that is well controlled. Father and mother are still alive; father and mother are both 79 years old. Has no siblings.

Safety: Care should be taken to make sure that the patient's condition does not cause safety concerns with his or her work or daily activities.

Distress: It is important to identify patients who are in acute distress during the visit with the provider. Care should be taken to elicit information from the patient that could suggest that this condition is affecting the patient's "activities of daily living" (ADLs).

Lifestyle: Lifestyle is very important to discuss if it is contributing to the patient's disease process. Take into account smoking, drug use, diet, and/or failure to exercise.

Nutrition and exercise: The patient's diet and exercise, or lack thereof, should be discussed, especially if it can help to alleviate or is contributing to the patient's condition and/or concerns.

PHYSICAL EXAMINATION

General: Awake and alert; oriented to person, place, and time; and in no apparent distress

Integumentary: Within normal limits. No cyanosis or pallor discovered.

Lungs: Has mild rhonchi to bilateral upper and lower lobes that clear with effective cough. No deformities discovered on palpation or percussion of chest and thorax.

Heart: Has regular rate and rhythm with no murmurs, rubs, or gallops discovered on auscultation.

Head: Normocephalic

Ears: Tympanic membranes are visible without erythema or drainage.

(continued)

(continued)

Sinuses: Frontal and maxillary sinuses are nontender to palpation.

Nose and mouth: Nasal and oral pharyngeal passages are nonerythematous and without drainage.

Neck: Thyroid within normal limits and lymph nodes are nontender and nonenlarged.

Extremities: No clubbing noted on fingers or toes.

Diagnosis: Early onset of bronchitis and/or bronchiectasis. Likely early onset chronic obstructive pulmonary disease.

ICD-10-CM Diagnosis Code: J20.9 Acute Bronchitis, Unspecified

ICD-10-CM Diagnosis Code: J47.9 Bronchiectasis, Uncomplicated

Assessment of Special Populations

 ### PEDIATRIC POPULATION

When evaluating infants, note that you will need to count the respirations for an entire minute because of the increased respiratory rate. Also note that an irregular respiratory rate and/or brief periods of apnea of about 10 to 15 seconds are common. Infants and children less than 5 or 6 years of age usually demonstrate broncho vesicular breath sounds.

Some disorders of childhood are listed in the text that follows, but the provider should be familiar with asthma, because it is one of the most common respiratory disorders of childhood. Always be suspicious of asthma when encountering a child or teenager with a cough. Some other disorders associated with children are as follows: Croup, epiglottis, bacterial tracheitis, tracheal-broncho malacia, and foreign body aspiration. Also on physical exam, the provider should be aware and familiar with: nasal flaring, accessory muscle use, and tripoding. These are all signs of respiratory distress.

 ### PATIENTS WITH DISABILITIES

Individuals with physical disability often have a narrow margin of safety or health because of the effects of their disabling condition. Thus, special attention should be given to the history and physical examination of those with disabilities that have the potential to affect respiratory function. For example, individuals with spinal cord injury, multiple sclerosis, or other disabilities that affect mobility can experience compromised respiratory status when they develop even a mild upper respiratory infection that would be merely inconvenient or annoying in someone without such disabling conditions. Cough, for example, can be ineffective in clearing the airways in individuals with expiratory muscle weakness, leading to aspiration and aspiration pneumonia. Asking a patient with such disabilities to cough to determine its strength and ability to clear the airways would be an example of modifying the examination to address the patient's health-related needs.

ELDERLY POPULATION

On routine physical examination of an elderly person, it is common to encounter an increased anteroposterior diameter. This deformity gives the chest an abnormally rounded appearance (also see Barrell Chest in "Abnormal Findings: Chest Inspection"). Clubbing is also a common finding to encounter in aging adults with respiratory disorders. This is commonly due to emphysema, but can be encountered with other pulmonary disorders. Some common pulmonary disorders of the elderly are as follows: Emphysema (chronic bronchitis), bronchiectasis, pulmonary hypertension, pneumonia, and tuberculosis.

VETERAN POPULATION

The provider should ask the patient if they served in the military, and if so, the dates and capacity in which they served (pilot, ground forces, medical services, etc.) should be ascertained. Based upon this information, the provider will be aware of what potential hazards or chemicals of warfare the patient may have been exposed to.

Diagnostic Reasoning

Common Differential Diagnoses: Respiratory System	
Diagnosis	**Key History or Physical Examination Differentiators**
Acute pulmonary embolism	Dyspnea that is a result of an occlusion of all or part of a pulmonary artery and has a sudden onset.
Angina pectoris	Chest pain that is pressing, squeezing, tight, heavy, or occasionally burning in quality that is secondary to ischemia. The location is usually retrosternal or across the anterior chest, sometimes radiating to the shoulders, arms, neck, lower jaw, or upper abdomen and is sometimes associated with dyspnea, nausea, and/or sweating. This type of chest pain is often associated with mild to moderate pain and is a result of temporary myocardial ischemia.
Anxiety	Chest pain that has a stabbing, sticking, or dull-aching type quality and is located below the left breast, or across the anterior chest. The cause of this type of chest pain is unclear.
Asthma	Cough that can be productive for thick mucoid sputum. Usually associated with history of allergies, episodic wheezing, and dyspnea
	Dyspnea that is associated with a reversible hyperresponsiveness of the airways that can also result in excess mucous production. Dyspnea is periodic with acute episodes that can be related to allergic triggers.

(continued)

Common Differential Diagnoses: Respiratory System (*continued*)	
Diagnosis	**Key History or Physical Examination Differentiators**
Bacterial pneumonia: *Klebsiella*	Productive cough with sticky, red, jelly-like or mucoid, purulent, blood-streaked, diffusely pinkish, or rusty-colored sputum usually seen in alcoholic men
Bacterial pneumonia: Pneumococcal	Productive cough with mucoid, purulent, blood-streaked, diffusely pinkish, or rusty-colored sputum with associated high fever, chills, dyspnea, and chest discomfort. An acute illness, usually preceded by an acute respiratory infection
Bronchiectasis	Usually encountered in patients with recurrent bronchopulmonary infections or sinusitis
Cancer of the lung	Dry productive cough that may be blood or blood streaked. Associated with a patient who has a long history of cigarette smoking, dyspnea, and weight loss
Chronic bronchitis	Chronic productive cough with purulent or blood-streaked/bloody sputum. Encountered in patients with recurrent lung infections and a long history of cigarette smoking
	Dyspnea that is a result of chronic airway obstruction, secondary to excess mucous production. Dyspnea is slowly progressive and related to a cough
Chronic obstructive pulmonary disease	Dyspnea that is associated with overdistension of airspaces that is due to airway obstruction. Dyspnea is slowly progressive and related to a subsequently mild cough
Costochondritis, chest wall pain	Chest pain that has a stabbing, sticking, or dull-aching type quality and is often located below the left breast or along the costal cartilages. This type of chest pain is usually associated with local reproducible tenderness with palpation.
Diffuse esophageal spasm	Chest pain that is usually squeezing in quality and is located in the retrosternal area and may radiate to the back, arms, and jaw. This type of chest pain is associated with dysphagia.
Diffuse interstitial lung diseases	Dyspnea that is associated with widespread infiltration of fluid into interstitial spaces that causes dyspnea that is progressive
Dissecting aortic aneurysm	Chest pain that is ripping or tearing in quality and is located in the anterior chest, radiating to the neck, back, or abdomen. This type of chest pain can be associated with hoarseness, dysphagia, syncope, hemiplegia, or paraplegia and is a result of a splitting of the aortic wall.
Gastroesophageal reflux	Chronic cough that is usually at night or early morning, associated with repeated attempts to clear throat and a history of heartburn and regurgitation

(*continued*)

Common Differential Diagnoses: Respiratory System (*continued*)

Diagnosis	Key History or Physical Examination Differentiators
Laryngitis	Dry cough with or without sputum that is associated with a minor illness or viral syndrome
Left-sided heart failure	Dyspnea, elevated pulmonary capillary transudates fluid, decreased compliance of the lungs, and increased work of breathing that is slowly progressive or sudden in onset
Left ventricular failure or mitral stenosis	Dry cough at night, which may progress to being productive with pink frothy sputum or frank hemoptysis. Usually associated with dyspnea, orthopnea, and paroxysmal nocturnal dyspnea
Lung abscess	Productive cough for purulent foul-smelling or bloody sputum. Usually associated with a patient who demonstrates poor dental hygiene and prior episodes of impaired consciousness. Usually associated with a febrile illness
Mycoplasma and viral pneumonias	Dry hacking cough that is associated with malaise, headache, and sometimes dyspnea. Usually associated with acute febrile illness
Myocardial infarction	Chest pain that is pressing, squeezing, tight, heavy, or occasionally burning in quality that is secondary to ischemia. The location is usually retrosternal or across the anterior chest, sometimes radiating to the shoulders, arms, neck, lower jaw, or upper abdomen and is associated with dyspnea, nausea, vomiting, sweating, and weakness. This type of pain is often associated with severe pain and is a result of prolonged myocardial ischemia.
Pericarditis	Chest pain that has a sharp, knifelike quality and is located in the retrosternal or left precordial areas and may radiate to the tip of the left shoulder. This type of chest pain is associated with autoimmune disorders, post myocardial infarction, viral infection, or chest irradiation and is a result of irritation of the parietal pleura.
Pleuritic chest pain	Chest pain that is sharp and knifelike in quality and is located on the chest wall of the right or left side of the chest. This type of chest pain is associated with inflammation of the parietal pleura that can be associated with pneumonia, pulmonary infarction, or neoplasm.
Pneumonia	Dyspnea that is a result of inflammation of lung parenchyma from the respiratory bronchioles to the alveoli. The dyspnea is the result of an acute illness that has yet to reveal a determining agent.

(continued)

Common Differential Diagnoses: Respiratory System (*continued*)	
Diagnosis	**Key History or Physical Examination Differentiators**
Postnasal drip	Chronic productive cough with mucoid or mucopurulent sputum that can sometimes be visualized in the posterior pharynx. Usually associated with inability to clear sputum after multiple attempts and in patients with allergic rhinitis, with or without sinusitis
Pulmonary emboli	Productive cough with dark, bright red, or mixed blood in sputum. Usually associated with a patient that exhibits dyspnea, anxiety, chest pain, fever, or factors that predispose him or her to deep vein thrombosis
Pulmonary tuberculosis	Chronic productive cough for mucoid, purulent, blood-streaked, or bloody secretions. Patient usually has no early symptoms but later experiences anorexia, weight loss, fatigue, fever, and night sweats.
Reflux esophagitis	Chest pain that has a burning or squeezing quality that is located in the retrosternal area and may radiate to the back.
Spontaneous pneumothorax	Dyspnea that is the result of a leakage of air into the pleural space that results in partial or complete collapse of the lung. Dyspnea is usually sudden in onset.
Tracheobronchitis	Dry or productive cough that is acute with retrosternal discomfort and is usually associated with a viral illness
	Chest pain that is burning in quality and is located in the upper sternal area or on either side of the sternum. This type of chest pain is associated with a cough and is a result of inflammation of the trachea and large bronchi.

BIBLIOGRAPHY

Bickley, L., Szilagyi, P., & Hoffman, R. (2017). *Bates' guide to physical examination and history taking* (12th ed.). Philadelphia, PA: Wolters Kluwer.

Gomella, L. G., & Haist, S. A. (2007). *Clinician's pocket reference* (11th ed.). New York, NY: McGraw-Hill.

Henderson, M., Tierney, L., Jr., & Smetana, G. (2012). *The patient history. An evidence-based approach to differential diagnosis* (2nd ed.). New York, NY: McGraw-Hill Medical.

Malanga, G. A., & Mautner, K. R. (Eds.). (2017). *Musculoskeletal physical examination: An evidenced-based approach* (2nd ed.). Philadelphia, PA: Elsevier Health Sciences.

Marcdante, K. J., M., & Kliegman, R. M. (2014). *Nelson essentials of pediatrics* (7th ed.). Philadelphia, PA: Elsevier Health Sciences.

Martini, F., Nath, J., & Bartholomew, E. (2018). *Fundamentals of anatomy & physiology* (11th global ed.). Harlow, England: Pearson.

Papadakis, M., McPhee, S., & Rabow, M. (2019). *Current medical diagnosis & treatment 2019* (58th ed.). New York, NY: McGraw-Hill Medical.

Smith, W. L., & Farrell, T. A. (Eds.). (2014). *Radiology 101: The basics and fundamentals of imaging* (4th ed.). Philadelphia, PA: Wolters Kluwer.

Tintinalli, J., Stapczynski, J., Ma, O., Yealy, D., Meckler, G., & Cline, D. (Eds.). (2015). *Tintinalli's emergency medicine: A comprehensive study guide* (8th ed.). New York, NY: McGraw-Hill.

ADVANCED HEALTH ASSESSMENT OF THE ABDOMEN, RECTUM, AND ANUS

Adrienne Small

(continued)

Overview of Anatomy and Physiology

THE ABDOMEN

The abdomen is bordered superiorly by the diaphragm; the inferior border is the pelvis. The abdominal cavity contains portions of the alimentary tract, the entire gastrointestinal system, and portions of the circulatory system (Figure 8.1). The alimentary tract extends from the mouth to the anus. Its structures are the esophagus, stomach, and large and small intestines. Other organs in the gastrointestinal system are the liver, gallbladder, pancreas, spleen, kidneys, and bladder. A membrane, called the peritoneum, provides a covering for these abdominal organs.

The anterior abdominal wall consists of four groups of muscles: the rectus abdominis, internal and external obliques, transversus abdominis, and the pyramidalis. The abdomen is usually divided into four quadrants, which are formed by drawing two lines that intersect at the umbilicus. The quadrants are the right upper quadrant (RUQ), left upper quadrant (LUQ), left lower quadrant (LLQ), and right lower quadrant (RLQ). For descriptive purposes, the abdomen can also be divided into nine sectors. Using this system, the region directly around the umbilicus is called the umbilical region. The epigastric region is superior to the umbilical region, while the hypogastric region lies inferior (Figure 8.2).

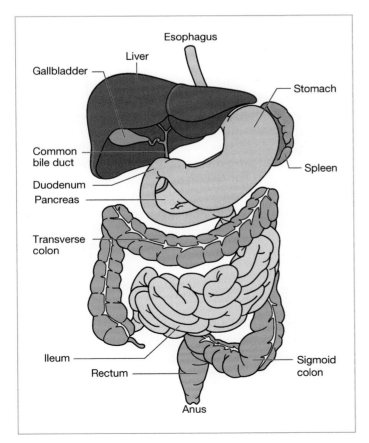

FIGURE 8.1 Anatomy of the abdominal cavity.

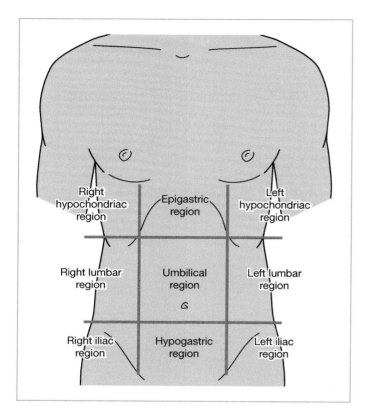

FIGURE 8.2 The four quadrants and nine sectors of the abdomen.

Visualizing the abdomen and its organs by quadrants is very helpful during assessment. The location of abdominal symptoms often gives key diagnostic clues:

- RUQ: Gallbladder, liver, pylorus, duodenum, and ascending colon
- LUQ: Stomach, spleen, pancreas, and transverse colon
- LLQ: Descending colon
- RLQ: Appendix, ascending colon, cecum

THE STOMACH

The stomach is a hollow organ that lies transversely in the upper abdomen, mostly in the epigastric region. The stomach is described in three sections: The fundus, the body, and the pylorus.

Food and liquid are propelled down the length of the esophagus through a series of coordinated peristaltic waves and enter the stomach through the lower esophageal sphincter. Digestion begins in the stomach. Cells in the stomach lining produce hydrochloric acid that digests food. The stomach also secretes gastric lipase and pepsin, which are enzymes that break down fats and carbohydrates, respectively. This mixture of partially digested food (called chyme) is propelled through the pylorus into the small intestine.

THE SMALL INTESTINE

The small intestine is approximately 20 feet long. In the small intestine, food is mixed with bile and pancreatic enzymes. Nutrients are then absorbed through the mucosal lining into the bloodstream. Matter that cannot be absorbed is propelled through the ileocecal valve into the large intestine.

THE LARGE INTESTINE

The large intestine is approximately 5 feet long and is composed of the ascending colon, the transverse colon, the descending colon, and the sigmoid colon. The cecum and appendix are part of the ascending colon. The function of the large intestine is to absorb water and transport waste. Water is absorbed in the ascending colon. Bacterial flora in the large intestine decompose undigested food and other waste, which is then expelled into the rectum.

LIVER

The liver is located primarily in the RUQ of the abdomen, beneath the diaphragm. It extends from the fifth intercostal space down to the costal margin (Figure 8.3). It consists of two large lobes and two smaller lobes, which are connected by branches of the hepatic artery, portal vein, and bile duct. The liver is covered by a fibrous capsule called *Glisson's capsule*. The liver secretes bile, which aids in the absorption of lipids and fatty acids. The liver also breaks down proteins into amino acids and converts the waste into urea, as well as plays a role in carbohydrate metabolism.

GALLBLADDER

The gallbladder is approximately 4 inches long and lies below the inferior surface of the liver (Figure 8.4). It is a sack-shaped organ, which is not palpable. The gallbladder stores bile from the liver, which it releases into the duodenum. In the small intestine, bile helps maintain the alkaline environment necessary for digestion and absorption of lipids.

PANCREAS

The pancreas lies posterior to the stomach and its tail rests on the spleen. This organ is a gland that has endocrine and exocrine functions. The islets of Langerhans, which are responsible for endocrine function, contain alpha and beta cells. After a meal, elevated blood glucose levels stimulate the alpha and beta cells in the pancreas. The alpha cells secrete glucagon, which stimulates glycogenolysis in the liver. Insulin is produced and secreted by the beta cells. Insulin is necessary for the metabolism of carbohydrates. The pancreatic duct intersects with the common bile duct from the gallbladder and travels down into the duodenum (Figure 8.5).

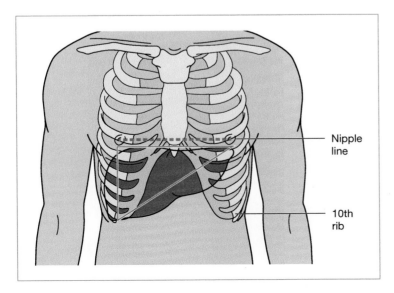

Nipple line

10th rib

FIGURE 8.3 Location of the liver. The liver is located primarily in the right upper quadrant of the abdomen, beneath the diaphragm. It extends from the fifth intercostal space down to the costal margin.

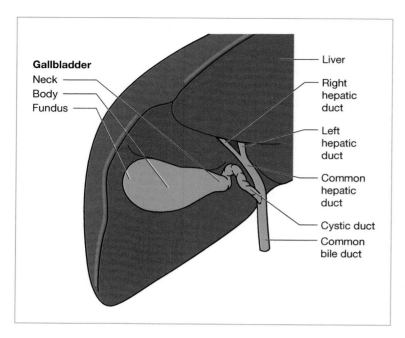

FIGURE 8.4 Location of the gallbladder. The gallbladder is approximately 4 inches long and lies below the inferior surface of the liver.

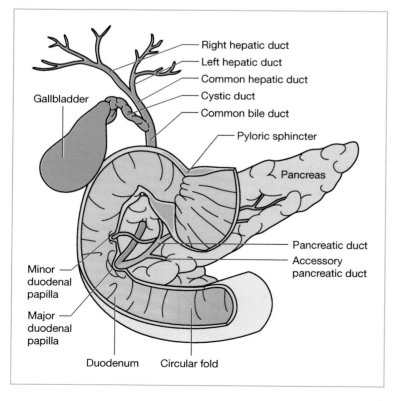

FIGURE 8.5 Anatomy of the pancreas.

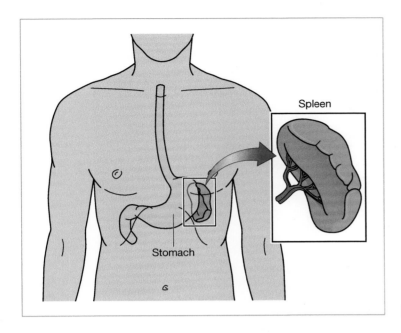

FIGURE 8.6 Location of the spleen.

SPLEEN

The spleen is the largest lymphatic organ in the body. It is located in the LUQ, behind the stomach and above the left kidney (Figure 8.6). It lies in an oblique orientation along the 10th rib. The spleen acts as a filter, removing bacteria and antibody-coated cells from the body. It also destroys aging and deformed red blood cells. Approximately one-third of the body's platelets are stored in the spleen at any given time.

THE KIDNEYS AND BLADDER

The kidneys are located in the posterior upper abdomen. They rest against the back muscles and are protected by the rib cage (Figure 8.7). They are shaped like beans; each is approximately 4 inches long. The right kidney sits slightly lower than the left kidney due to the liver.

The kidneys perform multiple functions. They are responsible for excretion of urea, uric acid, and creatinine in the form of urine. The kidneys regulate the fluid volume by filtering and resorbing sodium and balancing the levels of water and electrolytes. Erythropoietin, which stimulates red blood cell production, is produced by the kidneys. Vitamin D synthesis occurs in the kidneys, which also regulate serum calcium and phosphate levels. Additionally, the kidneys secrete hormones that manage blood pressure.

The bladder is a hollow organ, which is located in the pelvis. It is connected to the kidneys by two ureters. The function of the bladder is to collect urine, which is then excreted through the urethra. Urine travels through the ureters to the bladder by a series of peristaltic waves. The bladder holds between 500 and 1,000 mL of urine.

THE RECTUM AND ANUS

The rectum is the straight portion of the bowel between the sigmoid colon and the anal canal (Figure 8.8). The rectum is 12 to 15 cm in length and acts as a collection area for feces. It lies posterior to the urinary bladder. In women, the uterus lies just anterior to the rectum and can be palpated through the anterior wall of the rectum. The rectum is separated from the anus by the anorectal ring.

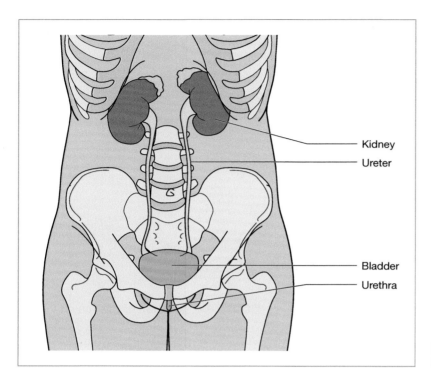

FIGURE 8.7 The location of the kidneys and bladder.

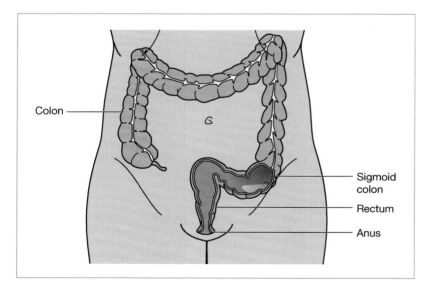

FIGURE 8.8 Location of the rectum.

The anus is the point where solid waste (feces) leaves the body. Located just below the rectum, it is the most distal part of the digestive tract. The anus is 2 to 3 cm long. It is surrounded by two layers of muscles: The internal and external sphincters (Figure 8.9).

The upper part of the anus is composed of columnar or epithelial cells. The lower portion of the anus is composed of squamous cells. The point where the upper and lower portions of the anus converge is called the squamocolumnar junction.

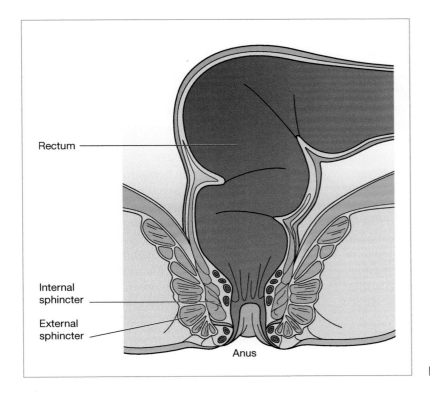

Rectum

Internal sphincter

External sphincter

Anus

FIGURE 8.9 Location of the anus.

Screening Health Assessment and Normal Findings

THE ABDOMEN

Assessment of the abdomen involves four basic techniques: Inspection, auscultation, percussion, and palpation. The provider should generally conduct the exam in this order. Prior to examining the patient, the provider should ask the patient to point to the painful area. In patients with abdominal complaints, palpation often causes severe pain and apprehension. If palpation is performed first, the resulting discomfort could limit patient cooperation with the remainder of the exam. Make several general observations about the patient, including:

- The degree of discomfort, particularly when the patient is unaware of being observed

- The patient's preferred position: a fetal position could indicate renal colic, while lying still with flexed knees is typical of peritonitis.

INSPECTION OF THE ABDOMEN

The abdomen should be inspected from different angles for size, shape, and color. Standing to the side of the patient, the provider should first observe the skin. Striae, which are commonly called "stretch marks," are lighter colored stripes on the skin. Striae are caused by rapidly expanding skin surface, as caused by weight gain or pregnancy. Scars on the abdomen give clues regarding the patient's previous surgical history.

The abdomen and flanks should also be assessed for distention and bruising. The shape of the abdomen should be noted. There are many factors that influence the contour of the abdomen. These include age, sex, weight, and muscle tone. The abdomen is typically described as distended or nondistended. Other descriptors include flat, protuberant, rounded, or concave. In addition to documenting the shape of the abdomen, the provider should also assess whether the contour is symmetrical. Asymmetry can be caused by masses or enlarged organs. Peristaltic waves are most often visible in thin patients or in patients with bowel obstructions. If surface vessels are present on the abdomen, they should be palpated in order to determine the direction of blood flow.

AUSCULTATION OF THE ABDOMEN

Use the diaphragm of the stethoscope to assess bowel sounds. Listen in all four quadrants. The presence and quality of bowel sounds should be noted. Normal bowel sounds are medium-pitched and occur up to 12 times per minute (every 5–15 seconds). If bowel sounds are hypoactive, the provider may have to listen for 2 to 5 minutes. If bowel sounds cannot be heard in this manner, it is sometimes helpful to place the stethoscope just to the right of the umbilicus, over the ileocecal valve.

The bell of the stethoscope should be used to listen for bruits in the abdominal vessels. Bruits are produced when blood flows through a narrowed artery, or when a large volume of blood is flowing from an area of high pressure to an area of lower pressure. Listen for bruits over the descending aorta, as well as the renal, iliac, and femoral arteries (Figure 8.10).

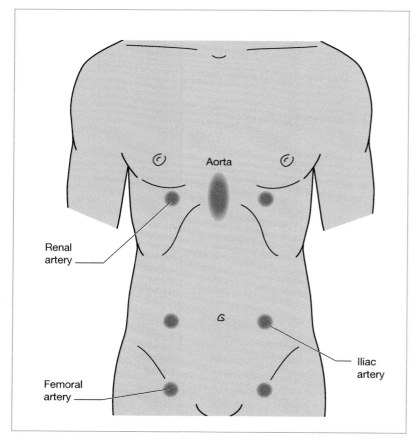

Aorta

Renal artery

Iliac artery

Femoral artery

FIGURE 8.10 Areas to auscultate for bruit.

PERCUSSION OF THE ABDOMEN

Percussion is used to measure and locate abdominal organs. It is also used to assess for the presence of masses and fluid collections. The provider should firmly press the middle finger of his or her nondominant hand flat against the abdomen. Using the pulp of the middle finger of the dominant hand, strike the middle finger that is pressing down on the abdomen. The entire abdomen should be percussed, taking care not to skip over any areas. Air-filled areas of the abdomen will have a hollow or tympanic sound. Solid areas, such as organs, masses, or stool, will have a dull sound. Fluid collections, like fluid-filled cysts and ascites, will also be dull on percussion. Percussion should not be performed if a patient has a transplanted organ, or if an abdominal aortic aneurysm (AAA) is suspected.

PALPATION OF THE ABDOMEN

The abdomen is palpated to assess for tenderness, resistance, abdominal wall defects, abdominal masses, organomegaly, and peritoneal irritation. Palpation should cover the entire abdomen. If the patient is experiencing pain, begin palpating in the area farthest away from the painful region. Begin with light palpation. Some patients, particularly children, are ticklish, which will cause them to tense their abdominal muscles and move around during the exam. Ticklishness can be diminished by having the patient place his or her hand over the provider's hand and palpate the abdomen with the provider.

During light palpation, the provider palpates the entire abdomen with the fingertips. Light palpation is useful for assessing the surface of the abdomen for tenderness, abdominal wall masses such as lipomas, and areas of resistance or *guarding*. After lightly palpating the entire abdomen, the patient should be asked to flex his or her knees. Knee flexion relaxes the abdominal muscles, allowing for more effective deep palpation. During deep palpation, the provider's hand remains fixed on one area of skin, while moving the fingers around to palpate the area under the skin. The provider repeats this until the entire abdomen has been palpated. Some providers prefer the two-handed method for deep palpation. In this method, the provider's hands are placed one on top of the other. The upper hand is used to press down on the abdomen, and the lower hand is used to feel for masses (Figure 8.11).

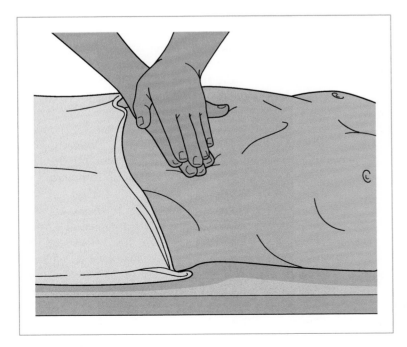

FIGURE 8.11 Two-handed method for deep palpation of the abdomen. The provider's hands are placed one on top of the other. The upper hand is used to press down on the abdomen, and the lower hand is used to feel for masses.

TABLE 8.1
Descriptors for Abdominal Tenderness

Diagnostic Clue	Descriptor
Location	Quadrant of the abdomen where encountered
Depth	Superficial or deep
Tenderness	Gauged by patient response; can be mild, moderate, or severe
Guarding	Present or absent
Referred tenderness (Rovsing's sign)	Present or absent
Rigidity	Present (note location) or absent

TABLE 8.2
Descriptors for Abdominal Mass

Diagnostic Clue	Descriptor
Size	Expressed in centimeters
Shape	Round, oval, or irregular
Consistency	Hard, soft, or rubbery
Location	Region of the abdomen where palpated
Mobility	Fixed or mobile
Tenderness	Degree of tenderness (nontender, slightly tender, or exquisitely tender)
Pulsation	Involving an artery

Guarding is an important diagnostic clue because the patient is contracting the abdominal muscles to avoid pain. *Rigidity* is a sign of underlying peritoneal inflammation. Guarding is a voluntary action and is frequently generalized to the whole abdomen. Rigidity is involuntary and can be unilateral, occurring over an inflamed area, such as appendicitis. Table 8.1 lists how to describe abdominal tenderness.

When an abdominal mass is discovered, it should be determined whether it is in the abdominal wall (intramural) or within the abdominal cavity. This can be done by having the patient tense the abdominal muscles (either by raising the head or raising both feet). An abdominal wall mass will become more prominent when the abdominal muscles are tensed. If an abdominal mass is discovered, the description should include the elements listed in Table 8.2.

THE ABDOMINAL WALL

Physical examination of the abdominal wall involves inspection, percussion, and palpation. The abdominal wall is inspected for distended abdominal wall vessels, protruding hernias, and distention. Abdominal wall distention can be due to muscle wall injury, hernia, organomegaly, and masses within the abdominal wall or the abdominal cavity.

Carnett's sign is useful in determining whether abdominal pain stems from the abdominal wall or from the viscera. To conduct this test, the patient is asked to contract the abdominal muscles. If the pain worsens, the pain is likely due to abdominal wall pathology. Carnett's sign has been shown to be 95% diagnostic for abdominal wall pain.

Aortic pulsations are visibly evident in children and thin adults. During the abdominal exam, the aortic pulsation can be felt in the epigastric region. The average width of the aortic pulsation in an adult is less than 3 cm.

The liver is assessed for size, tenderness, and consistency. Palpation gives information about the size and whether the liver border is smooth or nodular. Liver size is also assessed using percussion in the midclavicular line (MCL). In individuals with a lot of breast tissue, liver span can be measured in the anterior axillary line (AAL). The normal liver span is 6 to 12 cm in the MCL.

PERCUSSION OF THE ABDOMINAL WALL

The patient should be lying supine. In the MCL or AAL, begin percussing over the base of the right lung, where the sounds are tympanic. Continue percussing downward until dullness is heard. This is the upper border of the liver. To find the lower liver border, begin percussing a few centimeters below the costal margin and travel upward toward the ribs. The lower border of the liver is where dullness is first encountered. This is typically at or slightly above the costal margin (Figure 8.12).

Alternately, the provider can start percussing in the MCL below the umbilicus, then percuss upward in a straight line until dullness is encountered. This area should be marked as the lower border of the liver; it is usually at or above the costal margin. Continue percussing upward in the MCL until dullness ceases and tympany is first heard. This is the upper border of the liver, which is usually at the fifth intercostal space.

PALPATION OF THE ABDOMINAL WALL

The patient should be lying supine. The lower liver border was previously determined using percussion. The provider then places his or her hand below the lower liver border and asks the patient to take a deep breath. The liver lowers during inspiration and rises during expiration. Therefore, the provider's hand should remain stationary as the patient inhales, which allows the liver to be palpated as it passes under the provider's fingers. A normal liver is often unpalpable, except in thin patients. If palpable, the liver border should feel smooth.

Alternately, the liver can be palpated using the "hooking" method (Figure 8.13). With the patient supine, the examiner stands on the patient's right side, facing the patient's feet. The fingers of one or both hands are curled (or hooked) around the costal margin or just below the lowest area where liver dullness was percussed. As the patient takes a deep

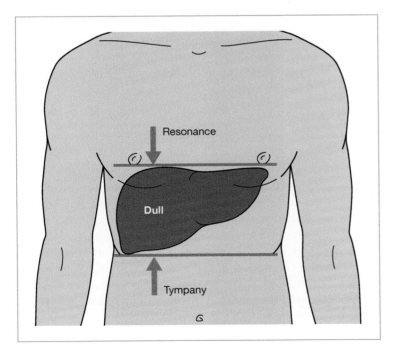

FIGURE 8.12 Percussion of the abdominal wall. The lower border of the liver is where dullness is first encountered.

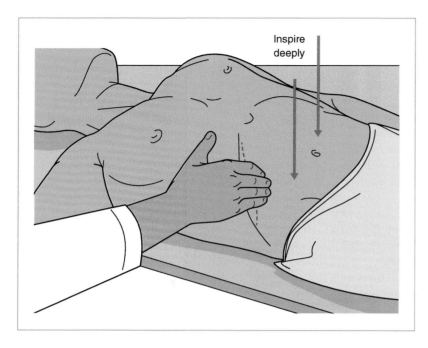

Inspire
deeply

FIGURE 8.13 Hooking method of liver palpation. The fingers of one or both of the provider's hands are curled (or hooked) around the costal margin. As the patient takes a deep breath, the provider's fingers hook inward and up, feeling for the edge of the liver.

breath, the provider's fingers hook inward and up, feeling for the edge of the liver.

It should be noted that palpation of a healthy liver is sometimes painful. However, an enlarged and tender liver can be caused by hepatitis, congestive heart failure, and cancer. The liver becomes painful when the capsule is distended due to infection or an inflammatory process. An irregular liver border or palpable nodules is indicative of cirrhosis.

THE SPLEEN

PERCUSSION OF THE SPLEEN

The patient should be lying supine. The provider percusses the lowest intercostal space in the left AAL. The sound will be tympanic. The patient takes a deep breath, and the provider percusses the same spot again. If the spleen is not enlarged, the area should remain tympanic. If there is dullness to percussion in this spot, there is a possibility that the spleen is enlarged. This is known as *Castell's sign*.

PALPATION OF THE SPLEEN

The normal spleen is usually not palpable; however, it may be palpated in young children and slender individuals. To palpate the spleen, the patient should be lying supine, with arms at the sides and knees slightly flexed to relax the abdominal musculature. The examiner should palpate for the spleen at the left costal margin in the MCL (Figure 8.14). An unpalpable spleen can sometimes be palpated if the patient lies on his or her right side.

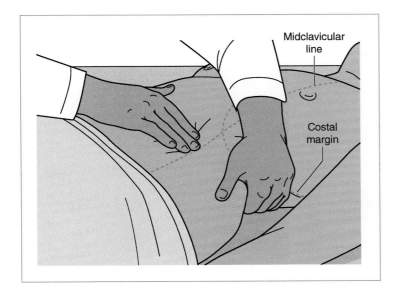

Midclavicular line

Costal margin

FIGURE 8.14 Palpation of the spleen.

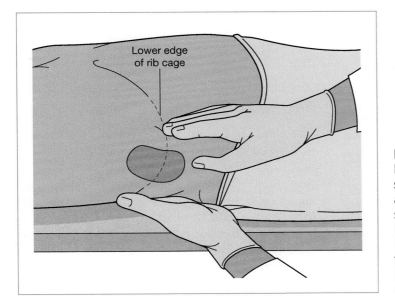

Lower edge of rib cage

FIGURE 8.15 Technique for palpation of the kidney. With the patient supine, one hand should be placed underneath the patient, at the costovertebral angle. The other hand should be placed on the abdomen just below the costal margin. As the patient inhales, the provider attempts to capture the kidney by lifting up with the bottom hand, while palpating deeply using the upper hand.

THE KIDNEYS AND BLADDER

PALPATION OF THE KIDNEYS

The technique for palpating the kidneys is similar to the technique for palpating the spleen. With the patient supine, one hand should be placed underneath the patient, at the costovertebral angle (CVA). The other hand should be placed on the abdomen just below the costal margin. As the patient inhales, the provider attempts to capture the kidney by lifting up with the bottom hand, while palpating deeply using the upper hand (Figure 8.15). This maneuver should be done on each side.

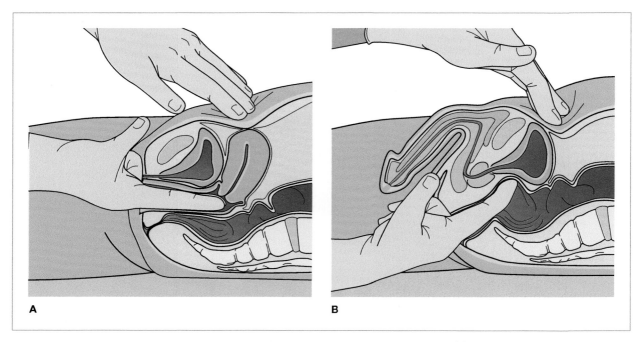

FIGURE 8.16 Bimanual palpation of the bladder in the female (**A**) and male (**B**).

PALPATION OF THE BLADDER

The bladder is not usually palpable. To palpate for an enlarged bladder, the provider palpates over the symphysis pubis. The bladder can also be palpated bimanually. In women, the provider inserts two gloved, lubricated fingers into the vagina while using the other hand to palpate the abdomen from above. The fingers in the vagina lift the bladder anteriorly so that it can be palpated more easily through the abdominal wall. This procedure is similar in males: The examiner inserts a gloved finger into the rectum while using the other hand to palpate the abdomen from above (Figure 8.16).

THE RECTUM AND ANUS

Examination of the rectum involves inspection and palpation, in the form of the digital rectal exam (DRE). This can be done with the patient in the lithotomy position or side-lying with one or both knees raised to the chest. A rectal exam should be conducted on patients presenting with abdominal or rectal complaints.

INSPECTION OF THE RECTUM AND ANUS

The provider begins by inspecting the anus, looking for tears, external lesions, and general sphincter tone. If necessary, the patient can be instructed to bear down (Valsalva maneuver) in order to assess for rectal prolapse. An *anoscope* is an instrument that is inserted into the anus, allowing the examiner to perform an internal examination of the anus (Figure 8.17). *Proctoscopes* and *rectoscopes* are longer versions of the anoscope and provide visualization of the anus and rectum.

PALPATION OF THE RECTUM AND ANUS

DRE is performed if the history or physical indicates that there may be a mass or infection in the rectum. When performing the DRE, the patient should lie on his or her left side (Sims position), stand and lean

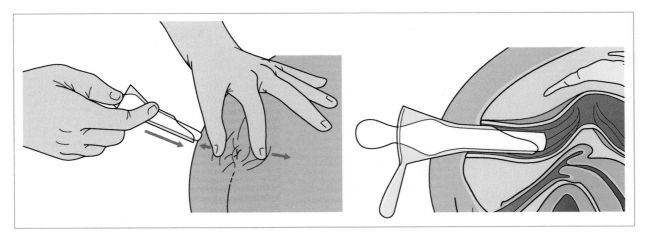

FIGURE 8.17 Internal examination of the anus using an anoscope.

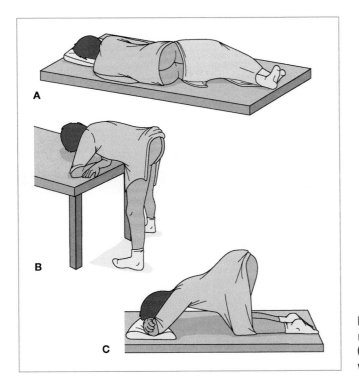

FIGURE 8.18 Positioning of patient for digital rectal examination. (**A**) Left-sided (Sims) position. (**B**) Standing position. (**C**) Kneeling position with weight resting on both elbows.

forward over the exam table, or kneel with weight resting on both elbows (Figure 8.18).

The provider inserts a gloved, lubricated finger into the anus (Figure 8.19). As the finger passes through the anus, the provider makes note of the tone and strength of the sphincter muscles and also palpates any internal hemorrhoid, rectal abscess, and impacted stool. After DRE, the gloved finger is inspected for blood. Stool that is on the glove can be used to test for occult blood.

A DRE is indicated for any patient complaining of abdominal pain. DRE is the only direct method of palpating the male prostate gland. A DRE is also performed as part of the bimanual gynecological exam, to allow better palpation of the uterus.

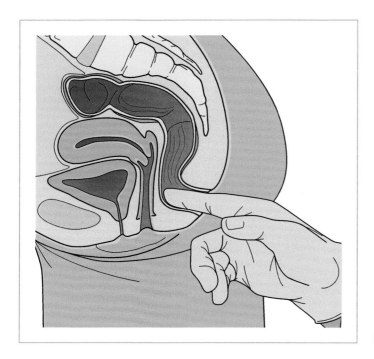

FIGURE 8.19 Digital rectal examination.

Focused Health Assessment and Abnormal Findings

INSPECTION OF THE ABDOMEN

Distention of the abdomen can be caused by obesity, pregnancy, constipation, bowel obstruction, organomegaly, uterine fibroid, or ascites. Table 8.3 lists the possible causes of a distention in relation to the area of the abdomen that is distended.

INSPECTION OF THE ABDOMINAL WALL

Bruising of the skin of the abdomen suggests internal bleeding caused by trauma to the abdominal wall or pancreatic disease. Cullen sign and Grey Turner sign are both caused by retroperitoneal bleeding associated with pancreatitis or ruptured aortic aneurysm. Cullen sign is an area of ecchymosis over the periumbilical region (Figure 8.20). Cullen sign is also associated with ruptured ectopic pregnancy. Patients with Grey Turner

TABLE 8.3 Causes of Abdominal Distention	
Area of the Abdomen	**Possible Causes**
Lower third of the abdomen	Full bladder Pregnancy Ovarian tumor Uterine fibroids
Lower half of the abdomen (below umbilicus)	Full bladder Pregnancy Ovarian tumor
Upper half of the abdomen (above umbilicus)	Splenomegaly Hepatomegaly Pancreatic cyst Gastric fullness
Distention of the entire abdomen	Obesity Ascites Pregnancy

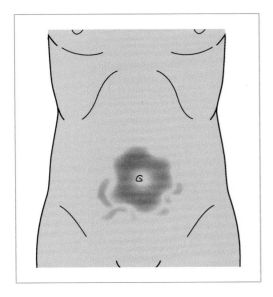

FIGURE 8.20 Cullen sign. An area of ecchymosis over the periumbilical region.

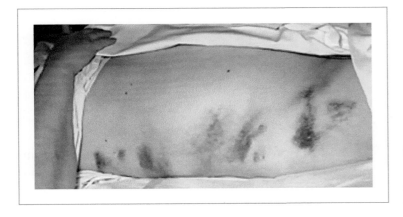

FIGURE 8.21 Grey Turner sign. Ecchymotic areas over flanks.

Source: Courtesy of Herbert L. Fred and Hendrik A. van Dijk.

sign have ecchymotic areas over both flanks (Figure 8.21).

The presence of prominent vessels on the abdominal wall is indicative of disease. Spider angiomas are typically found above the umbilicus and are associated with cirrhosis of the liver. Distended vessels, similar to varicosities, may also be present on the abdomen. These are usually indicative of hepatic disease, heart failure, or occlusion of other vessels.

HERNIAS

A hernia is an area where a body part is bulging through the muscles that contain it. Abdominal hernias can be either *congenital* or *acquired*. *Congenital hernias* are present from birth. *Acquired hernias* appear as a result of progressive weakening of the abdominal musculature. Hernias often come to the attention of the patient when they notice an unusual painless bulging or swelling in an area. A hernia can be visualized by asking the patient to perform the action that he or she is usually doing when he or she observes the bulging. Coughing and straining are the actions that most commonly aggravate a hernia.

When the provider palpates the area while the patient performs the action that produces the hernia, a palpable muscular defect is often appreciated. If a bulging hernia can be pushed back into place, the hernia is *reducible*. Incarceration occurs when

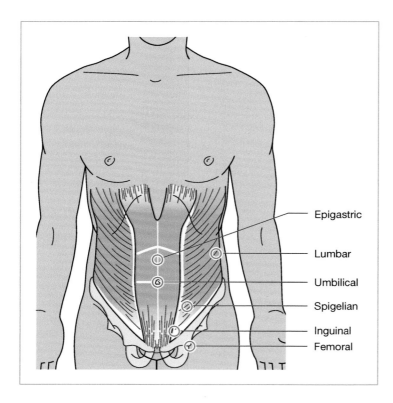

FIGURE 8.22 Hernia sites.

BOX 8.1   Risk Factors for Hernia

- Weight-lifting or straining
- Obesity
- Male gender
- Family history of hernias
- Abdominal surgery
- Abdominal wall injury

the contents of a hernia (usually a loop of bowel) bulge through a weak area of musculature, become entrapped in the area, and cannot be reduced. Circulation to the trapped bowel is diminished to the point that the affected area begins to die. This is called strangulation and is a surgical emergency. Hernias are labeled according to their anatomic location (Figure 8.22). Inguinal hernias are the most common type of groin hernia. Risk factors for hernias are listed in Box 8.1.

DIASTASIS RECTI

Diastasis recti is also called "Rectus abdominis diastasis" (RAD). This condition refers to a widening of the distance between the rectus abdominus muscles. This occurs because increased intraabdominal pressure stretches the linea alba, causing it to become lax (Figure 8.23). The linea alba is the area of the abdomen where the two rectus muscles are joined. RAD is most often an acquired condition and may occur with or without bulging of abdominal organs.

Conditions that contribute to the development of acquired RAD include previous abdominal surgery, pregnancy, and obesity. The typical patient with RAD is either an obese middle-aged man or a fit woman who has had a multiple-gestation pregnancy or delivered a large infant.

Diastasis recti is easy to diagnose. With the patient supine, the provider asks the patient to raise his or her head as though doing an abdominal crunch. When the abdominal wall is tensed, there

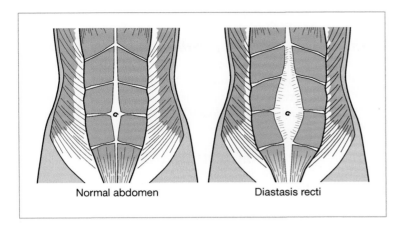

Normal abdomen   Diastasis recti

FIGURE 8.23 Diastasis recti. Widening of the distance between the rectus abdominis muscles.

is a classic midline bulge running the length of the patient's abdomen. The provider is able to palpate the "gap" between the rectus muscles. Although some patients with RAD may feel slight discomfort when they use their abdominal muscles, most patients experience no pain. Asymptomatic RAD requires no treatment. This condition is not a hernia and there is no risk of incarceration. It is certainly possible to have both an umbilical or an incisional hernia and a diastasis recti. Symptomatic RAD requires surgical intervention. Patients may also seek surgical repair for cosmetic reasons following weight loss or pregnancy.

AUSCULTATION OF THE ABDOMEN

BOWEL SOUNDS

There is a large degree of variation in normal bowel sounds. Although the practice of auscultating bowel sounds has been around for hundreds of years, the clinical value of this practice is the subject of much debate. Absent, high-pitched, and hyperactive bowel sounds have the most predictive value for bowel obstruction (Table 8.4). It is possible for bowel sounds in one portion of the abdomen to be hyperactive, while bowel sounds in another quadrant are absent.

TABLE 8.4
Bowel Sounds

Bowel Sounds	Possible Cause
Hyperactive (greater than 30 per minute)	Hunger (normal) Diarrhea Intestinal obstruction Bacterial or viral gastroenteritis
Hypoactive (less than 5 per minute)	Medications Bowel obstruction Postoperative paralytic ileus Peritonitis
Borborygmi	Normal digestion Gastric dilatation
Succussion splash	Delayed gastric emptying Gastric dilation Obstruction
High-pitched rushing sounds	Small bowel obstruction
Absent	Postoperative paralytic ileus Bowel obstruction

ABDOMINAL VESSELS

BRUITS

A bruit is also known as a vascular murmur. Bruits occur when blood flows through a tortuous vessel. It is often described as a "whooshing sound." Systolic bruits are not necessarily associated with disease, but bruits with systolic and diastolic components are associated with hypertension. The abdominal arteries should always be auscultated in patients with hypertension since renal disease is a common cause of secondary hypertension. Using the bell of the stethoscope, listen over the aorta, as well as the renal, iliac, and femoral arteries, as illustrated in Figure 8.10.

VENOUS HUM

A venous hum is a roaring noise. If dilated vessels are visible on the surface of the abdomen, the stethoscope should be lightly placed in the epigastric region. The presence of a venous hum is usually associated with portal hypertension and cirrhosis.

ABDOMINAL AORTIC ANEURYSM

The majority of AAAs occur distal to the renal arteries and are asymptomatic. A ruptured AAA may present as a pulsatile mass in the epigastric region (Figure 8.24). These patients also have back pain, abdominal pain, or pain radiating to the groin. This

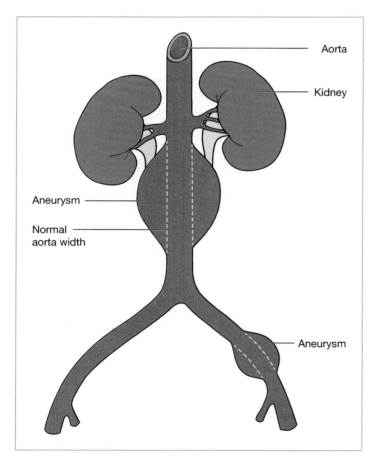

Aorta

Kidney

Aneurysm

Normal
aorta width

Aneurysm

FIGURE 8.24 Abdominal aortic aneurysms.

pain is caused by the bulging aneurysm compressing adjacent structures. Aortic pulsations greater than 3 cm warrant further investigation since manual palpation alone is insufficient to diagnose this condition.

THE GALLBLADDER

MURPHY'S SIGN

Gallbladder disease is often a cause of RUQ pain. Murphy's sign assesses for focal tenderness over the gallbladder. With the patient supine, the provider palpates in the subcostal region of the RUQ while the patient takes a deep breath. This deep inspiration pushes the gallbladder toward the provider's hand. If cholecystitis is present, the painful pressure on the inflamed gallbladder will cause the patient to stop breathing momentarily. This is documented as a positive Murphy's sign. Murphy's sign has been shown to be up to 97% sensitive and 48% specific for gallbladder disease. This test is less sensitive in elderly patients, and a negative Murphy's sign should not be used to exclusively rule out cholecystitis in these patients.

THE LIVER

HEPATOMEGALY

Liver enlargement (hepatomegaly) is diagnosed when the liver extends significantly past the costal margin (Figure 8.25). The most frequent cause of liver enlargement is portal hypertension, followed by viral infection and cancer. Categories of medical conditions that cause hepatomegaly are listed in Table 8.5.

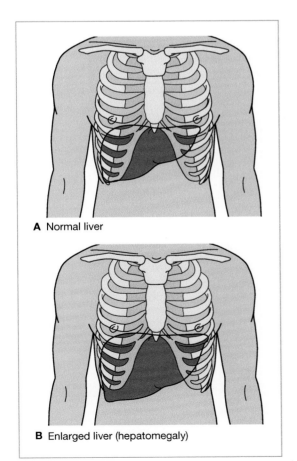

A Normal liver

B Enlarged liver (hepatomegaly)

FIGURE 8.25 Hepatomegaly. (**A**) Normal liver. (**B**) Enlarged liver (hepatomegaly) that extends past the costal margin.

FRICTION RUBS

Listen over the liver and the spleen for friction rubs. The stethoscope should be placed just below the sternal border. Friction rubs occur when there is friction or rubbing on the peritoneal surface of an inflamed organ. Since the liver and spleen are close to the abdominal wall, these organs produce a rub when enlarged. A rub sounds like two fingers rubbing together. Friction rubs can also be felt. If a rub is present, the provider may be able to detect it by placing a hand over the organ while the patient breathes. A friction rub over the liver is suggestive of liver cancer.

ASCITES

Ascites is a collection of fluid in the peritoneal cavity. The majority of cases of ascites are caused by advanced liver disease, such as cirrhosis or liver failure. Other causes of ascites include: malignancy, heart failure, pancreatic disease, and nephrotic syndrome. On examination, patients with ascites will exhibit dullness with percussion of their flanks, while the periumbilical region remains tympanic. This area of dullness will shift if the patient is turned on his or her side (Figure 8.26). Abdominal distention can be monitored by obtaining daily waist circumferences. Clinical signs of ascites are listed in Box 8.2.

Patients with ascites will always have other symptoms of fluid retention, such as hepatojugular reflux, jugular vein distention (RUQ), and lower extremity edema.

TABLE 8.5 Causes of Hepatomegaly (VINDICATE)	
V	Vascular
I	Inflammatory
N	Neoplasm
D	Drugs/Deficiency/Degenerative
I	Idiopathic
C	Congenital
A	Autoimmune
T	Trauma
E	Endocrine

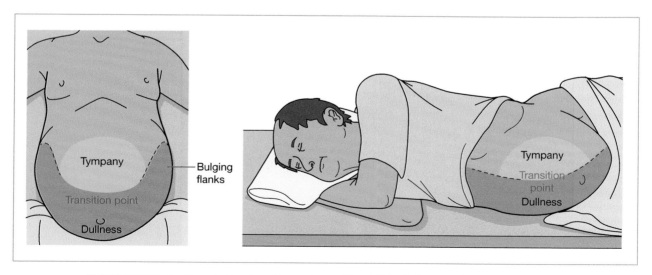

FIGURE 8.26 Ascites. Patients with ascites will exhibit dullness with percussion of their flanks, while the periumbilical region remains tympanic. This area of dullness will shift if the patient is turned on his or her side.

THE SPLEEN

SPLENOMEGALY

When percussing the abdomen, dullness in the LUQ is suspicious for splenomegaly. As the spleen enlarges, it tends to move anteriorly and to the right (Figure 8.27). In severe cases of splenomegaly, the spleen can be felt nearer to the RLQ. For this reason, the provider should begin palpating for an enlarged spleen near the right iliac fossa, moving upward diagonally to the patient's left a few centimeters at a time, so as not to miss an enlarged spleen. Patients with splenomegaly should be checked for hepatomegaly as well. Splenomegaly can be caused by alcoholic cirrhosis or portal hypertension.

A ruptured spleen is a life-threatening emergency. Therefore, vigorous palpation of the spleen should be avoided. Patients recovering from infectious mononucleosis should be checked for splenomegaly. If the spleen is enlarged, these patients should be advised to avoid contact sports for 4 weeks or until completely recovered.

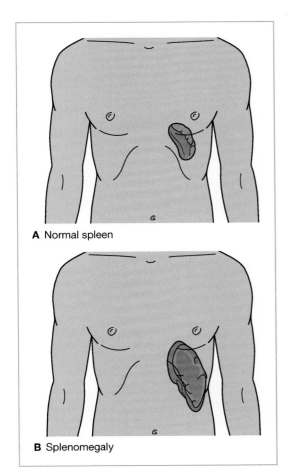

A Normal spleen

B Splenomegaly

FIGURE 8.27 (A) Normal spleen. **(B)** Splenomegaly. As the spleen enlarges, it moves anteriorly and to the right.

THE KIDNEYS AND BLADDER

COSTOVERTEBRAL ANGLE TENDERNESS

The CVA is the angle formed by the 12th rib and the adjacent lumbar vertebrae (Figure 8.28). To test for pyelonephritis, the provider places an open palm flat over the CVA and strikes the hand with the heel of a closed fist. The patient will experience extreme pain if pyelonephritis is present. This occurs because jarring is irritating to an inflamed kidney. Causes of CVA tenderness include renal abscess, pyelonephritis, and renal calculi.

BLADDER PALPATION AND PERCUSSION

A distended bladder might rise above the pubic bone and become palpable. The bladder will percuss as an area of dullness at or above the pubis. In women of childbearing age, the bladder should be differentiated from a gravid or fibroid uterus.

THE APPENDIX

REBOUND TENDERNESS

RLQ pain is the most commonly recognized symptom of acute appendicitis. To assess for peritoneal irritation caused by an inflamed appendix, the provider can check for *rebound tenderness*. The provider presses in the RLQ, then abruptly withdraws the hand. If the pain worsens when the hand is withdrawn, the test is positive for rebound tenderness. Rebound tenderness is a reliable indicator of peritoneal irritation.

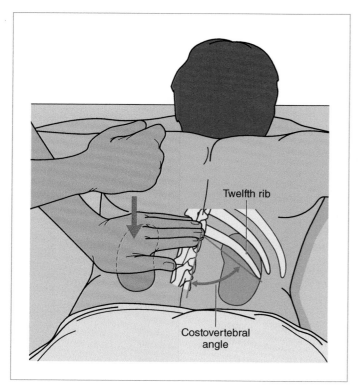

Twelfth rib

Costovertebral
angle

FIGURE 8.28 Testing for pyelonephritis. The examiner places an open palm flat over the costovertebral angle and strikes the hand with the heel of a closed fist.

OTHER TESTS FOR APPENDICITIS

Markle sign: Have the patient stand up on his or her toes, and then drop down to a regular standing position. If peritonitis is present, the patient will experience abdominal pain when his or her heels hit the floor.

McBurney's point: Tenderness at a point located at one-third of the distance between the umbilicus and the anterior superior iliac spine (Figure 8.29). This distance is approximately 2 inches.

Rovsing's sign: Patient experiences pain in the RLQ when the LLQ is palpated. This occurs because displacing the abdominal contents on the left side causes vibrations that migrate to the right and irritate the peritoneum surrounding the inflamed appendix.

Obturator sign: The patient experiences suprapubic pain when the examiner flexes the thigh and rotates the femur internally and externally. This occurs because the inflamed appendix is rubbing against the obturator muscle (Figure 8.30). This test is used to detect a pelvic appendix.

Psoas sign: The patient experiences pain when the right hip is passively extended. The patient flexes the hip in response to the pain. This occurs because the inflamed appendix is rubbing against the iliopsoas muscle (Figure 8.31).

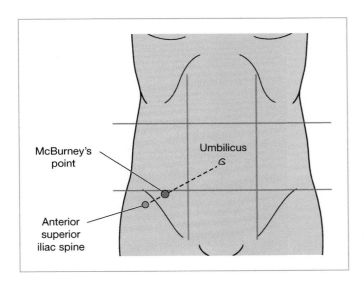

FIGURE 8.29 McBurney's point. Tenderness located one-third of the distance between the umbilicus and the anterior superior iliac spine.

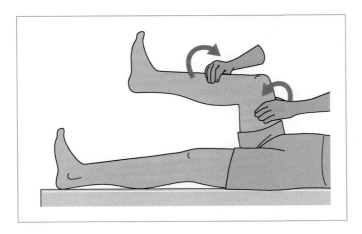

FIGURE 8.30 Obturator test.

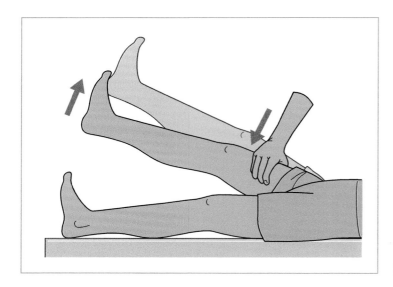

FIGURE 8.31 Iliopsoas test.

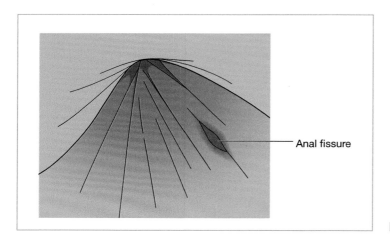

Anal fissure

FIGURE 8.32 Anal fissure.

THE RECTUM AND ANUS

ANAL FISSURES

Anal fissures are linear tears in the skin around the anus (Figure 8.32). Fissures are the most common cause of anal pain and rectal bleeding. This condition is usually caused by the passage of hard stool. Patients typically complain of rectal pain that worsens during defecation. Other causes of anal fissures are listed in Box 8.3. Although patients of all ages can get anal fissures, this condition occurs most frequently in infants and the elderly.

BOX 8.3 Common Causes of Anal Fissures
• Constipation/diarrhea
• Vaginal delivery
• Anal sex
• Malignancy
• Sexually transmitted disease

Those who suffer from fecal incontinence or hemorrhoids have an increased risk of developing fissures. Crohn's disease also causes anal fissures; therefore, patients with multiple, recurrent, or nonhealing fissures should be evaluated for Crohn's disease. Anal fissures can be acute or chronic. Acute fissures look similar to fresh linear wounds. Chronic fissures are whitish in appearance.

HEMORRHOIDS

A hemorrhoid is a swollen vein on the anus, very similar to a varicosity. Hemorrhoids can occur internally or externally (Figure 8.33). Approximately 90% of hemorrhoids are located on the medial, posterior region of the anus. Patients may be unaware that they have hemorrhoids. Symptoms of hemorrhoids include painless bright red rectal bleeding (hematochezia), constipation, perianal itching, rectal leakage, and skin tags. These symptoms are exacerbated by straining at stool. Thrombosed hemorrhoids are extremely painful. This condition occurs when a blood clot forms within the vessel (Figure 8.34).

Hemorrhoids are assessed by inspection and palpation. External hemorrhoids are easily visualized by parting the buttocks. Internal hemorrhoids may require the use of an anoscope to visualize the anal canal.

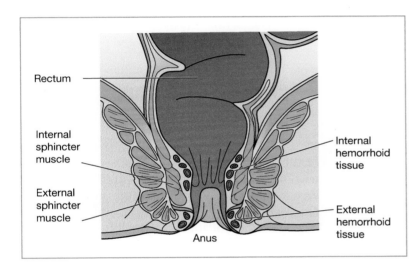

FIGURE 8.33 Internal and external hemorrhoid tissue.

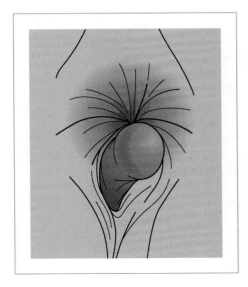

FIGURE 8.34 Thrombosed hemorrhoids.

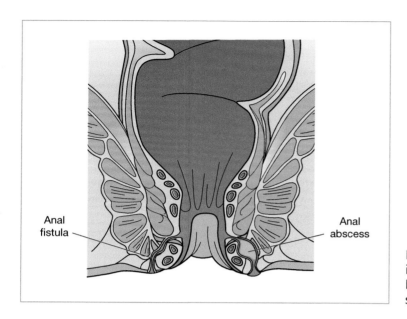

Anal
fistula

Anal
abscess

FIGURE 8.35 Complication of perianal infection. The development of a fistula between the abscess and perianal skin is shown.

PERIANAL INFECTIONS

Anorectal abscesses are most frequently caused by obstruction of an anal crypt gland. The obstruction is usually caused by debris such as fecal matter or decaying squamous cells, which leads to bacterial overgrowth and production of pus. Patients usually complain of a painful rectal mass with painful defecation and anal discharge. If the infection has progressed, the patient might also exhibit signs of systemic infection such as fever, chills, or malaise. Some anorectal infections will spontaneously drain on their own. If this does not occur, incision and drainage are indicated. Untreated abscesses can cause sepsis. Another complication is the development of fistulas between the abscess and the perianal skin (Figure 8.35).

RECTAL PROLAPSE

Rectal prolapse, also called rectal procidentia, occurs when the rectum protrudes from the anus.

This usually occurs as a result of a weakening of the pelvic floor muscles, with accompanying weakness of the internal and external sphincter muscles. Rectal prolapse occurs most often in older women, but it can occur in men as well. On physical exam, it looks as though a pink donut is coming out of the anus (Figure 8.36). This is actually concentric rings of the rectum bulging outward. It is also possible to have an internal rectal prolapse, in which the rectum telescopes or folds onto itself (see Figure 8.36). Associated symptoms of rectal prolapse include sensation of a mass in the rectum, incomplete bowel evacuation, abdominal pain, fecal incontinence, and mucous-like discharge from the rectum.

If the rectal prolapse is not evident during the physical examination, it can be reproduced by having the patient squat and bear down. Administration of an enema will also induce prolapse. Most prolapses are intermittent and can be reduced. In some cases, surgical repair is necessary to correct fecal incontinence or to prevent incarceration of the prolapsed area.

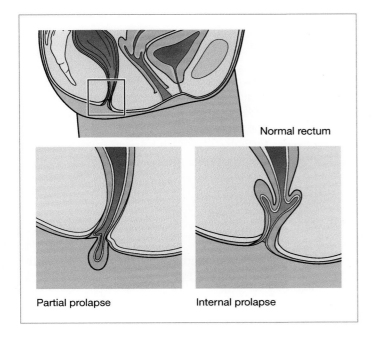

Normal rectum

Partial prolapse

Internal prolapse

FIGURE 8.36 Rectal prolapse.

Holistic Assessment

DIET AND EXERCISE

Dietary assessment should be done on every patient with a gastrointestinal complaint. Although not all abdominal complaints arise from the digestive system, a gastrointestinal cause must be excluded. When feasible, a 24-hour diet recall should be conducted on patients presenting with acute abdominal complaints. For recurrent or chronic gastrointestinal complaints, a food diary is useful for documenting a timeline of symptoms triggered by certain foods. Recent studies have linked the consumption of high amounts of animal protein with fatty liver disease. Dietary information can be used to form differential diagnoses. The food diary also allows the provider to identify nutritional deficiencies in the diet. Patients should also be questioned about recent weight gain or loss, intentional and unintentional.

All patients should be asked about their exercise activities and sports involvement. An enlarged spleen is at risk for rupture during contact sports and activities that increase intra-abdominal pressure. Therefore, adolescents and young adults with splenic enlargement should be counseled to avoid contact and high-impact sports such as football, field hockey, hockey, basketball, and gymnastics. Infectious mononucleosis and sickle cell disease are illnesses that commonly cause splenomegaly in young people.

IMMUNIZATION HISTORY

A thorough immunization history should be obtained. In the United States, the childhood immunization schedule now includes hepatitis A, hepatitis B, and human papillomavirus infection (HPV) vaccines. Hepatitis A and B are infectious agents that cause liver disease. Hepatitis A vaccine was recommended for all children beginning in 1996. Hepatitis B vaccine was recommended for infants beginning in 1991. Older individuals would not have received either of these vaccines during childhood and are at risk for contracting these illnesses.

SOCIAL HISTORY

Alcohol consumption can exacerbate gastrointestinal disorders and is toxic to the liver. In suspected liver or pancreatic disease, the social history should include detailed questions about alcohol consumption, such as amount and type. In patients whose alcohol consumption exceeds the recommended daily amount, the CAGE (cut down, annoyed, guilty, and eye-opener) questions can be used to assess for alcoholism.

CULTURE

There is a strong connection between culture and diet. When addressing gastrointestinal complaints, the patient's culture must be considered. In addition to diet, cultures have unique remedies for illnesses. Patients should be questioned regarding the use of herbal remedies.

LIVING SITUATION

The patient's living situation can shed light on the nature of an illness. For instance, if a patient has diarrhea, it is useful to know whether other members of the household are similarly ill. Providers should find out about the patient's water source since well water can be contaminated with microbes and parasites. In developing nations that lack adequate sewage systems, gastrointestinal disease and hepatitis can be spread from improperly treated human and animal waste.

CASE STUDY: ABDOMEN

DOCUMENTATION

Chief complaint: "Indigestion" off and on for the past 6 weeks

History of the present illness: GW is a 38-year-old male who complains of indigestion off and on for the past 6 weeks. He describes the symptoms as a "slight burning in the middle of his chest," accompanied by the feeling that his "food is coming back up." He rates this burning as 2/10 pain. Symptoms typically start within 30 minutes after a meal and are worse at night when he is lying down. He recalls having similar symptoms when he was in college, and he used "antacid pills" with complete relief of symptoms. He has tried using over-the-counter antacid pills for the past week, with slight relief of symptoms.

Medications: Over-the-counter antacid pills

Allergies: No known allergies

Past Medical History: Overweight

(continued)

(continued)

Past Surgical History: No prior surgeries or hospitalizations

Family History: No relevant family history

SOCIAL HISTORY

Alcohol: Consumes approximately 24 oz. of beer on Sundays

Tobacco: Cigarettes—½ pack per day, for the past 20 years

Drugs: Denies illicit drug use

Marital Status: Married, two children

Occupation: Car salesman; works 10 to 12 hours/day

Diet: Eats fast food for breakfast and lunch. Snacks on baked goods at work throughout the day. Has dinner at 9 or 10 p.m. Goes to bed at 11 p.m; wakes at 7 a.m.

REVIEW OF SYSTEMS

Constitutional: No complaints of fever, chills, or malaise

Cardiovascular: Denies chest pain, denies palpitations. Denies peripheral edema. Denies shortness of breath. Denies dyspnea on exertion.

Gastrointestinal: Denies nausea/vomiting. Denies diarrhea. Reports daily formed stools; denies constipation.

PHYSICAL EXAMINATION

Vital signs: Temperature: 98.2°C; pulse: 74; respirations: 16; blood pressure: 128/76 (sitting)

Height: 70"; weight: 200 lbs.

General: Alert, in no apparent distress

Mouth/throat: Posterior pharynx is clear; no dental erosion noted

Integumentary: Skin is warm and dry

Heart: Regular rate and rhythm, S1, S2

Lungs: Clear to auscultation; no wheezes

Abdomen: Soft and nondistended; bowel sounds present in all four quadrants. Nontender to light and deep palpation. No epigastric tenderness. No palpable masses. No hepatomegaly.

Diagnosis: Gastroesophageal reflux disease

ICD-10-CM Diagnosis Code: K21.9 Gastroesophageal Reflux Disease Without Esophagitis

CASE STUDY: RECTUM AND ANUS

DOCUMENTATION

Chief complaint: Constipation, rectal pain, and occasional rectal bleeding

History of Present Illness: TW is a 37-year-old female who complains of difficulty passing stools for the past 2 weeks. She usually has daily formed stools. Lately, she has had to strain during bowel movements and has been experiencing rectal pain while stooling. She has noticed small amounts of bright red blood on the toilet paper when she wipes herself after bowel movements. She reports having a hemorrhoid a few years ago. The patient started a low-carb diet 3 weeks ago and has not been taking any fiber supplements.

Medications: OTC multivitamin daily; hydrochlorothiazide 25 mg daily

Allergies: Penicillin (hives)

Past Medical History: Hypertension

Past Surgical History: C-section

Family History: Hypertension, both parents; negative for cancer; negative for inflammatory bowel disease; negative for colon polyps

SOCIAL HISTORY

Alcohol: Rarely drinks alcohol; one glass of wine with dinner, twice a month

Tobacco: Denies tobacco use

Drugs: Denies illicit drug use

Marital Status: Divorced, one child

Occupation: Commercial truck driver

Diet: Drinks approximately four glasses of fluids a day. Does not drink caffeinated beverages. Follows a 1,200-calorie low-carb diet; each meal consists of a protein shake or a 4-ounce serving of meat protein.

Exercise: Does not exercise

REVIEW OF SYSTEMS

Constitutional: No complaints of fever, chills, or malaise. Denies unintentional weight loss

Gastrointestinal: Denies nausea/vomiting. Denies diarrhea. Passing hard brown stools every 3 to 4 days. Strains at stool.

Rectal: Denies pain during bowel movements. Has noticed drops of blood on toilet paper and in the toilet water after passing stool.

(continued)

(continued)

PHYSICAL EXAMINATION

Vital signs: Temperature: 97.6°C; pulse: 78; respirations: 16; blood pressure: 110/70 (sitting)

Height: 64"; weight: 150 lbs

General: Alert, in no apparent distress

Integumentary: Skin is warm and dry.

Abdomen: Soft, nondistended; hypoactive bowel sounds noted in all four quadrants. Nontender to light and deep palpation. No palpable masses.

Rectum: 2 cm tender, thrombosed external hemorrhoid noted; no active bleeding. Digital rectal exam: Good sphincter tone; no palpable masses in rectal vault.

Diagnosis: Constipation; hemorrhoids

ICD-10-CM Diagnosis Code: K59.00 Constipation, Unspecified

ICD-10-CM Diagnosis Code: K64.9 Unspecified Hemorrhoids

Assessment of Special Populations

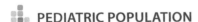 PEDIATRIC POPULATION

Infants and young children are unable to verbalize the location of abdominal discomfort. The provider must obtain a detailed history of the illness. Changes in feeding behavior and stool consistency often provide valuable clues regarding the nature of the illness. Caregivers should also be queried regarding the presence of similar symptoms in other family members. Vomiting and changes in stool amount and consistency are also symptoms of gastrointestinal disease. Gastroesophageal reflux disease (GERD), pyloric stenosis, umbilical hernia, and intussusception are common gastrointestinal disorders found in the pediatric population.

UMBILICAL HERNIA

Umbilical hernias are common in infants and children. The umbilical ring is the opening through which the fetal umbilical vessels connect to the placenta. After birth, this ring gradually closes as the rectus abdominis muscles develop. However, an umbilical hernia presents as a bulging at the umbilicus. This bulge occurs because a portion of the bowel is protruding through the open umbilical ring (Figure 8.37) and is less likely to close spontaneously. African American children have a higher occurrence of umbilical hernias.

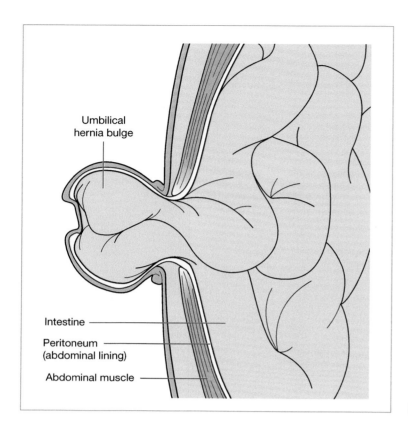

Umbilical
hernia bulge

Intestine

Peritoneum
(abdominal lining)

Abdominal muscle

FIGURE 8.37 Umbilical hernia.

PYLORIC STENOSIS

Pyloric stenosis should be considered in infants less than 3 months old who present with nonbilious postprandial projectile vomiting. In pyloric stenosis, the pylorus is hypertrophied (Figure 8.38), causing varying degrees of gastric obstruction. Patients present with a history of forceful vomiting. On palpation, an olive-shaped mass is present in the RUQ.

INTUSSUSCEPTION

In intussusception, the bowel folds in on itself, like the portions of a collapsible telescope (Figure 8.39). Intussusception should be considered in children under age 4 who present with intermittent spells of crying accompanied by severe abdominal pain. Symptoms may progress to constant pain and inconsolable crying. A sausage-shaped mass is palpable

in the RLQ. Patients may also have the classic "currant jelly stools" which are bloody and filled with mucus. This, when present, is a late finding.

FEMALE POPULATION

In women with lower abdominal pain, a pelvic etiology should be explored. A thorough menstrual history should be conducted on women of childbearing age. This includes, but is not limited to:

- Last menstrual period—(the first day of bleeding)
- Length of menstrual cycle
- Length of an average menstrual period
- History of dysmenorrhea
- History of menorrhagia
- History of uterine fibroids

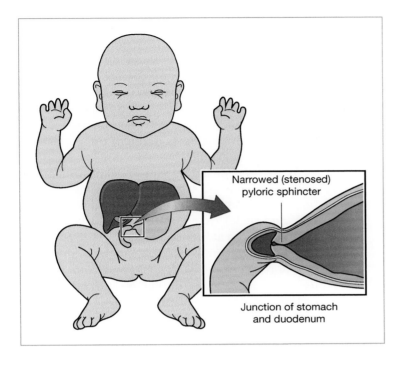

Narrowed (stenosed)
pyloric sphincter

Junction of stomach
and duodenum

FIGURE 8.38 Pyloric stenosis.

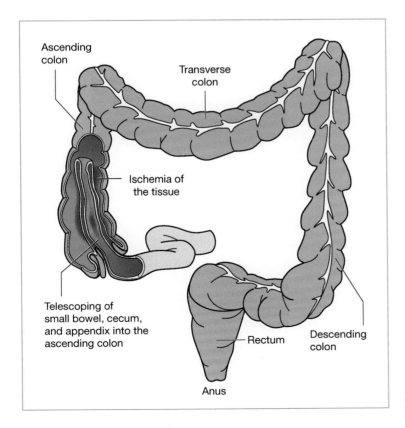

Ascending
colon

Transverse
colon

Ischemia of
the tissue

Telescoping of
small bowel, cecum,
and appendix into the
ascending colon

Rectum

Descending
colon

Anus

FIGURE 8.39 Intussusception.

A sexual history is obtained to assess the patient's risk of sexually transmitted infection. This should minimally include:

- Current and past sexual partners
- Use of contraception and barrier methods
- History of dyspareunia
- Past and current physical and/or sexual abuse
- History of sexually transmitted infection
- History of abnormal vaginal discharge

ELDERLY POPULATION

Abdominal pain in the elderly is misdiagnosed 50% of the time, and the mortality rate of these patients is high. Assessing abdominal complaints in the elderly is a challenge because they often present with atypical symptoms. Therefore, great care must be taken when assessing older adults with abdominal complaints. Constipation is a problem in as many as 50% of elderly patients. It can be due to primary, secondary, or idiopathic causes. Slowed colonic transit and pelvic floor dysfunction are the primary causes of constipation. Constipation can also be caused by poor fluid intake, inactivity, and inadequate dietary fiber.

Polypharmacy is common among older patients, who frequently have multiple chronic illnesses. It is important to do a complete medication reconciliation, considering all known drug interactions and side effects. Opioids, taken for pain, mask abdominal symptoms and also cause constipation. Anticoagulant use places these patients at higher risk for gastrointestinal bleeds. Anticholinergics can cause urinary retention. The rectal exam should assess for stool impaction, hemorrhoids and fissures, sphincter tone, vaginal masses, and enlarged prostate.

TRANSGENDER AND GAY PATIENTS

When addressing abdominal and anorectal complaints in transgender patients, the examiner must consider the patient's biological sex and the patient's declared gender. It is important to know whether the patient has undergone sexual reassignment surgery (SRS). Knowing which organs the patient has will narrow the list of differential diagnoses and prevent dangerous omissions during the physical exam. For example, a transgender man with abdominal pain would need a pelvic exam to rule out a gynecological source, if the patient has not yet undergone SRS.

All patients should be questioned regarding their sexual preferences. A transgender female who participates in receptive anal sex is at a higher risk for HPV and rectal cancers. Men who have sex with men (MSM) are at increased risk for HPV and squamous cell cancer. These patients should receive annual rectal exams with anal Papanicolaou (Pap) tests. Lesions detected during the DRE may require further examination using high-resolution anoscopy. Women who have sex with women (WSW) should be asked about recent sexual encounters with men, in order to rule out pregnancy and sexually transmitted pelvic infections as a source of abdominal pain.

Healthcare providers should base their treatment choices and necessary screenings on a combination of factors such as biological sex, surgical status, declared gender, and past or current use of hormone replacement therapy (HRT). For example, a transgender man who has not undergone SRS might still need a pap smear, and a transgender woman, depending on the patient's age, might need a prostate exam.

PATIENTS WITH DISABILITIES

PHYSICAL DISABILITY

A number of patients with disabilities, such as spinal cord injury or spina bifida, may have undergone surgery that has altered the normal anatomy and physiology of the lower gastrointestinal (GI) tract. For example, these patients may have a revision of the bladder and bowel resulting in alterations in evacuation of either the bladder, the bowel, or both. Therefore, it is important to ask how the patient carries out bowel and bladder management and to ensure that the patient has no difficulty maintaining bowel and bladder function. Patients with disabilities whose normal patterns of mobility are altered with hospitalization and illness are at increased risk of issues associated with immobility; changes in their usual mobility and their effects should be part of the assessment of these patients.

INTELLECTUAL DISABILITY

Depending on the degree of impairment, patients with intellectual disability might be unable to verbalize their symptoms. Caregivers should be carefully questioned regarding the patient's medications, diet, and toileting. As many as 5% of patients with intellectual delay also have some degree of dysphagia. Dysphagia can cause gastrointestinal problems and malnutrition. Additionally, these patients are very prone to constipation. Causes of constipation in this population are:

• Poor dentition

• Sedentary lifestyle

• Medications

Gastrostomy tubes are frequently placed in patients who have significant feeding issues. Individuals with gastrostomy tubes can experience complications such as infections, fistulas, and chronic abdominal wall pain.

The provider should be mindful of the fact that these patients, male and female, are extremely vulnerable to physical and sexual abuse. Pelvic and rectal etiologies for lower abdominal pain should be explored. Blunt trauma should be suspected in patients who present with abdominal bruising, tenderness, distention, or splenomegaly.

VETERAN POPULATION

The provider should ask the patient if they served in the military. If so, the dates and capacity in which they served (e.g., pilot, ground forces, medical services) should be ascertained. Based upon this information, the provider will be aware of what potential hazards or chemicals of warfare the patient may have been exposed to.

Diagnostic Reasoning

Common Differential Diagnoses: Abdominal and Rectal Conditions

Condition	Differential Diagnoses	Symptoms
Acute bowel obstruction	Constipation	Absence of flatus; nausea/vomiting; constipation; abdominal distention; crampy abdominal pain
Acute gastroenteritis	Infectious colitis Protozoal infection Foodborne illness *Clostridium difficile* infection Irritable bowel syndrome Malabsorption syndromes Medication-induced diarrhea Laxative abuse	Diarrhea; nausea/vomiting; fever; diffuse abdominal tenderness

(continued)

Common Differential Diagnoses: Abdominal and Rectal Conditions (*continued*)

Condition	Differential Diagnoses	Symptoms
Anal fissures	Hemorrhoids Colorectal cancer Proctitis	Severe rectal pain that is exacerbated by defecation; hematochezia
Appendicitis	Ovarian cyst Tubo-ovarian	Pain in the periumbilical region that eventually migrates to the right lower quadrant; rebound tenderness; nausea/vomiting; fever; anorexia
Cholecystitis	Pancreatitis Peptic ulcer disease	Positive Murphy's sign; right upper quadrant pain; epigastric pain; fever
Crohn's disease	Appendicitis Ulcerative colitis	Weight loss; colicky right lower quadrant pain; right lower quadrant tenderness; palpable right lower quadrant mass; diarrhea; bloody stools; steatorrhea
Diverticulitis	Appendicitis Inflammatory bowel disease	Left lower quadrant pain and tenderness; palpable left lower quadrant mass; low-grade fever; nausea/vomiting; previous diagnosis of diverticulitis; constipation; ribbon-like stools
Ectopic pregnancy	Tubo-ovarian abscess Appendicitis	History of pelvic inflammatory disease; previous tubal pregnancy or tubal surgery; vaginal bleeding
Gastroesophageal reflux disease	Myocardial infarction Angina pectoris Peptic ulcer disease Gastritis Esophagitis Functional chest pain	Retrosternal burning sensation; chest pain; regurgitation; odynophagia; cough; hoarseness; wheezing

(*continued*)

Common Differential Diagnoses: Abdominal and Rectal Conditions (*continued*)

Condition	Differential Diagnoses	Symptoms
Hemorrhoids	Anal fissures Colorectal cancer Proctitis Rectal prolapse	Bright red, painless bleeding associated with bowel movements; sensation of anal fullness; perianal itching; perianal pain or irritation
Hepatitis (viral)	Cholecystitis	Itching; jaundice; dark urine; right upper quadrant tenderness; nausea/vomiting; fatigue, malaise
Inflammatory bowel disease	Irritable bowel syndrome	History of diarrhea for several months; absence of abdominal pain
Irritable bowel syndrome		Recent stressful events; lower abdominal cramping, relieved by passage of flatus or defecation; pain 1–2 hours after meals; diarrhea alternating with constipation
Pancreatitis	Gastritis Biliary disease Peptic ulcer disease	Acute pain in the upper abdomen that radiates to the back; epigastric tenderness; upper abdomen distention
Peptic ulcer disease	Pancreatitis Cholecystitis Gastric malignancy Dyspepsia GERD	Pain that occurs 2–4 hours after a meal; pain in right or left upper quadrant; GERD symptoms; history of NSAID use; history of *Helicobacter pylori* infection; unexplained iron deficiency anemia
Ulcerative colitis	Crohn's disease	Bloody diarrhea containing mucus and pus; rectal urgency; abdominal cramping; weight loss; anemia

GERD, gastroesophageal reflux disease; NSAID, nonsteroidal anti-inflammatory drug.

BIBLIOGRAPHY

Akram, J., & Matzen, S. H. (2014). Rectus abdominis diastasis. *Journal of Plastic Surgery and Hand Surgery, 48*(3), 163–169. doi:10.3109/2000656X.2013.859145

Baid, H. (2009). A critical review of auscultating bowel sounds. *British Journal of Nursing, 18*(18), 1125–1129. doi:10.12968/bjon.2009.18.18.44555

Bharucha, A. E., Chakraborty, S., & Sletten, C. D. (2016). Common functional gastroenterological disorders associated with abdominal pain. *Mayo Clinic Proceedings, 91*(8), 1118–1132. doi:10.1016/j.mayocp.2016.06.003

Cotter, T. G., Buckley, N. S., & Loftus, C. G. (2017). Approach to the patient with hematochezia. *Mayo Clinic Proceedings, 92*(5), 797–804. doi:10.1016/j.mayocp.2016.12.021

Floyd, S. R., Pierce, D. M., & Geraci, S. A. (2016). Preventive and primary care for lesbian, gay and bisexual patients. *American Journal of the Medical Sciences, 352*(6), 637–643. doi:10.1016/j.amjms.2016.05.008

Fritz, D., & Weilitz, P. B. (2016). Abdominal assessment. *Home Healthcare Now, 34*(3), 151–155. doi:10.1097/NHH.0000000000000364

Hatch, Q., & Steele, S. R. (2013). Rectal prolapse and intussusception. *Gastroenterology Clinics of North America, 42*(4), 837–861. doi:10.1016/j.gtc.2013.08.002

Magidson, P. D., & Martinez, J. P. (2016). Abdominal pain in the geriatric patient. *Emergency Medicine Clinics of North America, 34*(3), 559–574. doi:10.1016/j.emc.2016.04.008

Robinson, A. (2010). The transgender patient and your practice: What physicians and staff need to know. *The Journal of Medical Practice Management, 25*, 364–367. Retrieved from https://greenbranch.com/store/index.cfm/product/630/the-transgender-patient-and-your-practice-what-physicians-and-staff-need-to-know.cfm

Zens, T., Nichol, P. F., Cartmill, R., & Kohler, J. E. (2017). Management of asymptomatic pediatric umbilical hernias: A systematic review. *Journal of Pediatric Surgery, 52*(11), 1723–1731. doi:10.1016/j.jpedsurg.2017.07.016

9

ADVANCED HEALTH ASSESSMENT OF THE MALE GENITOURINARY SYSTEM

Susanne A. Quallich

CHAPTER CONTENTS

(continued)

ASSESSMENT OF SPECIAL POPULATIONS
  Adolescent Population
  Transgender Population
  Elderly Population
  Patients With Disabilities
  Veteran Population
  Elite Athlete Population

DIAGNOSTIC REASONING
  Common Differential Diagnoses: Male Genitourinary System

Overview of Anatomy and Physiology

In the male, several organs serve as parts of both the urinary tract and the reproductive system. Disorders in the male reproductive organs may interfere with the functions of one or both of these systems. As a result, diseases of the male reproductive system are usually treated in collaboration with a urologist, as there is no one specific "men's health specialist." The structures in the male reproductive system include the testes, the vas deferens (ductus deferens) and seminal vesicles, the penis, and accessory glands such as the prostate gland and Cowper's gland (bulbourethral gland; Figure 9.1).

THE TESTES

The testes are formed early in embryological development within the abdominal cavity, near the kidneys. During the last month of fetal development, they descend posterior to the peritoneum and pierce the abdominal wall in the groin, then progress along the inguinal canal into the scrotum. In this descent, they are accompanied by blood vessels, lymphatics, nerves, and ducts, all of which become the structures of the spermatic cord. This cord extends from the internal inguinal ring

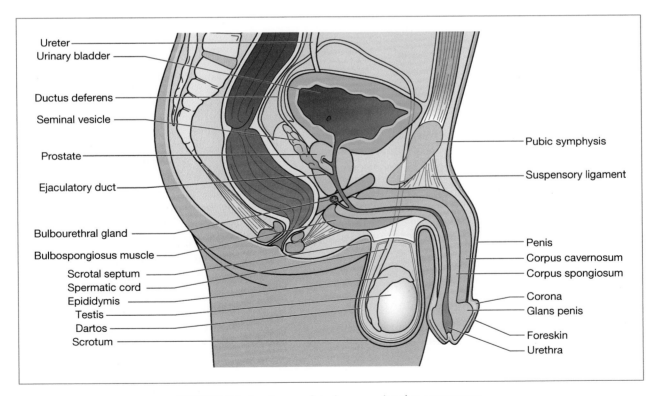

FIGURE 9.1 Anatomy of male reproductive structures.

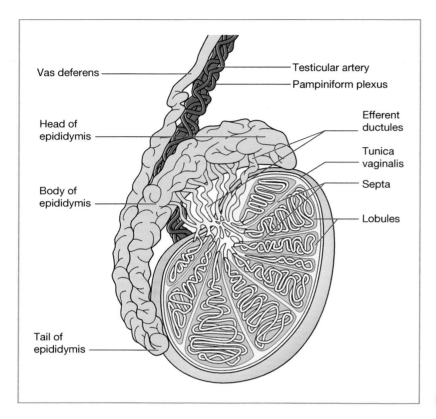

Vas deferens

Testicular artery
Pampiniform plexus

Head of
epididymis

Efferent
ductules

Tunica
vaginalis

Septa

Body of
epididymis

Lobules

Tail of
epididymis

FIGURE 9.2 Anatomy of the testis.

through the abdominal wall and the inguinal canal to the scrotum. As the testes descend into the scrotum, a tubular extension of peritoneum accompanies them. This tissue is obliterated during fetal development; the only remaining portion is that which covers the testes, the tunica vaginalis (Figure 9.2).

The testes are encased in the scrotum, which keeps them at a slightly lower temperature than the rest of the body to promote spermatogenesis. The testes have a dual function: Spermatogenesis (production of sperm) and secretion of the male sex hormone testosterone, which induces and maintains male sex characteristics. The testes consist of numerous seminiferous tubules in which the spermatozoa form; these are divided into segments within the testicle itself.

VAS DEFERENS AND SEMINAL VESICLES

Collecting tubules transmit the spermatozoa into the epididymis, a structure lying on the testes and which contains winding ducts that coalesce into the vas deferens. The vas is a firm, tubular structure that passes upward through the inguinal canal as part of the spermatic cord, entering the abdominal cavity behind the peritoneum. It then extends downward toward the base of the bladder. The vas ends in an elongated structure, the seminal vesicle, which can store some sperm short term and provides almost 50% of the ejaculate fluid volume. The tract is continued as the ejaculatory duct, which passes through the prostate gland to enter the urethra. Secretions from the seminal vesicles join secretions from the prostate and exit the penis during ejaculation.

THE PENIS

The penis has a dual function: It is the organ for copulation and for urination. Anatomically, it consists of the glans penis, the body, and the root (Figure 9.3). The glans penis is the soft, rounded portion at the distal end of the penis, and the urethra opens at the tip of the glans (meatal opening). The glans is naturally covered by elongated penile skin—the foreskin—which may be retracted to expose the glans. However, many men have had the foreskin removed (circumcision) as newborns. The body of the penis is composed of erectile tissues containing numerous blood vessels that become distended, leading to an erection during sexual excitement. The rigidity for the erection is due to blood distending the paired penile corpora, which are chambers that are covered with very tough connective tissue, the tunica albuginea. The urethra, which passes through the penis, extends from the bladder through the prostate to the distal end of the penis, ending at the meatal opening.

THE PROSTATE AND COWPER'S GLANDS

The prostate gland lies just below the neck of the bladder (see Figure 9.3). It surrounds the urethra and includes the ejaculatory duct, a continuation of the vas deferens. This gland produces a secretion that is chemically and physiologically suitable to the needs of the spermatozoa in their passage from the testes. The Cowper's gland lies below the prostate, within the posterior aspect of the urethra (see Figure 9.3). This gland empties its secretions into the urethra prior to and during ejaculation, providing lubrication.

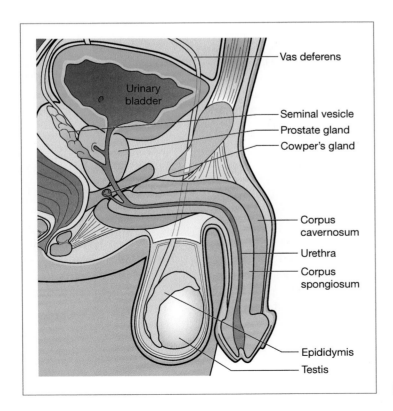

FIGURE 9.3 Anatomy of the penis.

Ejaculation requires a coordination of neurological impulses that close the bladder neck and contract the pelvic floor to promote the forward expulsion of semen. Erection and ejaculation are controlled by two distinct spinal cord reflex arcs; this contributes to the reflex erections seen in men with spinal cord injuries and men who had retroperitoneal surgery having a preserved ability to ejaculate without erections.

Screening Health Assessment and Normal Findings

Assessment of the male genitalia is accomplished with inspection and palpation; there is rarely a need for percussion or auscultation. The provider may need water-soluble lubricant and a penlight for examination of the scrotum. The penlight would be used to transilluminate the scrotum during an evaluation for a possible hydrocele or other mass. A stethoscope can be used to listen for bowel sounds if there is uncertainty about a hernia that has descended into the scrotal sac. Prior to any exam, the provider may want to measure his or her index finger for use as a ruler to measure the penis, testes, and prostate.

Examination of the male patient is best done in a warm room in order to avoid exaggeration and activation of the cremaster reflex. The genital examination includes inspection and palpation of the male genitalia. The genitourinary (GU) examination is a routine genital examination plus a digital rectal examination (DRE). Specialized examination maneuvers are indicated as needed. Facilities may differ in their chaperone policy for the male genital examination; the provider may wish to document that a chaperone was offered and/or declined for the male GU examination.

INSPECTION

The providers should observe for age-appropriate development of male secondary sex characteristics and Tanner stage (Table 9.1); lesions or scarring of the penis, scrotum, or groin; discoloration of the penis, scrotum, or groin; asymmetry of testicles; gynecomastia; hirsutism; location and size of the opening of the meatus; and presence of scars in the abdomen, groin, or inguinal areas. The tone of the dartos muscle governs the size of the scrotum; in a cool environment, it causes the scrotum to contract.

AUSCULTATION

Auscultate the abdomen as indicated based on suspected etiology for presentation complaint(s). Auscultation is rarely indicated in the evaluation of male reproductive complaints, except with a suspected herniation of bowel into the scrotum or as part of a complete physical.

PERCUSSION

Percuss the abdomen as indicated based on suspected etiology for presentation complaint(s). Percussion is rarely indicated in the evaluation of male reproductive complaints, except as part of a complete physical.

TABLE 9.1
Tanner Stages in Males

Stage	Characteristics		Testicular Size
I	Prepubertal		Volume: <4.0 mL Dimension: <2.5 cm
II	Scrotum: Growth and change in texture and color (reddens) Testes: Growth		Volume: >4.0 mL Dimension: 2.5–3.2 cm
III	Penis: Growth in length Testes: Growth		Volume: >10.0 mL Dimension: <3.6 cm
IV	Penis: Growth in breadth; development of glans Scrotum: Growth and darkening Testes: Growth		Volume: >16.0 mL Dimension: 4.1–4.5 cm
V	Adult genitalia		Volume: >25.0 mL Dimension: >4.5 cm

PALPATION

Palpation is the most important part of the male GU physical examination. This examination requires palpation of all suspected intrascrotal masses; these are masses that may arise from the surface of the testicle, adjacent to, or separate from the testis(es). Each testis must be assessed individually; in fact, each side of the scrotum is palpated separately (Figure 9.4). See Table 9.2 for examination maneuvers that can help assess the scrotal structures and aid in diagnosis.

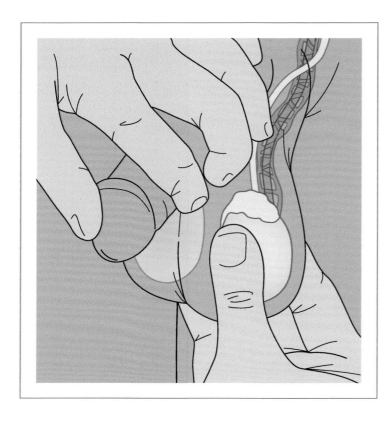

FIGURE 9.4 Palpation of the scrotum. Each side of the scrotum must be palpated separately.

TABLE 9.2
Physical Examination Maneuvers for Assessment of Male Reproductive System Complaints

Maneuver	Description	Demonstration
Cremasteric reflex	• Brushing or touching the skin of the scrotum in a downward direction can result in elevation of the testicle on the same side. • Reaction can be aggravated by a cool room; the reflex may engage prior to contact from examiner.	
Digital rectal examination	• Gloved, lubricated finger is inserted into the anus and swept from one side to the other across surface of the prostate. • Prostate should be symmetrical, nontender, free of nodules; approximately the size of a walnut; smooth, rubbery consistency. • Examination also involves estimation of anal sphincter tone. • Seminal vesicles are almost never palpable.	Bladder Prostate

(continued)

TABLE 9.2
Physical Examination Maneuvers for Assessment of Male Reproductive System Complaints (*continued*)

Maneuver	Description	Demonstration
Examination for hernia	• Index finger is inserted into scrotum from below, and scrotal skin is invaginated into the external inguinal ring. • Fingertips of opposite hand are placed over internal inguinal canal; patient should be asked to Valsalva or cough. • A hernia will be felt as a bulge that descends against the index finger with Valsalva maneuver/cough.	
Neurological examination	• Superficial anal reflex (perianal sensation): Stroking anus with a cotton swab will result in reflexive contraction of external anal sphincter ("anal wink"). • Bulbocavernosus reflex: Inserting gloved finger into anus and squeezing glans penis will result in contraction of anal sphincter and bulbocavernosus muscles. • These tests are most relevant if evaluating complaints of erectile and ejaculatory dysfunction.	
Transillumination of hydrocele	• Light source is shined through mass. • Hydrocele will glow reddish or orange. • May feel as though it surrounds testis. • May feel turbid or tense; rarely painful to exam.	
Transillumination of spermatocele	• Light source is shined through mass. • Testis palpated as separate from spermatocele. • Epididymis may not be palpated separately from a spermatocele. • Mass feels connected to testis at superior aspect.	
Valsalva maneuver to evaluate for varicocele	• Performed with patient standing and in a warm room. • Valsalva will reverse the flow into the pampiniform plexus of the scrotum. • Results in palpable distention of veins, "bag of worms," if varicocele is of sufficient size.	

Focused Health Assessment and Abnormal Findings

If this examination is part of a complete physical examination, progressing to the GU last allows time for the patient to become comfortable with the clinical interaction. Patient privacy should always be a primary concern; men should always be given the option for a companion to remain in the room during the exam.

Certain questions establish a direction for the male GU physical examination. The provider must ask about the presence of similar GU or functional complaints in the past, regardless of the presenting complaint and its apparent duration. Establish the start of puberty; asking if the patient started shaving at about the same time as classmates helps confirm normal physiological and endocrine development. Asking about previous paternity helps confirm that the patient's endocrine status was normal in the past (use their judgment about this line of questioning with younger men). Men should be asked about any activity that may put the groin at risk (contact sports, all-terrain vehicles, and cycling) and any potential exposure to environmental toxins.

Any presentation of GU complaints should involve a brief sexual history, including number and gender of partners and the history of using protection for sexual activity, as sexually transmitted infections (STI) can have a period of latency in men. Ideally, any history of unprotected sex should be disclosed, as well as new partners, onset of signs and symptoms of pain and/or discharge, and new lesions or skin abnormalities. Testing, evaluation, treatment, and reporting will proceed according to current Centers for Disease Control and Prevention guidelines.

Family history is also important in the context of GU complaints. Inquire about testicular and other GU malignancies specifically, a general history of any cancers, prostate or bladder problems in other family members (including female relatives with bladder conditions), and other members of the family with similar complaints to the patient's presenting complaint.

PAST SURGICAL HISTORY

Previous procedures may change the physical examination findings. Even in a young man, the history should include investigation of any procedures he may have had as an infant or small child and any surgery that may have compromised the structure or function of his reproductive or GU system. Surgeries when the patient was young can include orchidopexy, hernia repair (ask age at repair), and hypospadias or epispadias repair. In adult men, ask about hernia repair and presence/absence of mesh used for the repair, as well as previous prostate procedures. Always ask about a history of vasectomy, as many men do not consider this surgery, but it can help sort out any findings in the scrotum, such as an indurated epididymis.

PALPATION

See Table 9.3 for a guide to palpation of male reproductive structures, normal/abnormal findings, and possible etiology.

TABLE 9.3
Palpation of Male Reproductive Structures: Normal and Abnormal Findings

Structure	Normal Findings on Palpation	Abnormalities and Possible Etiology
Penis	• Soft and pliable along the length of the shaft • Average flaccid length 6 cm • Meatus midline and central to glans • Foreskin should retract and draw forward easily • Always remember to replace the prepuce back over glans when exam is complete	• Areas of fibrous plaque along shaft—Peyronie's disease, previous injury • Difficulty with foreskin retraction—phimosis, edema, balanitis, balanoposthitis • Difficulty moving foreskin forward—paraphimosis, edema • Entire shaft of penis fibrous and with reduced pliability—previous priapism • Meatus not midline, not central to glans, or positioned along length of shaft—hypospadias, epispadias • Firmness to glans may indicate malignancy, especially if uncircumcised male
Scrotum	• Loose sac of skin partially covered with hair; contains testes	• Areas of erythema or nodularity—infected sebaceous glands or hair follicles • Unilateral, uncomfortable swelling of the scrotum—testicular mass, hydrocele, hematoma, spermatocele, varicocele
Testes	• Two testes, freely movable within scrotum • Palpate between thumb and first two fingers of the hand • Firm, smooth, rubbery consistency • Average 6 cm × 4 cm in size • Rarely symmetrical, but should be close in size • Separate from epididymis	• Mass associated with testis—tumor, hydrocele, spermatocele • Solitary testes—nondescent of testis or previous surgical removal • Small, soft testis(es)—Klinefelter disease, history of infection/trauma, late orchidopexy
Epididymis	• Soft ridge of tissue longitudinally posterior to testis • Separate from testis	• Cystic or nodular—spermatocele, previous or current infection, history of vasectomy • Fluctuant or tense mass—spermatocele • Localized pain—epididymitis, epididymal cyst, postvasectomy pain syndrome

(continued)

TABLE 9.3
Palpation of Male Reproductive Structures: Normal and Abnormal Findings (*continued*)

Structure	Normal Findings on Palpation	Abnormalities and Possible Etiology
Vas deferens and spermatic cord	• Firm, rubbery consistency • Smooth along its length • Present from epididymis to inguinal canal	• Absence of vas bilaterally or unilaterally—cystic fibrosis or a variant • Sperm granuloma—postvasectomy • Congested veins unilaterally or bilaterally over spermatic cord—varicocele • Beading/nodularity of the cord—obstruction of epididymis, tubercular infection of the epididymis

Holistic Health Assessment

It is vital to note that no single speciality has claim to the arena of "men's health." Many specialties are involved in the emerging field of men's health from urology, cardiology, internal medicine, family practice, and psychology. This means that different providers will have different foci when examining and evaluating men, but also that the field is rich with multidisciplinary approaches to the care of men.

As with any body system, providers should establish duration and severity of the presenting complaint. Providers should also specifically ask about men's attempts at self-care and self-management of their concern, as it is well established that men are poor consumers of preventative care, and may turn to the Internet as their primary source of information. Providers should also address safety/distress, financial implications, and spiritual considerations with patients as needed.

CASE STUDY

DOCUMENTATION

Chief Complaint: Unilateral testicular swelling

History of Present Illness: Present to right scrotum for several years, but recently seems to have increased in size. Denies sexually transmitted infection risk, denies fever/chills/trauma to site. Some increased discomfort with prolonged sitting, standing, or tight clothing.

(continued)

(continued)

REVIEW OF SYSTEMS

Constitutional: No fever, chills, or malaise

Integumentary: Denies rashes or lesions to scrotum/groin

PHYSICAL EXAMINATION

General: Well appearing, no acute distress

Integumentary: No erythema or ecchymosis or open areas noted to scrotum/groin

Genitourinary: Nontender scrotal swelling noted. Unable to palpate right testis; left easily identified. + transillumination. Some retraction of the penis due to size of fluid collection.

Diagnosis: Right Hydrocele

ICD-10-CM Diagnosis Code: N43.3 Hydrocele, Unspecified

Assessment of Special Populations

ADOLESCENT POPULATION

Providers should be aware of the particular needs of the male adolescent within the anticipated developmental stage, as they work to establish an individual identity. While a lengthy discussion is beyond the scope of this chapter, providers should be ready to assess mental health, substance abuse, sexuality, family planning, immunizations, transition from the family home, unintentional injury and violence, and relationship issues as needed. This should also include an assessment of social media use, as teens may be more likely to use social media platforms for health information. Providers may also consider obesity screening and suicide risk assessment.

TRANSGENDER POPULATION

Transgender men (biological females who identify as male) require consideration in regard to their specific health needs, especially relative to genital complaints and reproductive health needs. This includes a transgender-welcoming clinic environment and focus on safety and education, including education regarding egg or embryo cryopreservation. Genital examination should not be completed unless it is relevant to the presenting complaint. Health maintenance and screening are the same as for other patients. Transgender men should be empowered by the clinical environment and feel that providers are open to all questions and concerns. This is especially important with sexual health concerns, as they may have partners of both sexes and may require access to a reliable provider for hormone management and birth control. Assessment of high-risk sexual practices is vitally important in this population.

Not all transgender men proceed with full reassignment surgery; in addition to hysterectomy, many will seek testosterone management and breast reduction, along with possible aesthetic procedures such as liposuction.

Transgender women (biological males who identify as female) can present with issues such as testicular pain or prostate infection. Cryopreservation of sperm may be of interest to this population. Not all transgender women proceed with full reassignment surgery, but many will undergo breast implants and bilateral orchiectomy. Some will also pursue thyroid cartilage reduction and electrolysis. Health maintenance and screening are the same as for other male patients, including monitoring prostate-specific antigen (PSA) as they age.

Transgender youth also require special considerations, as their specific health needs are superimposed on emerging personal identity and sexual identification. Management of these patients can be quite complex, as they may be seen as a particularly vulnerable population that may need the consent of a parent for hormone management.

SEXUAL FUNCTION ASSESSMENT

Male sexuality is a complex phenomenon that is strongly influenced by personal, cultural, and social factors; some men will not be comfortable discussing these domains with female providers. Sexual function can become altered in the presence of illness and comorbidities such as diabetes and cardiovascular disease.

Providers should also be aware that standard men's health questionnaires represent a heterosexual, heteronormative perspective, and do not offer the opportunity to assess sexual function concerns for LGBTQ (lesbian, gay, bisexual, transgender, and queer) patients.

ELDERLY POPULATION

As men age, the prostate gland enlarges, prostate secretion decreases, the scrotum may hang lower, the external portion of the penile shaft may become less pronounced, the testes become smaller and less firm, and pubic hair becomes sparser. The sexual response cycle slows, attaining an erection takes longer, and full erections may not be attained until climax, although sexual function is also affected by any comorbidities that may be present. Reproductive capacity is maintained until death, although sperm production may suffer with weight gain and other comorbidities. Older men may also have functional or cognitive issues that contribute to urinary urgency and possible continence issues.

PATIENTS WITH DISABILITIES

Men with disabilities may present with disorders that affect their mobility or cause weakness or sensory changes in the lower extremities, which may create challenges with transfer to the examination table, as well as changes in bladder control. These may occur in patients with spinal cord injury, spina bifida, multiple sclerosis, or other neurological disorders. It is important to ask these patients about how they manage bladder control, and if the bladder management strategy is effective. The patient in a wheelchair or one who uses assistive devices, such as a cane, walker, or crutches, should be transferred to the examination table and have an exam as thorough as that of any other patient. If a patient has cognitive impairment and impaired recall, family members or caregivers may be able to provide details of the patient's voiding history.

VETERAN POPULATION

A detailed military history is vital, especially in the context of an endocrine or fertility evaluation; note should be made of known or suspected exposure to chemicals that are known to be spermatotoxic (e.g., hydrocarbons) or radiation exposure. The Veterans Administration mandates some coverage for fertility care for men, so men with suspected or confirmed fertility issues should be encouraged to check with their local Veterans Affairs medical center (VAMC).

ELITE ATHLETE POPULATION

Complaints in this population are more the result of the specific type of activity. Marathon runners can have issues with groin and pelvic floor complaints and can have exacerbations of varicocele pain. Distance cyclists may also report pelvic floor numbness and numbness to the penis due to pressure from the horn of the bicycle seat. Elite athletes are at risk for a paradoxical hypogonadism; their extreme exercise regimen can result in such a significant physiological stress that the hypothalamic-pituitary-gonadal axis becomes suppressed. Men who engage in mixed martial arts and competitive weight lifting may also "cycle" anabolic steroids, but the true incidence of this is unknown.

Diagnostic Reasoning

Common Differential Diagnoses: Male Genitourinary System	
Diagnosis	**Key History or Physical Examination Differentiators**
Balanitis	• Increased incidence with uncircumcised males, very obese males with a retracted penis, and men with poorly controlled diabetes mellitus
	• Commonly caused by *Candida albicans*
	• Penile edema, erythema, and pain of the glans; dysuria; urethral discharge; history of discharge from between foreskin and glans
	• GU exam: Will confirm edema, erythema, and exudates; examine for any inguinal adenopathy
Epididymitis (Figure 9.5)	• Spread of an infection from the bladder or urethra
	• Increased risk with uncircumcised men, men with indwelling catheters, men with BPH
	• Heterosexual men younger than 35: Causative organisms—*Neisseria gonorrhoeae* and *Chlamydia trachomatis*
	• Homosexual men: Causative organism—*Escherichia coli*
	• Sudden onset (over 24–48 hours) of painful swelling in the scrotum
	• Urethral discharge and/or fever, complaints of urethritis/cystitis
	• GU exam: Pain will localize to the affected epididymis with palpation; spermatic cord tender and swollen
Erectile dysfunction	• Underlying causes: Arteriogenic, venogenic, endocrinologic, neurological, psychological, medicinal
	• History of declining erectile function
	• GU exam: With recognized chronic conditions, the focus should be on the routine genital examination along with a cardiovascular examination

(continued)

Common Differential Diagnoses: Male Genitourinary System (*continued*)	
Diagnosis	**Key History or Physical Examination Differentiators**
Hydrocele	• Collection of fluid between the layers of the tunica vaginalis • Often occurs unilaterally • Origin idiopathic in adult men • Not usually painful • Heaviness or discomfort during prolonged standing/sitting • GU exam: Confirmed with transillumination
Hypogonadism	• Possible fatigue, truncal obesity, atrophic testes, loss of facial and pubic hair, decreased muscle bulk • GU exam: Typically unhelpful; full examination may demonstrate some regression of secondary sexual characteristics, decline in muscle bulk
Klinefelter syndrome	• Incidence of 1:500 male births • Delayed completion of puberty, delayed virilization • GU exam: Lack of development of secondary sexual characteristics (small [<3 cm] atrophic testes, small phallus, diminished body hair, diminished muscle bulk) and feminine (i.e., truncal), rather than male, fat distribution
Orchitis	• Extension of an infection from the epididymis to the testis • Increased risk with uncircumcised men, men with indwelling catheters, men with BPH • Heterosexual men younger than 35: Causative organisms—*Neisseria gonorrhoeae* and *Chlamydia trachomatis* • Homosexual men: Causative organism—*Escherichia coli* • Occurs in up to 30% of prepubertal male patients with mumps • May be urethral discharge and/or fever, complaints of urethritis/cystitis; reactive hydrocele may form
Peyronie's disease	• Progressive curvature of the shaft of penis with erection • May be a history of trauma to penile shaft that occurred during intercourse • GU exam: Evidence of palpable plaque that involves tunica albuginea
Phimosis (Figure 9.6)	• Uncircumcised males only • History of progressive difficulty at retracting the foreskin • Possible setting of recurrent UTIs • GU exam: Opening of foreskin has contracted to the point at which the actual opening is quite small

(continued)

Common Differential Diagnoses: Male Genitourinary System (*continued*)

Diagnosis	Key History or Physical Examination Differentiators
Spermatocele	• Painless mass in the head of the epididymis • Contains fluid and sperm • May complain of scrotal mass—"like a third testicle" • GU exam: Nontender mass, clearly distinct from and above testis on palpation
Testicular mass	• Acute onset of a painful or tender testis or swelling; possible discomfort for several months • GU exam: Pain or tenderness on examination; may localize to affected testis
Testicular or scrotal pain	• Trauma may precede complaint of pain • Acute pain or progressive pain • History of recurrent scrotal infections and current constitutional symptoms • GU exam: May reveal generalized tenderness of scrotum and its contents, unilateral scrotal swelling, localized tenderness to one or more scrotal structures
Testicular torsion (Figure 9.7)	• Most commonly seen in early puberty; no established risk factors • Swelling and tissue necrosis after 6–8 hours • Acute and sudden onset of pain that localizes to affected testis • Abdominal discomfort, nausea, and vomiting • GU exam: Traditional landmarks within the scrotum may be difficult to assess because of edema • **Urological emergency**
Varicocele	• Palpable or visible dilation of vessels of pampiniform plexus • More common on the left; due to greater distance, internal spermatic vein must traverse to the left renal vein • No specific risk factors; present in 15%–20% of men • Asymptomatic • GU exam: Can be exaggerated during physical examination with Valsalva maneuver while standing; distention of pampiniform plexus should disappear when the patient lies down; long-standing varicocele may cause testicular atrophy • If varicocele is large, it may be visible during inspection (classic "bag of worms" description).

BPH, benign prostatic hypertrophy; GU, genitourinary; UTI, urinary tract infection.

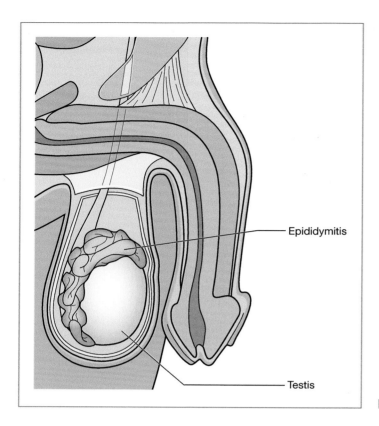

FIGURE 9.5 Epididymitis.

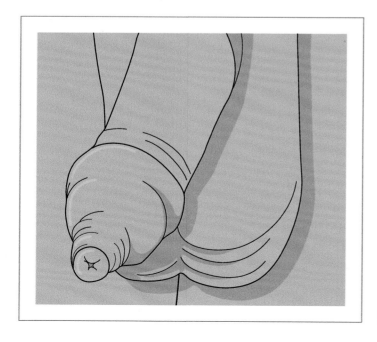

FIGURE 9.6 Phimosis.

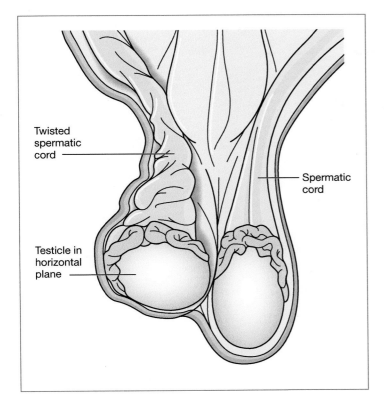

Twisted
spermatic
cord

Spermatic
cord

Testicle in
horizontal
plane

FIGURE 9.7 Testicular torsion. Note side-lie presentation.

BIBLIOGRAPHY

Burns, J. (2019). Adolescent males and the media. In S. A. Quallich (Ed.), *Manual of men's health: A practice guide for APRNs and PAs* (pp. 57–74). New York, NY: Springer Publishing Company.

Fleming, P. J., Lee, J. G., & Dworkin, S. L. (2014). "Real men don't cry": Constructions of masculinity and inadvertent harm in public health interventions. *American Journal of Public Health, 104*(6), 1029–1035. doi:10.2105/AJPH.2013.301820

Workowski, K. A., & Bolan, G. A. (2015). Sexually transmitted diseases treatment guidelines, 2015. *Morbidity and Mortality Weekly Report: Recommendations and Reports, 64*(3), 1–140. Retrieved from https://www.cdc.gov/std/tg2015/tg-2015-print.pdf

10

ADVANCED ASSESSMENT OF THE FEMALE REPRODUCTIVE SYSTEM

Angela Richard-Eaglin
Jacquelyn McMillian-Bohler

CHAPTER CONTENTS

(continued)

ASSESSMENT OF SPECIAL POPULATIONS
Transgender Population
Elderly Population
Pregnant Population
Pediatric Population
Patients With Disabilities
Veteran Population

GENOMICS AND GENETICS

DIAGNOSTIC REASONING
Common Differential Diagnoses: Female Genitourinary Complaints

Overview of Anatomy and Physiology

Accurate assessment of female reproductive system–related complaints is highly contingent on provider familiarity with the structures and functions of the female anatomy. Examination skills and recognition of abnormal findings is enriched when providers are knowledgeable about female anatomy. Comprehensive evaluation of the female patient must include a thorough and relevant history, followed by accurate assessment of relevant structures within the female reproductive system. This not only assists providers with differential diagnosis and diagnostic reasoning, but also guides formulation of a definitive diagnosis.

The female reproductive system is a sophisticated and unique system that has several functions, including interaction with other body systems that help to regulate and aid proper reproductive function. It is composed of internal and external structures, and includes the urinary system; hence, it is often referred to as the female genitourinary system. While the basic structures within the female reproductive system are often the same as a result of developmental dysfunctions that occur in utero, there may be variants in the appearance of the anatomical structures in some women. As a whole, the primary functions of the female reproductive system are reproduction, hormone balance, elimination of waste products, and aiding regulation of body fluid composition and volume.

EXTERNAL GENITALIA

The visible external structures of the female reproductive system are commonly referred to as the vulva or pudendum (Figure 10.1) and are identified by inspection. These structures include the mons pubis, labia (labia majora and labia minora), clitoris, vestibule, Skene and Bartholin glands, hymen, and the vaginal orifice. Vulva varies in size and appearance from woman to woman based on the volume of adipose tissue, length, and color of the labia. Pigmentation may be pink, brown, gray, or black.

MONS PUBIS

The mons pubis is the pad-like area of the vulva located over the symphysis pubis. During puberty, a triangular pattern of hair growth occurs in this area. It is comprised of fatty tissue and its function is to protect the symphysis pubis during sexual intercourse.

LABIA

LABIA MAJORA

During the embryonic stage, labia majora are homologous to the scrotum in males. The labia majora are the two fused longitudinal skin folds that extend anteriorly from the base of the mons pubis to the anterior perineum, where they form the posterior commissure. The inner aspects of the labia are smooth and hairless, while the outer edges are covered with hair. Variants in appearance may be present due to the amount of fat within the tissue. Other causes for variations in appearance are related to childbirth. In nulliparous women, the labia are close together. In multiparous women, the labia become less prominent. The labia majora help to keep the vaginal introitus closed, thus aiding in infection prevention.

LABIA MINORA

The labia minora are two smaller, nonfatty, smooth, and hairless skin folds that are located between the labia majora and the vaginal introitus. They form the enclosure for the urinary meatus and the vaginal opening. The superior aspect of the labia minora is divided into two lamellae, which fuse to form the prepuce of the clitoris. The inferior lamellae join to form the frenulum of the clitoris. The fourchette, which is located just above the perineum, is formed by the fusion of the lower ridges of the labia minora. The size and shape of the labia minora vary among women. Visualization of the labia minora in nulliparous women may not be apparent without separation

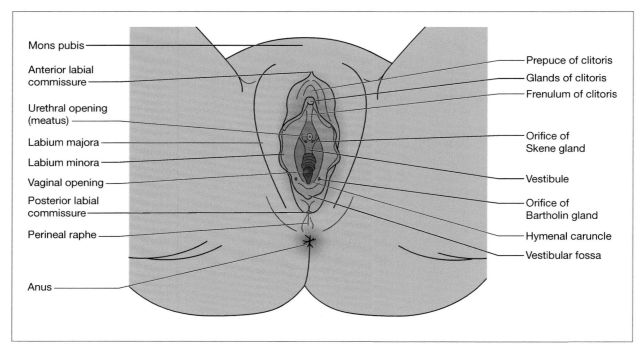

Mons pubis

Anterior labial commissure

Urethral opening (meatus)

Labium majora

Labium minora

Vaginal opening

Posterior labial commissure

Perineal raphe

Anus

Prepuce of clitoris

Glands of clitoris

Frenulum of clitoris

Orifice of Skene gland

Vestibule

Orifice of Bartholin gland

Hymenal caruncle

Vestibular fossa

FIGURE 10.1 Female vulva or pudendum. External vaginal structures include the mons pubis, labia (majora and minora), clitoris, urethral meatus, vestibule, Skene and Bartholin glands, hymen, and vaginal orifice.

of the labia majora. However, in multiparous women, the labia minora may protrude through the labia majora.

CLITORIS

The clitoris is the female equivalent of the male penis. It contains erectile tissue and is the primary erogenous organ within the female reproductive system. It is located in the superior aspect of the vulva, just above the frenulum. The clitoris varies in size from 1.5 to 2 cm in length. While it is composed of three types of tissue—the glans, a corporus, and two crura—the glans is the only visible portion. Along with those on the labia majora and labia minora, the clitoris has several nerve endings that work together during sexual arousal and sexual activity.

VESTIBULE

The vestibule is a triangular-shaped area that is located between the clitoris and the introitus of the vagina, and extends to the fourchette. The urethra (urinary meatus), vagina, Bartholin gland ducts, and the Skene glands are located within the vestibule. The urethral meatus is located immediately anterior to the vaginal orifice. The two Skene glands, also referred to as the paraurethral ducts, are usually located on each side of the urethral opening. They release mucus that aids in vaginal moisture. Bartholin glands also contain two ducts that are bilaterally located outside of the posterior aspect of the vaginal orifice. During sexual arousal, Bartholin glands secrete mucus that provides lubrication to the vagina. Bartholin glands may become blocked and develop infection and cyst and/ or abscess formation. In such cases, surgical intervention for incision and drainage may be necessary.

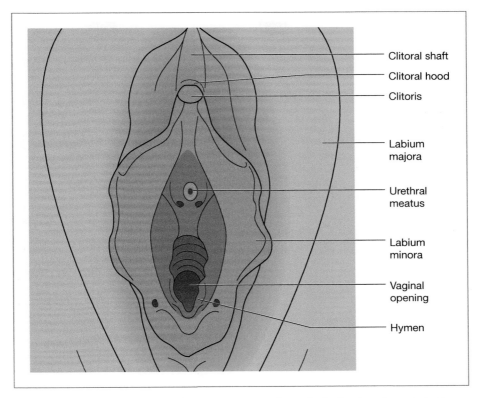

FIGURE 10.2 External vaginal structures. These include the clitoral shaft and hood, clitoris, labia majora, labia minora, urethral meatus, vaginal opening, and hymen.

VAGINAL ORIFICE AND HYMEN

The vaginal orifice (opening, introitus) is located behind the urethra and is enclosed within the labia minora in most virginal women. The hymen is located at the vaginal entrance (Figure 10.2). It is a thin membrane that is made mostly of collagenous connective tissue. The hymen varies in shape and thickness among females.

INTERNAL GENITALIA

The vagina, uterus, cervix, fallopian tubes, and ovaries make up the internal genitalia (Figure 10.3).

VAGINA

The vagina begins at the external vulva and extends to the uterine cervix. The vagina canal is composed of musculomembranous, connective, and erectile tissue. The uppermost portion of the vagina lies horizontally and terminates around the cervix to form the anterior and posterior fornix. It measures approximately 9 to 10 cm in length and lies posterior to the bladder and anterior to the rectum. The vaginal mucosa is pink and is situated within the transverse folds that are also commonly referred to as rugae. These rugae, along with the high elasticity of the vagina, allow vaginal distention during sexual intercourse and vaginal childbirth. Postmenopausal women who are multiparous may have smooth rugae. Estrogen and the

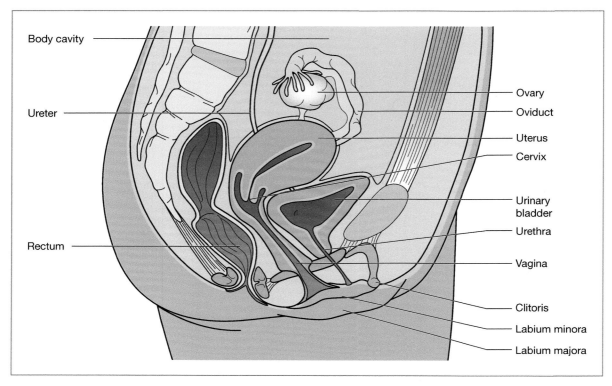

Body cavity

Ureter

Rectum

Ovary
Oviduct
Uterus
Cervix
Urinary bladder
Urethra
Vagina
Clitoris
Labium minora
Labium majora

FIGURE 10.3 Internal female genitalia (sagittal view). These structures include the ovaries, fallopian tubes, uterus, cervix, and the vagina.

mucous-producing cells of the vagina aid in vaginal lubrication during intercourse. The balance of normal vaginal flora and prevention of infections is the result of its acidic pH.

UTERUS

The uterus is a thick, hollow fibromuscular reproductive organ that resembles the shape of an inverted pear (Figure 10.4). It is made of connective and smooth muscle tissue and is located within the pelvis between the urinary bladder and the rectum. The uterus is divided into two main parts: The globe-shaped upper portion, which is the body, also known as the corpus; and the cervix, which is the lower part that opens into the vagina. The uppermost part of the corpus, known as the fundus, is composed mainly of muscle. The corpus composition allows for expansion to hold a growing fetus

during pregnancy, and it allows for adequacy of contractions during labor and delivery.

The corpus (body) of the uterine wall is made of three layers: Serosal, muscular, and mucosal. The outermost layer covering the uterus is the serosal layer, which is formed by the peritoneum. This layer keeps the uterus separate from the abdominal cavity. The muscular middle layer is known as the myometrium, and it makes up the largest portion of the uterus. It is composed of smooth muscle and connective tissue. The third and innermost mucosal layer is known as the endometrium. The normal endometrium is a thin, pink layer of tissue that lines the uterine cavity in nonpregnant women. During the reproductive years, part of the uterine lining is shed with menstruation and pregnancy. Endometriosis is an aberration that occurs when endometrial tissue grows outside of the uterus. Endometrial thickness varies and is dependent on the amount of estrogen and progesterone influence on the individual woman.

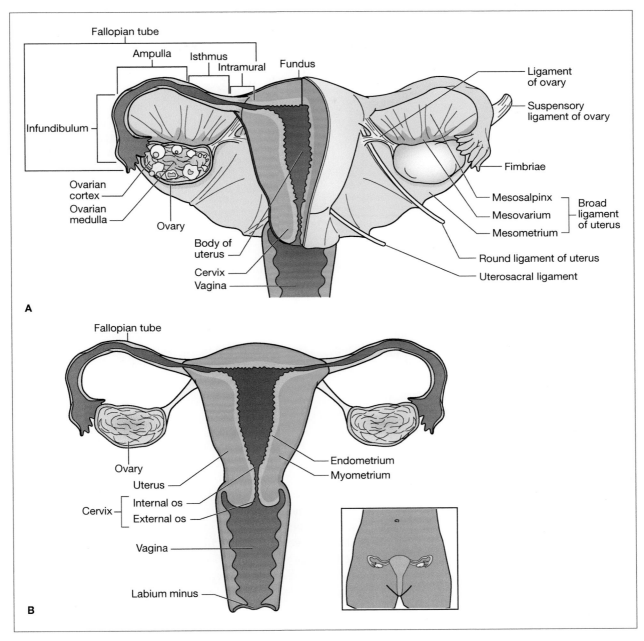

FIGURE 10.4 Uterine structures. (**A**) Sagittal view of the uterine fundus, ovaries, fallopian tubes, cervix, and vagina. (**B**) External and frontal views of uterine structures. External and frontal views of portions of the uterus, fallopian tubes, ovaries, cervix (internal and external os), and vagina.

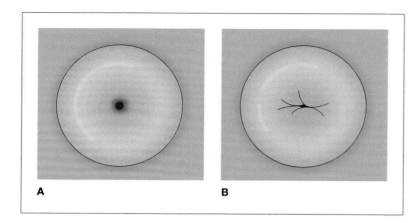

FIGURE 10.5 The cervical os. A nulliparous cervix (**A**) is smooth and pink with a round os. A multiparous cervix (**B**) is pink with a thin, narrow os, and is not as smooth as a nulliparous cervix; it may be described as resembling a "fish mouth."

CERVIX

The inferior portion of the uterus is called the cervix. The average length of the cervix is 3 to 5 cm. The opening of the cervix that is visualized through the vagina is called the external cervical os. During labor and delivery, the internal os dilates to allow the passage of the fetus. The endocervix is the canal that connects the uterus and vagina and allows sperm penetration for potential reproduction and blood evacuation during menstruation. In nulliparous women, the cervical os is round (Figure 10.5A); in multiparous women, it is a transverse slit (Figure 10.5B).

FALLOPIAN TUBES

The fallopian tubes, also referred to as oviducts, average in length from 8 to 14 cm. They are located bilaterally at the superior aspect of the uterine body. The ovaries are encircled by the fimbriae, which are located at the distal ends of the fallopian tubes. The main function of the fallopian tubes is transportation of ovum for fertilization and transport of fertilized ova to the uterus for implantation. The three parts of the fallopian tube are the isthmus, ampulla, and infundibulum.

OVARIES

Ovaries are female reproductive glands located on each side of the uterus, encircled by the fimbria of the fallopian tubes. The ovaries are responsible for the production of ova (eggs). The ovaries are oval shaped and appear to be grayish in color. The actual size of an ovary varies based on age and hormonal levels. During childbearing years, ovarian size is approximately 3 to 5 cm in length. During menopause, the ovaries become smaller and atrophic.

Screening Health Assessment and Normal Findings

HEALTH HISTORY

A detailed and relevant history is one of the most important components of any provider visit because it guides accurate diagnosis and treatment. Prior to beginning a gynecological exam, the provider should attempt to establish a trusting relationship by making her feel comfortable and relaxed. Assumptions should not be made about the patient's sexual orientation or level of sexual activity based on appearance. Introduction to the patient and obtaining the history should be done prior to asking the patient to disrobe. The patient should be interviewed privately (alone) unless circumstances requiring assistance are present, such as communication barriers (language or hearing). Inform the patient that you will be asking questions that may seem personal or intimate and explain the reasoning for this. Questions should be straightforward, open ended, and phrased using nonjudgmental language and should progress from broad to focused, more sensitive and intimate. It is essential for the provider to maintain self-awareness (body language, verbal responses to patient answers) during the interview. This promotes a supportive and trusting patient–provider relationship that facilitates honest transfer of information.

ESSENTIAL ELEMENTS OF A FEMALE REPRODUCTIVE HEALTH HISTORY

There are essential leading and follow-up questions that must be asked. The questions in the list that follows are examples and not exhaustive. Detailed and specific questions related to the chief complaint (CC) should be asked to elicit adequate information to arrive at a diagnosis and formulate a treatment plan.

MENSTRUAL HISTORY

- **Age at menarche:** How old were you when you got your first period?
- **Days bleeding:** How many days does your period last?
- **Length of cycle:** How often do your periods occur (i.e., days between cycles)?
- **Regularity:**
  - Are your periods regular (i.e., occur at the same time each month)?
  - Have you ever had irregular periods?
  - Describe your menstrual flow.

OBSTETRIC HISTORY

- How many times have you been pregnant?
- How many babies did you carry to term?

- How many preterm births have you had?
- How many live births have you had? How many living children do you have?
- Have you had any stillbirths?
- Have you had any miscarriages? How many?
- Have you had any elective abortions? How many?
- Were your babies delivered vaginally or via cesarean (C-section)?
- Are you still able to get pregnant? Did you have a tubal ligation?

SEXUAL HISTORY

- Do you have any concerns regarding sex?
- Have you ever had sexual intercourse? Are you currently sexually active?
- **Recent activity:** When was your last episode of sexual intercourse?
- **Relationships:** Are you currently in a relationship? If so, is it monogamous?
- **Practices:**
  - Do you have sex with men, women, or both?
  - Do you have sex with men who have sex with men?
  - What types of sexual practices do you engage in—oral, vaginal, anal, or all three?
- **Partners:**
  - How many partners have you had in your lifetime?
  - How many partners have you had in the last 3 months?
  - How many partners have you had in the last month?
  - How many partners do you currently have?
  - Do you have any new sexual partners?
- **Family planning and prevention:**
  - Are you trying to conceive?
  - Are you using contraception? If so, what type of contraception do you use?

- ○ What measures are you using to prevent pregnancy?
- ○ Are you interested in starting a method of contraceptive?
- ○ What measures are you taking to prevent sexually transmitted diseases (STDs)?

SCREENING HISTORY (IF APPROPRIATE)

- **Cervical:**
  - ○ When was your last Papanicolaou (Pap) smear? Was it normal?
  - ○ Have you ever had an abnormal Pap smear? If so, what was the result?
- **Breasts:**
  - ○ When was your last mammogram? Was it normal?
  - ○ Have you ever had an abnormal mammogram? If so, what was the result?
  - ○ Have you ever had a breast ultrasound, biopsy, or needle aspiration? If so, what was the result?
- **Sexually transmitted diseases/infections:**
  - ○ Have you ever had any sexually transmitted diseases? If so, what were you diagnosed with? Did you get treated? Was your partner treated? Did you and your partner abstain from intercourse until you both completed the entire course of treatment or for at least a total of 7 days following a single-dose treatment?
  - ○ Were you ever screened for HIV? If so, what was the result? When was your last screening?
  - ○ Are you interested in sexually transmitted infection (STI)/HIV screening?

GYNECOLOGICAL AND BREAST HISTORY

Do you have a past history of any of the following?

- Ovarian cysts or uterine masses (benign [fibroids] or malignant)
- Endometriosis
- Polycystic ovarian syndrome (PCOS)

- Infertility
- Breast cysts or nodules/masses (fibroadenomas)
- Gynecological procedures for abnormal findings—laparoscopic procedures, biopsies, or hysterectomy

PAST MEDICAL HISTORY

- Do you have any chronic medical conditions/diseases?
- Do you take medications for any chronic illnesses?

FAMILY HISTORY

- Have any of your first-degree relatives been diagnosed with breast cancer, cervical cancer, ovarian cancer, or uterine cancer?

PAST SURGICAL HISTORY

- What, if any, surgical procedures have you had? When (date/year)?

SOCIAL HISTORY

- How often do you drink alcohol? What type of alcoholic beverages do you consume? How many drinks do you usually have?
- Do you smoke cigarettes or use any other type of tobacco products? How long have you been a smoker? How many cigarettes or packs of cigarettes do you smoke per day?
- Do you use marijuana or any other illicit drugs?
- Do you take medications that are not prescribed to you, such as opioid/narcotic medications, pain relievers, anxiety medications, attention deficit disorder/attention deficit hyperactivity disorder (ADD/ADHD) medications, and so forth?

REVIEW OF SYSTEMS

As part of a focused exam, the following systems should also be reviewed:

- **General:** Fever, chills, fatigue, malaise
  - ○ Rationale: May indicate underlying infection (e.g., pelvic inflammatory disease [PID]), cancer, or hormonal alterations

- **Cardiovascular:** Chest pain or discomfort, palpitations
  - ○ Rationale: Cardiovascular disease is the leading cause of death in women in the United States. Every opportunity for early detection and treatment should be seized.
- **Respiratory:** Dyspnea, shortness of breath, orthopnea
  - ○ Rationale: Underlying infectious condition or respiratory disease
- **Gastrointestinal:** Nausea, vomiting, abdominal pain.
  - ○ Rationale: May be a result of pregnancy in women of reproductive age; may indicate underlying infection or disease process
- **Genitourinary:** Abdominal pain, vaginal discharge, dysuria, urinary urgency, urinary frequency, flank pain
  - ○ Rationale: May indicate urinary tract infection (UTI), STI, nephrolithiasis
- **Neurological (elderly patients):** Mental status
  - ○ Rationale: Altered mental status may indicate a UTI in elderly patients

PHYSICAL EXAMINATION

Clinical breast examination is a key component of a well-woman exam. The exam should begin with careful inspection of the breasts, followed by systematic palpation.

INSPECTION OF THE FEMALE BREASTS

With the patient standing or sitting up with her arms at her sides, inspect the breasts for the following (Figure 10.6):

- **Symmetry:** It is normal for one breast to be slightly larger than the other, but the provider should note any gross differences.
- **Size:** Inspect the size of the breasts in terms of appropriateness for developmental stage.
- **Shape:** The normal breast is typically round. Note any distortions from the norm.
- **Skin characteristics:** Note color. Inspect for dimpling, lesions, erythematous areas, or other aberrations.
- **Nipples:** Note size, shape, position (inverted, everted, or flat), and presence of discharge.

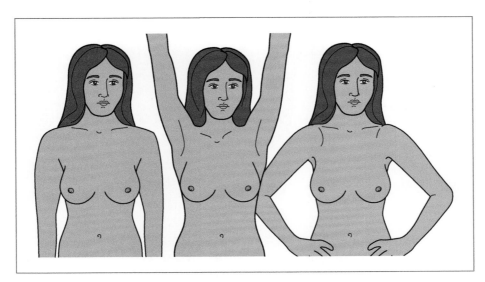

FIGURE 10.6 Positions for breast inspection. Inspection of breasts for symmetry requires specific positioning, including arms at sides, both arms raised, and hands on hips.

Next in the inspection phase of the exam, the provider will assess for breast aberrations that occur with movement. As the patient raises her arms above her head, observe for tethering of breast tissue to the chest wall. The provider may also observe for the movement of the breast tissue by asking the patient to place her hands on her hips and arch her back.

PALPATION OF THE FEMALE BREASTS

There are three different palpation techniques that can be used during the clinical breast exam (Figure 10.7). The provider's primary responsibility is to ensure that the exam includes palpation of all breast tissue, bilaterally. This includes palpation of the areola and the nipple. The proper technique for palpation is to use the pads of the middle three fingers, rather than the finger tips. During palpation, the provider should apply steady pressure, moving the fingers in a spiral motion. Different levels of pressure should be applied from superficial down to the level of the chest wall to ensure comprehensive evaluation of the tissue.

Due to the combination of lobular, ductal, and other supporting tissue, normal breast tissue feels lumpy in consistency. Aside from these normal findings, the breast should not contain any masses or nodules. The provider should note any nodules, masses, or lymphadenopathy. Often, lumps palpated during the clinical breast exam are benign fibroadenomas or cysts, which are mobile and have clearly defined borders. Firm, immobile/fixed masses with irregular or difficult to define borders are of concern and warrant further evaluation (i.e., diagnostic mammogram). It is also important to note that as women age, lobular tissue is replaced with fatty tissue, which decreases density of the breasts. For this reason, breast masses are easier to identify in older women.

VERTICAL STRIPS TECHNIQUE

With the patient sitting up, begin palpating in a spiral motion at the medial portion of the chest wall and end just below the posterior aspect of breast

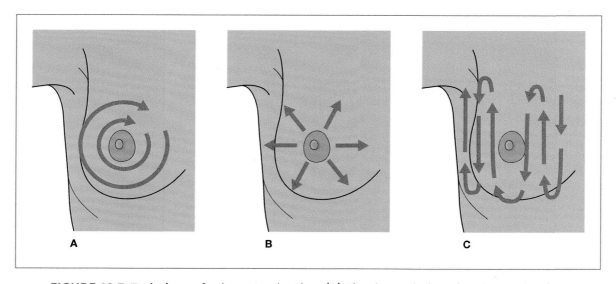

FIGURE 10.7 Techniques for breast palpation. (**A**) Circular technique involves palpation of the breast in a circular pattern. (**B**) Wedge technique involves separation of the breast into wedges or slices and palpation of each wedge. (**C**) Vertical strip technique involves palpation of the breast in a vertical pattern moving up and down the breast.

tissue. Using the dominant hand, palpate downward and then upward without lifting the fingers from the breast. For larger breasts, place the nondominant hand under the breasts to hold it up and enhance ability to palpate effectively. Palpate with the dominant hand. It is important to note that this technique may not be ideal for a woman with larger breasts, as it may be difficult to ensure effective examination of the entire breast tissue. Next, using the same spiral motion, palpate the tail of the breast and the axilla. Repeat the technique with the opposite breast.

CIRCULAR TECHNIQUE

With the patient lying flat, ask her to raise the arm of the breast being examined behind the head to stretch the breast tissue against the chest wall. Starting at the nipple, palpate the breast using spiral motions, moving in a circular pattern toward the periphery until all breast tissue is examined, including the tail.

WEDGE OR "SPOKES" OF A WHEEL TECHNIQUE

With the patient in a lying or sitting position, the breast is separated into quadrants resembling the spokes in a wheel or wedge, with the nipple at the center of the "wheel."

Starting at the nipple, palpate outward toward the periphery of the wedge (section of the breast) that is being examined. Using the spiral motion with the pads of the fingers, palpate a few centimeters at a time in each wedge until the entire section is palpated. Move to the next wedge after the entire breast, its tail, and its outer edges have been palpated.

GYNECOLOGICAL EXAMINATION

Prior to the patient entering the exam room, equipment should be gathered and set up in a way that ensures a systematic exam (Table 10.1).

Because of the intimate nature of the pelvic examination, preparation is one of the most crucial elements. Make sure that the temperature in the room is comfortable and gather and assemble all equipment before the patient enters the exam room. This ensures that the examination is efficient and timely, and that the provider is compassionate and considerate. Before beginning the exam, have the patient go to the restroom to empty her bladder.

TABLE 10.1
Equipment Used in a Pelvic Gynecological Exam

Equipment	Rationale
An adequate light source	A light source should be bright enough to allow adequate visualization of the internal vagina and cervix.
A portable table or stand	Provides a place to organize equipment to ensure systematic examination and collection of specimens. Although a chaperone should be present, if an exam must be performed alone, the portable table allows placement of equipment within reach.

(continued)

TABLE 10.1
Equipment Used in a Pelvic Gynecological Exam (*continued*)

Equipment	Rationale
Nonsterile gloves (optional: two pair)	Wearing gloves is a part of universal precautions. Nonsterile gloves are appropriate for a routine female exam on a nonpregnant woman. Many providers choose to double-glove so that the outer pair may be removed after the examination to prevent contamination of specimen collection tubes.
A metal or plastic speculum of appropriate size (You may use the patient's weight and height measurements to approximate the size. If necessary, you may change the size. Make sure to have more than one size available in the exam room.)	It is necessary to use the appropriately sized speculum to prevent and/or limit discomfort associated with speculum insertion/placement.
Water-soluble lubricant	Water-soluble lubrication eases discomfort during the digital vaginal exam.
Large cotton-tipped swabs	These are used for cleaning mucus, discharge, or any other fluids from the cervix to ensure adequate visualization.
If performing a Pap smear: ○ Media for preparing cervical cytological samples: Liquid-based solution ○ Sample collection tools: Spatula, cytobrush or broom, sample collection bag	Special media are necessary for collecting endocervical cells for cervical cancer screening.
Gonorrhea and chlamydia test kit (if applicable)	The USPSTF recommends screening sexually active women at age 24, as well as younger and older women who are at high risk for infection.

USPSTF, United States Preventive Services Task Force.

It is important to establish rapport with the patient prior to beginning the examination. Explain the purpose of the procedure and assure the patient that you will be as gentle as possible during the examination. This is especially important in patients who have never had this exam before and those who have experienced sexual trauma or sexual assault. After the patient interview is completed, provide the patient with a drape and a gown and ask her to remove all clothing, put the gown on with the opening in the front, then have a seat on the exam table and cover with the drape.

A chaperone should be present during the exam to assist the provider and, due to legal implications, to serve as a witness. Ask the patient when her last episode of intercourse was and if she douches. Neither of these should occur for at least 24 hours prior to the exam. If the patient used a douche or had sexual intercourse within 24 hours of the exam, the integrity of exam findings and test results may be compromised, especially if a Pap test is being done at this visit.

To begin the examination, have the patient lie supine. Assist her to the lithotomy position (Figure 10.8) by having her place her feet in the stirrups, then ask her to slide to the end of the exam table until her buttocks are slightly off of the end of the table. A good frame of reference is to place your hand at the end of the table and ask the patient to slide down until her buttocks touch your hand. This positioning allows the cervix to become more visible. The provider should adjust the exam-room stool to a comfortable height and sit at the foot of the exam table.

EXTERNAL GENITALIA EXAMINATION

Tell the patient what is going to happen prior to each step of the exam and explain each component of the examination and each procedure. Inspect the following:

- **Mons pubis:** Assess hygiene, the pattern of hair distribution based on developmental stage, and condition of the skin.

  - Rationale: The mons pubis should be clean. Generally, pubic hair should cover the surface of the mons pubis. Hair distribution varies based on age and developmental stage. The skin should be flesh colored, smooth, and devoid of lesions. Note the presence of any alopecia, erythema, swelling, lesions, or masses.

- **Clitoris:** Assess the condition of the skin, as well as the size.

  - Rationale: Skin should be intact and free of lesions, swelling, discharge, and erythema.

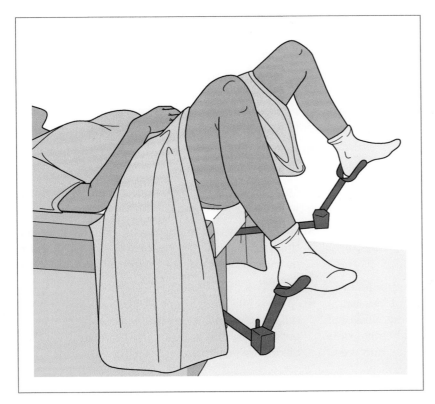

FIGURE 10.8 Lithotomy position. Patient lies supine with the hips and knees flexed, the legs abducted, and the feet placed in stirrups. This position is used for pelvic examination and childbirth.

The usual size of the clitoris is 1.5 to 2 cm in length. If the clitoris is enlarged, patients should be evaluated for elevated testosterone levels.

- **Vulva:** Assess the labia majora for skin condition, color, erythema, inflammation, discharge, and lesions. Using the index finger and the middle finger of the dominant hand, separate the labia majora to expose the labia minora and inspect the condition and color of the skin.

  - Rationale: The color of the labia majora varies but is most often the color of the woman's skin; however, it may be darker pigmented than the skin of the rest of the body. The labia minora should be moist and pink. The skin should be smooth, and devoid of lesions and nodules. A scant amount of normal clear or thin, white discharge may be present on the labia minora.

- **Urethral meatus:** Assess for color, ulceration, inflammation, nodule, discharge, or lesions.

  - Rationale: The urethral meatus should be pink and free of ulcerations, inflammation, nodules, lesions, and discharge.

- **Vaginal introitus:** Assess for erythema, lesions, tears, and discharge.

  - Rationale: A scant amount of normal clear or thin white discharge may be present. Tearing may indicate vaginal trauma and the provider should explore this through the patient interview.

- **Bartholin glands:** Assess the Bartholin gland by inserting the index finger into the vagina at the posterior end of the vaginal introitus. Palpate the tissue between the thumb and forefinger on each side. Note any swelling, tenderness, masses, or discharge.

  - Rationale: The Bartholin glands should be smooth, nontender, and devoid of masses or discharge. If tenderness, swelling, and/or discharge is noted, this may be indicative of an abscess. The presence of a mass may be suggestive of cancer. If any abnormality is discovered, the patient should be referred to a specialist.

- **Anus:** Assess for erythema, irritation, and for the presence of hemorrhoids.

  - Rationale: The anus should be rugated, nonerythematous, and free of lesions and swelling.

- **Palpatation:** Palpate the inguinal/groin area bilaterally or for the presence of lesions, masses, or lymph nodes. The area should be smooth and free of lesions, palpable lymph nodes, and masses.

PROCEDURE FOR A SPECULUM EXAMINATION

Step 1: Using the patient's size and stature as a guide, select the appropriately sized metal or plastic speculum (Figure 10.9).

Step 2: Show the speculum to the patient and explain the examination process.

Step 3: Ask the patient to open her legs as widely as possible and relax her leg and buttocks muscles. Explain that this positioning will promote ease of speculum insertion and lessen discomfort during insertion.

Step 4: Lubricate the speculum under a stream of warm water prior to insertion. Other forms of lubrication may compromise Pap test and culture results.

Step 5: Hold the speculum in your dominant hand at a 45-degree angle.

Step 6: Using the nondominant hand, spread the labia to open the vaginal introitus.

Step 7: Slowly and gently insert the speculum into the vagina with the tip of the blades pointing downward toward the posterior surface of the vagina.

Step 8: While gently depressing the perineal body, fully insert and rotate the speculum clockwise until the handle is in a vertical position and the blades are in a horizontal position.

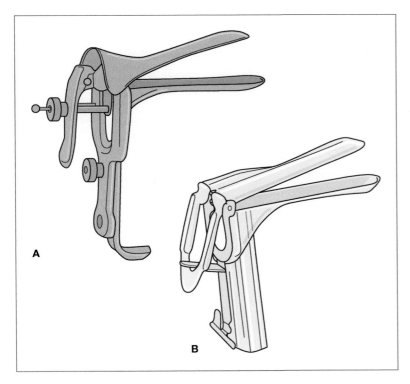

FIGURE 10.9 Types of specula. **(A)** Metal speculum. Metal specula are sterilized and reused. **(B)** Plastic speculum. Plastic specula are disposable and intended for one-time use only.

Step 9: Slowly open the speculum blades until the cervix is visible (Figure 10.10A).

Step 10: For specimen collection: Once the cervix is fully visualized, lock the speculum in place. Obtain specimens as indicated by the purpose of the examination (Figure 10.10B and C).

INTERNAL GENITALIA EXAMINATION

After speculum insertion, inspect the following:

- **Vaginal vault:** Inspect the vaginal vault and vaginal walls for color, inflammation, discharge, and lesions. Inspect the mucosa for moisture and dryness.
  - ○ Rationale: The vaginal walls should be pink and free of lesions and inflammation. Thin, clear or white, odorless discharge is normal. The mucosa should be moist.

- **Cervix:** Inspect the cervix for color, lesions/masses, and discharge. Note the shape of the cervical os.
  - ○ Rationale: The cervix should be pink and free of lesions, masses, and discharge. During early pregnancy, the cervix may be bluish in color. During certain periods of the menstrual cycle, a mucous-like discharge may be present and is a normal finding. The cervical os is round in nulliparous females and a slit in multiparous females (see Figure 10.5).

BIMANUAL EXAMINATION

A bimanual examination includes systematic palpation of the uterus, cervix, and adnexa (Figure 10.11). This procedure is usually performed after removal of the speculum; however, in circumstances where the cervix is difficult to view after speculum insertion, a bimanual exam may be performed to locate the

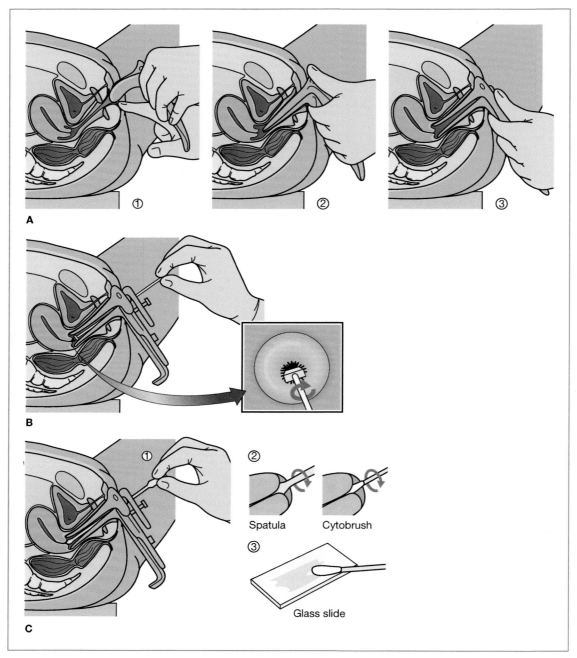

FIGURE 10.10 Speculum examination. (**A**) Speculum insertion steps: (**1**) Hold speculum at a 45-degree angle; (**2**) once the blades are inside the vaginal vault, rotate the speculum to a horizontal position; and (**3**) once the speculum is fully inserted, slowly open the blades until the cervix is visualized. When the cervix is positioned between the anterior and posterior blades, lock the speculum in place. (**B**) Pap smear procedure with broom. Insert the broom through the opening of the speculum to collect endocervical cells for Pap smear. (**C**) Pap smear procedure with spatula, brush, and slide. (**1**) A wooden spatula is inserted into the cervical os through the speculum opening, (**2**) the spatula is rotated clockwise to collect exocervical and endocervical cells; the cytobrush is inserted into the cervical os to collect endocervical cells, (**3**) the sample is affixed to a glass slide.

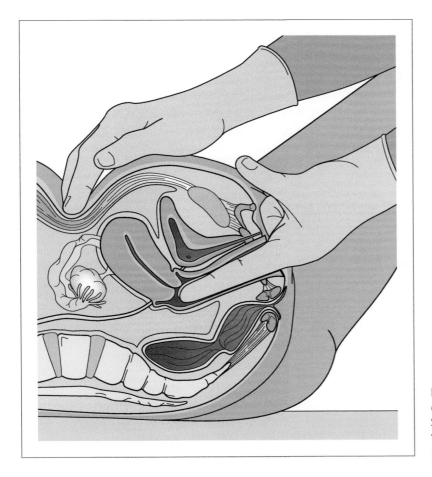

FIGURE 10.11 Bimanual examination of the reproductive structures. Simultaneous external palpation of the uterus and ovaries and internal palpation of the vagina and cervix.

position of the cervix prior to the speculum exam. The purpose of a bimanual examination is to assess the internal reproductive organs. Explain the procedure to the patient before beginning.

Procedure for Bimanual Examination

Step 1: Don clean nonsterile gloves. Apply the water-soluble lubricant to the index and middle fingers of the dominant hand. Cross-contamination is prevented by using clean gloves. The lubricant reduces friction and lessens discomfort when inserting fingers into the vagina.

Step 2: With the thumb abducted and the ring and fifth fingers flexed into the palm, gently insert the middle and index fingers of your gloved, lubricated hand into the vagina. Place your nondominant hand midway between the umbilicus and the symphysis pubis and press downward toward the hand that is inside the pelvis. This allows ease of palpation of the vagina and cervix.

Step 3: Palpate the vaginal walls. The vagina should be nontender and free of masses or lesions.

Step 4: Palpate the cervix and note the following: Position, shape, consistency, mobility, and tenderness. The cervical position may be anterior, midline, or posterior. It should be round, smooth, firm, mobile, and nontender.

Step 5: Slightly move your intravaginal hand forward to push the cervix anteriorly and, with the palmar surface of your nondominant hand, palpate the fundus (anterior portion) of the uterus.

Note the following: Size, position, consistency, tenderness, and mobility. This technique aids in lifting the fundus anteriorly so that it can be palpated. The uterus should not be enlarged and should be smooth, free of masses, nontender, and mobile.

Step 6: Palpate the adnexa (ovaries): While pushing inferiorly on the abdomen, gently move your intravaginal fingers into the lateral vaginal fornix. This should be done bilaterally. This procedure aids in placing the ovaries between the abdominal hand and the intravaginal hand. Note the size, shape, consistency, masses, mobility, and tenderness. Normal ovaries are almond shaped or ovoid and vary in size from 3 to 5 cm. They should be smooth, mobile, nontender, and free of masses.

Focused Health Assessment and Abnormal Findings

Some of the most commonly seen urogynecological complaints are pelvic pain, vaginal discharge, vaginal bleeding, lesions, urinary tract–related symptoms (dysuria, frequency, and urgency), hematuria, and urinary incontinence. When a woman presents with specific complaints, the provider is responsible for obtaining detailed information through a focused history and by performing a focused exam related to the patient's complaint; see example in Figure 10.12.

CHIEF COMPLAINT

Ascertain the reason for the visit by asking an open-ended question that allows the patient to describe her concern in her own words. The provider should restate the concern expressed to ensure clarification and assure the patient that her stated issue will be addressed. Some patients may not notice or may be too embarrassed to admit experiencing symptoms that may be associated with an infection; therefore, it is important for the provider to also ask very specific questions about the presenting symptoms.

HISTORY OF PRESENT ILLNESS

A. Did the symptoms begin gradually or suddenly?

B. If the symptoms are related to a lesion, mass, or pain, ask "Where is it located?"

C. How long have you had these symptoms?

D. Ask the patient to describe the lesions, mass, pain, and discharge as follows:

○ *Lesions:* Size, color, drainage, if multiple or single are present

○ *Mass:* Size, painful/tender

○ *Pain:* Character (sharp, stabbing, throbbing, radiation), severity, alleviating/aggravating factors, and timing (worse at any time of day, intermittent, or constant)

○ *Discharge:* Amount, consistency, color, odor, burning with urination, and presence of fever

INFECTIOUS DISORDERS

PEDICULOSIS PUBIS (CRABS, LICE)

Pediculosis pubis is a parasitic insect infection. The insects are usually found in the pubic hair; however, they can also be found anywhere on the body where coarse hair is located (axilla, legs, facial hair). The patient will typically complain of intense itching. The patient may see the louse moving along the hair shaft or see the louse eggs (nits) attached to the hair shaft. The provider may note the louse or nits. It is also possible to see areas of excoriation in the genital areas from tiny louse bites.

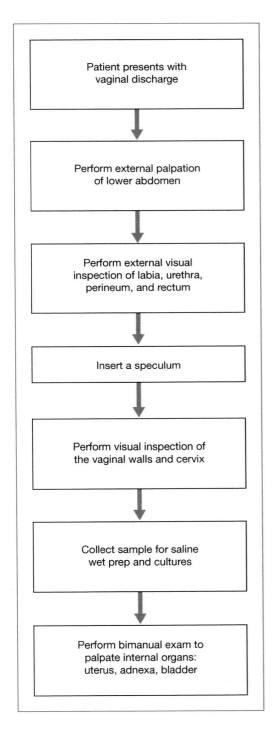

FIGURE 10.12 Algorithm for management of chief complaint of vaginal discharge.

HERPES SIMPLEX VIRUS

Herpes simplex virus (HSV) can infect the vulva, vagina, or the cervix. Most genital infections are caused by HSV-2, but HSV-1 (associated with oral herpes) can also infect the vulva. Patients will most often present with painful or tingling blisters or open lesions. They may also complain of dysuria or malaise. The lesions will appear as blisters or open ulcerative sores (Figure 10.13). Tender lymphadenopathy may be noted in the inguinal areas. The sores will usually be painful to the touch.

SYPHILIS

Syphilis is an STI caused by the bacterium *Treponema pallidum*. The bacterium is transmitted through a lesion called a chancre. The chancre can appear in the vagina or rectum, or on or near the external genitals, anus, or mouth. Syphilis can also be transmitted from a pregnant woman to her unborn fetus. The incubation period from time of exposure can be up to 21 days. Patients may present with a complaint of a sore, which appears on the part of the body that was exposed to the syphilis bacteria. The lesion is usually painless, and patients may not notice the lesion before it disappears. The chancre (the sore that is associated with syphilis) may be present for up to 6 weeks. A chancre may start as a single small round lesion that erupts into a flat ulcer. The lesions, as well as inguinal lymph nodes, are usually nontender. Even in the absence of treatment, the chancre will disappear and the infection will progress to secondary syphilis. Secondary syphilis may present as a squamopapular rash on the palms of the hands and soles of the feet. Confirmatory diagnosis of syphilis is made using nontreponemal and treponemal tests—blood tests.

HUMAN PAPILLOMAVIRUS

Human papillomavirus (HPV) is the most commonly occurring STI in the United States. HPV infections can be caused by one of 100 different strains of the virus. Low-risk strains cause about 90% of genital warts. Persistent HPV infections on the cervix can lead to cervical cancer, so identification and treatment is paramount. High-risk strains are responsible for 95% of cervical cancers. Patients may report wart-like growths that may have a "gritty feel." The warts

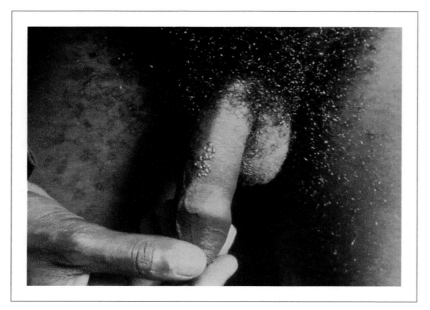

FIGURE 10.13 Herpetic lesions. Small vesicles on an erythematous base may appear as singular or clusters of lesions.

Source: Photo courtesy of CDC/Dr. Paul Wiesner.

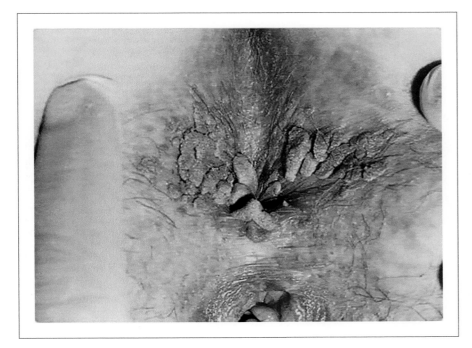

FIGURE 10.14 External genital warts. Single or multiple papular eruptions with a pearly, filiform, cauliflower, or plaque-like appearance may be observed.

Source: Image courtesy of SOA-AIDS Amsterdam.

are usually flesh colored, painless, and may be flat or pedunculated (Figure 10.14). The provider may note solitary warts or cauliflower-like clusters on the labia or in the vaginal canal, the perineum, the anus, or the rectum. Lesions on the cervix can be enhanced for visualization with 3% to 5% acetic acid solution, which will temporarily turn the HPV lesion(s) white.

CHLAMYDIA

While HPV is the most commonly occurring STI, chlamydia is the most commonly reported STI in the United States. Diagnosis can be made through collection of a urine sample, DNA findings through a Pap test, or via an endocervical swab. Chlamydia is typically asymptomatic; however, the patient may present with postcoital bleeding or dysuria. The provider may note a small amount of cloudy or yellowish mucopurulent discharge from the cervical os (Figure 10.15). The cervix

may be friable when touched with a cotton swab. On bimanual examination, cervical motion tenderness may be noted.

GONORRHEA

Gonorrhea is the second most commonly reported STI in the United States. This infection can be masked by a chlamydial infection; therefore, if the diagnosis of chlamydia is made, it is recommended that the provider automatically treat for gonorrhea. Women are usually asymptomatic. Some patients may present with a complaint of dysuria. A small amount of mucopurulent discharge may be noted (Figure 10.16). If the infection progresses to PID or salpingitis, the patient may present with fever, lower abdominal pain, adnexal discomfort, or cervical motion tenderness. Diagnosis is made through endocervical and vaginal cultures, urine testing, or it may be detected incidentally through Pap testing.

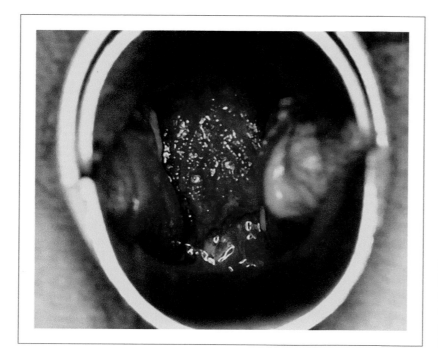

FIGURE 10.15 Chlamydial infection. Mucopurulent discharge and cervical erythema result from a chlamydial infection.

Source: Photo courtesy of CDC/Dr. Lourdes Fraw; Jim Pledger.

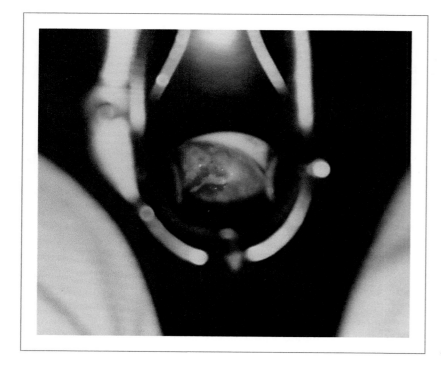

FIGURE 10.16 Gonorrheal infection. Mucopurulent cervical discharge with cervical irritation is observed.

Source: Photo courtesy of CDC.

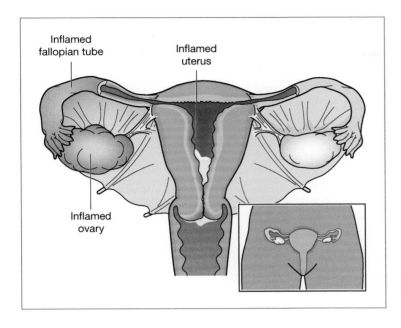

Inflamed
fallopian tube

Inflamed
uterus

Inflamed
ovary

FIGURE 10.17 Pelvic inflammatory disease (PID). Inflammation of the uterus, ovaries, and fallopian tubes are associated with PID.

PELVIC INFLAMMATORY DISEASE

PID is the result of an STI that spreads beyond the vagina and cervix into the uterus, fallopian tubes, abdomen, and/or ovaries (Figure 10.17). Patients may present with complaints of the following: Lower abdominal pain, vaginal discharge, unpleasant odor, abnormal uterine bleeding, fever, chills, or dysuria. On physical exam, the provider may note cervical motion tenderness or adnexal pain. The patient may have a fever and an elevated white blood cell count.

BACTERIAL VAGINOSIS

A bacterial vaginosis (BV) infection is the result of overgrowth of many anaerobic bacteria in the vagina. BV can occur in women engaged in heterosexual or same-sex relationships. The patient may report a watery dis-charge and odor, often described as "fishy." Oftentimes, the odor is most prominent after intercourse or during menses.

On inspection of the vaginal walls, the provider may note a thin greyish discharge. One of the methods for confirmation of BV is potassium chloride (KOH) testing, which is done by collecting a sample of the discharge with a cotton swab and placing the swab in a test tube with KOH. If an amine odor is released, the test is considered positive. A microscopic examination is another method of diagnosis for BV. A sample of the discharge is applied to a slide and set with normal saline. Microscopic examination will reveal clue cells (Figure 10.18), which is consistent with the diagnosis of BV. Testing a sample with nitrazine paper applied to the discharge will reveal an increased PH greater than 5. Special considerations for patients with BV include the following: (a) prolonged BV infections may lead to PID, and (b) BV in pregnancy has been linked to preterm delivery.

CANDIDIASIS

Candidiasis is a fungal infection resulting from the overgrowth of yeast in the vagina. *Candida albicans*, *Candida glabrata*, and *Candida tropicalis* are the most common organisms. Pregnancy or any condition that weakens the immune system predisposes women to a candida infection. A severe candida infection can spread to the vulva and cause significant swelling.

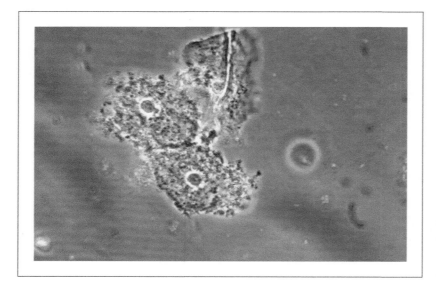

FIGURE 10.18 Wet mount. This saline smear shows "clue" cells, which are vaginal epithelial cells that have a peppered appearance due to the presence of *Coccobacilli.*

Source: Photo courtesy of CDC/M. Rein.

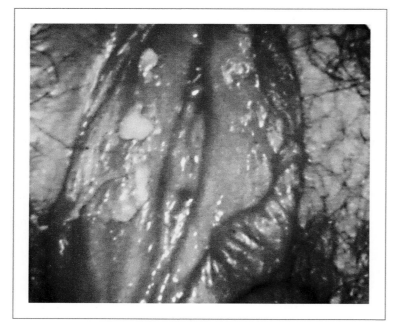

FIGURE 10.19 Candidiasis infection. Purulent discharge is present on the right labium minorum.

Source: Photo courtesy of CDC/Susan Lindsley.

If the vulva is scratched for relief, a secondary infection related to the broken skin may occur. Patients may also complain of dysuria or dyspareunia. While the hallmark symptom is severe itching, some patients with a candidal infection will not have any complaints. The provider will usually note a white clumpy, "cottage cheese"–like discharge (Figure 10.19). In severe cases, the labia may appear edematous and excoriated from scratching.

TRICHOMONIASIS

Trichomoniasis is caused by an infectious parasite called *Trichomonas vaginalis*. This infection is usually 100% transmissible. Patients often present with a musty odor, tenderness, dyspareunia, and/or dysuria. On examination, the discharge may appear green and frothy. The cervix may have petechiae, often called a "strawberry cervix" (Figure 10.20), and the vaginal PH may be greater than 4.5.

NONINFECTIOUS DISORDERS

CERVICITIS

Cervicitis is an inflammation of the cervix and the lower uterine segment. The etiology of the inflammation may be an infection or a hormone imbalance.

The patient may present with discharge, postcoital bleeding, itching, burning, and/or dysuria. The provider may note significant erythema on the cervix (Figure 10.21). The cervix may be friable when touched with a cotton swab or during specimen collection.

BARTHOLIN CYST/ABSCESS

A Bartholin abscess can occur when one of the Bartholin glands, located on either side of the vaginal opening, becomes infected. If the gland becomes blocked, a cyst can form, which can lead to an abscess if the cyst becomes infected. The causative bacterial organism of Bartholin abscesses may be *Escherichia coli*, chlamydia, or gonorrhea. Bartholin cysts may be up to an inch in diameter and usually cause significant pain.

Patients will present with complaints of a tender unilateral cyst on the labia. The provider will note a large unilateral, labial, fluid-filled cyst (Figure 10.22).

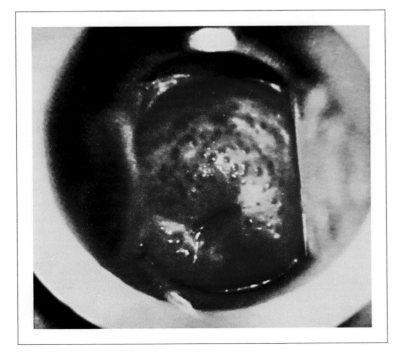

FIGURE 10.20 "Strawberry" cervix from a trichomoniasis infection. Cervical erythema with petechiae creates the appearance of an overripe strawberry.

Source: Photo courtesy of CDC.

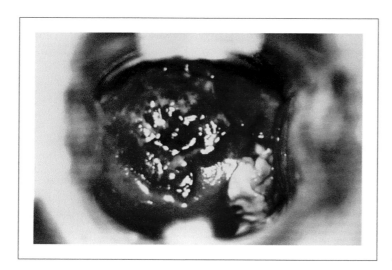

FIGURE 10.21 Cervicitis. Cervical inflammation and erythema are shown.

Source: Photo courtesy of CDC/Dr. Paul Wiesner.

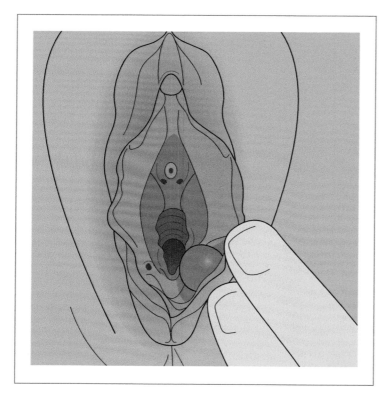

FIGURE 10.22 Bartholin cyst. The cyst is a tender, painful lump appearing near the vaginal orifice.

CERVICAL POLYPS

Up to 5% of women with a cervix may present with a cervical polyp, which appears as a benign tumor protruding from the cervical os (Figure 10.23). The polyps may appear as red, gray, or purplish in color.

The patient may complain of bleeding after intercourse; however, usually polyps are unknown to the patient. The provider may note a pedunculated growth from the cervical os. The polyp may be friable to the touch.

ATROPHIC VAGINITIS

Estrogen keeps the vagina lubricated. When estrogen levels are decreased because of hormonal dysfunction or menopause, the vagina will appear dry and friable.

The patient may present with complaints of vaginal dryness, burning, vaginal itching, vaginal bleeding, or dyspareunia. The provider may note decreased vaginal rugae and a shiny appearance to the vaginal walls. Due to the vaginal dryness and possible irritation, it may be difficult to introduce a speculum or a finger into the vagina during a bimanual examination.

ENDOMETRIOSIS

Retrograde bleeding during menses may lead to the migration of endometrial tissue into the pelvis (Figure 10.24). This tissue may attach to the intestine and lead to the development of scar tissue, which may subsequently cause pelvic adhesions, pelvic pain, obstruction of the fallopian tubes, and decreased ovarian function.

The patient may present with complaints of severe pain during menses, which often becomes progressively worse over time. The patient may also report dyspareunia, which occurs because of adhesion formation. On physical exam, the uterus may feel fixed and abdominal pain may be noted. In most cases, the examiner will not palpate any nodular masses.

UTERINE FIBROIDS

Fibroids (also known as leiomyomatas, leiomyomas, or myomas) are noncancerous growths of the uterus (Figure 10.25). Fibroids are almost always benign.

The patient may complain of a myriad of symptoms including heavy bleeding during menstruation, irregular bleeding, lower abdominal pain, pressure, dyspareunia, urinary frequency, anemia (from heavy

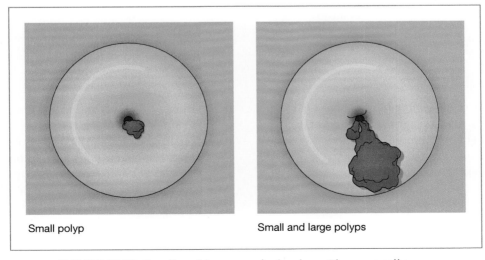

Small polyp

Small and large polyps

FIGURE 10.23 Small and large cervical polyps. These usually benign, fingerlike growths of tissue protrude into the cervical os.

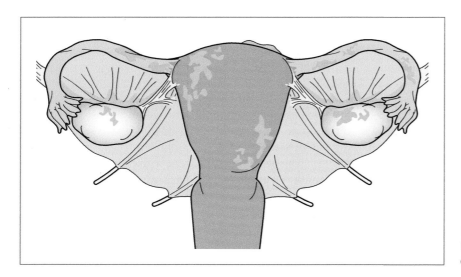

FIGURE 10.24 Endometriosis. Endometrial tissue is implanted outside of the uterine cavity.

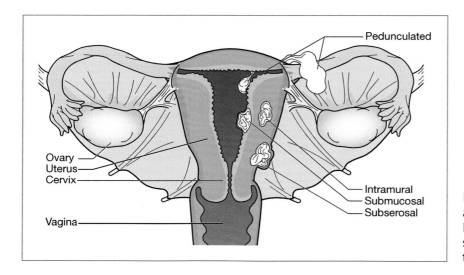

FIGURE 10.25 Uterine fibroids, also called leiomyomas, are benign tumors caused by smooth muscle and connective tissue overgrowth in the uterus.

menses and irregular bleeding), enlarged uterus, infertility, and miscarriages. On examination, the uterus may feel very firm, misshapen, and enlarged. Some fibroids can expand the uterus to the size of a fetus at 20 weeks' gestation.

ECTOPIC PREGNANCY

An ectopic pregnancy is any pregnancy that implants outside of the endometrium. In most cases, implantation will take place in the distal portion of the fallopian tube, but implantation may also occur in the abdominal cavity or the cervix (Figure 10.26). Any woman of childbearing age who could be pregnant should be given a pregnancy test with a presentation of irregular spotting or lower abdominal pain. The patient may present with abnormal bleeding. Late signs are consistent with a rupture of the ectopic pregnancy, including decreased blood pressure, tachycardia, diaphoresis, referred shoulder pain, fever, and shock. The patient may be unaware she is pregnant. An ectopic pregnancy is not usually palpable; however, a large tubal pregnancy may be

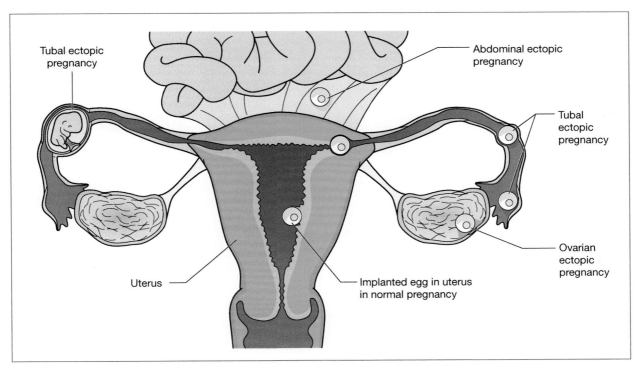

FIGURE 10.26 Implantation site for an ectopic pregnancy. Embryonic implantation may occur in the abdomen, fallopian tube, and ovary.

noted as an adnexal mass. The patient may report adnexal pain on examination. Ectopic pregnancy is usually diagnosed with a combination of serial qualitative human chorionic gonadotropin (BhCG) testing and ultrasound.

URINARY TRACT INFECTION

The gold standard for the diagnosis of a UTI is the detection of the pathogen in the presence of clinical symptoms. The pathogen is detected and identified by urine culture (using midstream urine). This also allows an estimate of the level of the bacteriuria.

Symptoms of a UTI may include dysuria, nocturia, polyuria, incontinence, hematuria, and malodorous or cloudy urine. The provider may note suprapubic pain, hematuria, or cloudy urine. Costovertebral angle (CVA) tenderness may be

noted in cases where the UTI has advanced to pyelonephritis.

COMMON ABNORMAL FINDINGS OF THE BREASTS

Benign breast abnormalities include lumps/masses, fibroadenomas, fatty tissue (lipomas), fibrocystic changes, abscesses, and nipple discharge. Lumps (masses) are either benign or cancerous. It is important for women to become familiar with the feel of their breast tissue for early detection through self-breast examination (SBE) and follow-up with a healthcare provider. Patient education regarding the difference between normal, lobular tissue and findings that require further examination is paramount. All abnormal findings should be further investigated.

FIBROADENOMAS

Fibroadenomas are among the most common benign breast lumps and are most often found in young women between the ages of 15 and 35 but may occur up to the time of menopause onset. They vary in size and shape and may either shrink, enlarge, or disappear on their own. They may be round, oval shaped, or lobular. Fibroadenomas are singular and are usually nontender, firm, smooth, mobile, and have well-defined borders. They may feel either hard or rubbery.

Treatment might include monitoring to detect changes in size or feel, a biopsy to further evaluate the lump, or surgical removal.

FATTY TISSUE (LIPOMAS)

A lipoma is a benign tumor composed of a pocket fatty tissue encapsulated by a thin fibrous capsule (Figure 10.27). It is usually painless, slow growing, and feels like dough.

FIBROCYSTIC CHANGES

Fibrocystic change, formerly known as fibrocystic breast disease, is a common benign breast condition that mostly occurs in premenopausal women. Since it is not a disease or disorder, it is now referred to as fibrocystic breast changes. It results

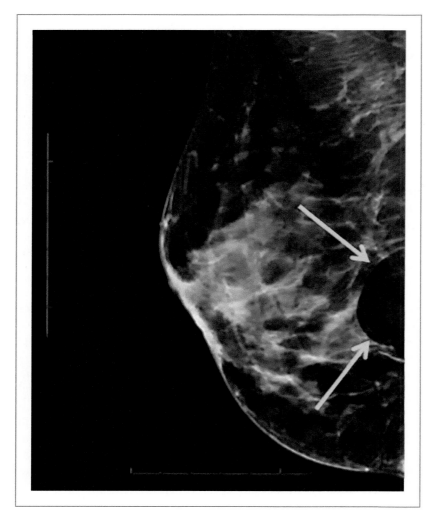

FIGURE 10.27 Fatty lipoma. This benign tumor is composed of fatty tissue.

in tender breast cysts with well-defined borders that are usually described as round, mobile, and elastic. The occurrence of breast cysts associated with fibrocystic breast changes may be constant or cyclical (corresponding to estrogen changes during the menstrual cycle).

ABSCESSES

A breast abscess is a localized inflammatory condition involving exudate formation in breast tissue. While rare, the most common causes are mastitis or cellulitis. Breast abscesses can be primary or occur when mastitis or cellulitis does not respond to antibiotic treatment.

NIPPLE DISCHARGE

Nipple discharge is one of the most common breast complaints and is usually the result of a benign condition. A thorough clinical history aids in distinguishing whether the cause is of a benign or pathological origin. Most often, benign nipple discharge is bilateral, involves more than one duct, and occurs when the breasts are manipulated. Spontaneous discharge that is unilateral, bloody, and involves one duct is usually indicative of a breast mass that is high risk for cancer.

Holistic Assessment

A holistic assessment of the reproductive system should include a discussion of intimate partner violence (IPV), screening for sexual dysfunction, cultural considerations, developmental considerations, and social determinates of health that could impact reproductive outcomes.

- **IPV:** More than 1 million women are sexually assaulted each year in the United States. IPV may contribute to gynecological disorders, unwanted pregnancies, and STI. The U.S. Preventive Services Task Force (USPSTF) recommends that clinicians screen women of childbearing age for IPV. It may take time for a patient to disclose IPV; therefore, providers should inquire about a possibility of IPV during each visit.

- **Screening for sexual dysfunction:** Sexual dysfunction is often missed or providers are reluctant to initiate a conversation about this topic. Patients should be asked about discomfort during sex. Underlying physiological disorders such as atrophic vaginitis, vaginismus or a uterine prolapse, relationship issues, or IPV may contribute to dyspareunia.

- **Preconception or family planning needs:** Discussing a reproductive plan with a woman can help to align her desire regarding conception with medical recommendations and treatment. A preconception visit should include discussions about nutrition, exercise, environmental exposures, substance use, chronic health conditions, support systems, and medications. Assessment of whether a woman desires contraception or requires referral for infertility may also be noted in the history obtained during routine physical exam.

- **Cultural considerations:** Patients should be asked about cultural preferences that may guide the physical examination and healthcare recommendations. Cultural preferences may impact a patient's decisions about contraception or reproduction.

- **Social determinates of health:** It has been shown that the social determinates of health, including education, childhood trauma, discrimination, food security, and socioeconomic status, can contribute to a person's overall health. Women should be screened for history of trauma and for current challenges that contribute to poor health outcomes. Women who lack the necessary resources for achieving or maintaining optimal health may require that the provider serve as the liaison for collaborating with other disciplines and community stakeholders in assisting the patient to obtain these resources.

CASE STUDY

Gina is a 24-year-old who calls the office with complaints of abdominal pain and urinary frequency and discomfort throughout the day and evening. She has been sexually active for the past 2 years and says that lately she finds sexual activity uncomfortable. She reports no other chronic conditions or remarkable medical history. On physical examination, suprapubic tenderness is noted.

Differential Diagnoses:

- UTI

- PID

- Sexually transmitted disease

- Vaginal infection

Most Likely Diagnosis: UTI

Labs/Diagnostic Tests:

- Urine analysis and urine culture

- Wet prep

- Vaginitis culture (Bacterial vaginitis [BV], gonorrhea [GC], and chlamydia)

Follow-up Plan: The provider should review the findings of the culture to ensure the appropriate antibiotics are prescribed. Depending on the results, the patient may need to return for a test of cure.

ICD-10-CM Diagnosis Code: R10.30 Lower Abdominal Pain, Unspecified

ICD-10-CM Diagnosis Code: R30.0 Dysuria

ICD-10-CM Diagnosis Code: N39.0 Urinary Tract Infection, Site Not Specified

Assessment of Special Populations

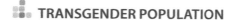 **TRANSGENDER POPULATION**

Women who have transitioned to men face many unique physiological and psychosocial challenges. There is limited research on the specific healthcare needs of the female to male transgender population. There is evidence to support that transgender men are at a greater risk of developing PCOS, contracting HIV, experiencing violence, and committing suicide. In addition to the physical considerations, the provider must also consider the psychological factors that impact transgender patients and address those needs as part of a holistic assessment. To that end, creating a safe environment and establishing a trusting relationship with the patient is paramount.

- Ask the patient whether the preferred pronouns are his or her, or he or she. Do not assume that because a patient is transgender that the pronoun preference aligns with physical, biological, or physiological appearance.

- Make the patient feel comfortable by projecting a nonjudgmental attitude.

- Explain the exam and procedures in the same way that you would with a nontransgender female. Allow the patient to participate in decisions regarding care.

- Due to the increased risk for suicide and violence, be sure to screen for depression and violence. The most effective way to screen is to use an approved, widely recognized tool.

- The assessment and physical examination of patients who identify as and are biologically female is the same as for those who identify as male but are biologically female.

ELDERLY POPULATION

Physiological changes occur as a result of the normal aging process. In general, as women age, estrogen levels decrease and cause gynecologic changes, including muscle atrophy and weakness, vaginal dryness, and hair thinning. The following should be considered when assessing this population:

- **Mons pubis:** Sparse, gray pubic hair
- **Labia majora and minora:** Atrophy, thinned skin
- **Vagina:** Pale, dry, atrophied (decreased elasticity)
- **Cervix:** Pale; absent after hysterectomy

PREGNANT POPULATION

The goal of the prenatal assessment is to determine normal growth of the fetus and stability of the mother. Assessment of the pregnant patient is done to:

- Confirm pregnancy
- Document normal pregnancy progression
- Identify risk factors for complication
- Diagnose complications early

CONFIRMATION OF PREGNANCY

Pregnancy can be confirmed by a pregnancy test. A qualitative measurement of human gonadotropin (HCG) is accomplished through urine pregnancy test. A qualitative urine pregnancy test may be performed by the patient at home. The urine test or a qualitative blood test may be performed by the provider in the office to confirm pregnancy. A quantitative measure of HCG is taken through the blood. In a normal pregnancy, a serum HCG will double every 36 hours for the first 8 weeks.

INITIAL INDICATORS OF PREGNANCY

The cervix softens at 4 to 6 weeks (Goodell's sign). The softening extends into the lower uterine segment from 6 to 8 weeks (Hegar's sign). Upon visualization, the cervix may appear cyanotic (Chadwick's sign). These changes are the result of increased blood flow, hyperplasia, and hypertrophy of the cervical glands. The patient may report other symptoms of pregnancy including breast tenderness, nausea, or fatigue. A patient experiencing an abnormal pregnancy may present with severe nausea and vomiting, uterine cramping, or vaginal bleeding.

UTERINE CHANGES

Uterine sizing (Figure 10.28) is performed to monitor progressive fetal growth and assess normal fetal development. The uterus will remain a pelvic organ until about 12 weeks' gestation. It is important to note that even in the case of an ectopic pregnancy, the uterus will feel enlarged. At 20 weeks, the uterine fundus will reach the level of the umbilicus. At 36 weeks, the uterine fundus will reach the level of the xiphoid process. The amount of amniotic fluid, the number of fetuses, or the size of the fetus may affect the measurement.

PROGRESSION OF PREGNANCY

For normal pregnancy, the American College of Obstetrics and Gynecology (ACOG) recommends an office visit at the following intervals:

- Every 4 weeks until 28 weeks
- Every 2 weeks from 28 to 36 weeks
- Every week from 36 weeks

Table 10.2 details the assessments that should be performed during these visits.

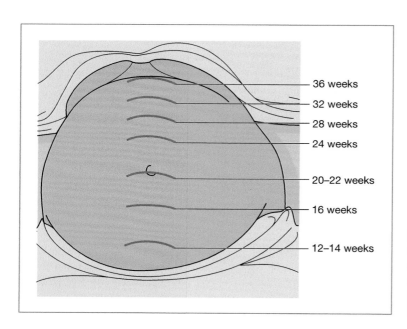

FIGURE 10.28 Fundal height measurements. Measurements of the distance from the symphysis pubis to the uterine fundus are used to determine gestational age in weeks; illustration from 12 to 36 weeks' gestation.

TABLE 10.2
Assessments Performed During Normal Prenatal and Postpartum Visits

Gestation	Initial Visit	20 Wk	24–28 Wk	35–36 Wk	>41 Wk	Postpartum
Vitals	BP Weight	BP Weight	BP Weight	BP Weight	BP Weight	BP Weight
Physical assessment	Full physical Uterine size Fetal heart tones	Fundal height Fetal heart tones	Fundal height Fetal heart tones	Fundal height Fetal heart tones	Fundal height Fetal heart tones	Full physical

(continued)

TABLE 10.2
Assessments Performed During Normal Prenatal and Postpartum Visits (*continued*)

Gestation	Initial Visit	20 Wk	24–28 Wk	35–36 Wk	>41 Wk	Postpartum
Labs	Urine culture Hemoglobin/ Hematocrit Type and screen Hemoglobin electrophoresis* HIV Pap (if needed) HBSaG 1–hr glucose† TSH	Urine (protein and glucose)	Urine (protein and glucose) Gestational diabetes screen Hemoglobin/ Hematocrit	Urine (protein and glucose) Group beta strep culture	Urine (protein and glucose)	Hemoglobin/ Hematocrit Glucose screening Pap (if needed)
Other testing		Fetal anatomy scan			Biophysical profile	Depression screening

*Recommended for patients of color.
†Recommended for women with body mass index (BMI) >35.

BP, blood pressure; HBSaG, hepatitis B surface antigen; TSH, thyroid-stimulating hormone.

ANTEPARTUM VISIT

During the antepartum visit, the provider performs a McDonald assessment (Figure 10.29). With the patient on her back, the measurement is taken from the symphysis pubis to the top of the fundus. In a normal pregnancy, the fundal measure is consistent with the gestation + 2 cm.

POSTPARTUM VISIT

The goal of the postpartum visit is to assess the status of recovering from the delivery, noting any physical or psychological complication in need of follow up, as well as to reassess and discuss family planning desires. A postpartum visit may be scheduled at 2 to 3 weeks postpartum and again at 6 weeks postpartum. The visit should include questions regarding infant feeding, including whether the mother has any concerns related to breast- or bottle feeding. Screening should be included for postpartum depression, and concerns related to sex and sexual health should also be discussed.

▦ PEDIATRIC POPULATION

When assessing pediatric patients, in addition to the stage of physical development, psychosocial developmental stages should be considered.

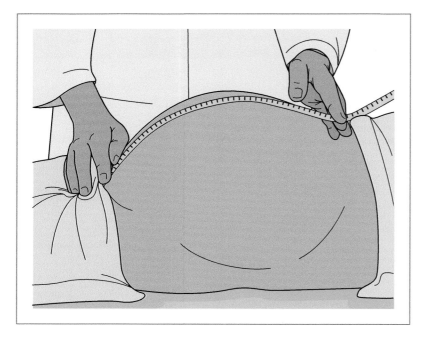

FIGURE 10.29 McDonald measurement. Measurement of uterine size to assess fetal growth; measures the distance from the symphysis pubis to the uterine fundus to determine gestational age in weeks.

- Carefully explain assessment/physical exam processes and procedures to the patient in language that is understandable and aligns with the patient's developmental stage. This may ease or decrease any anxiety that the patient may have.

- Obtain a comprehensive sexual history; this is important to determine the need for and schedule of pelvic examinations and Pap smears.

- Breast development and pubic hair distribution vary based on the Tanner stage of development.

- Choose a speculum based on the size and stature of the patient. Use the smallest speculum possible to ease discomfort associated with speculum insertion.

- Inspect the vagina for any signs of sexual trauma, including bruising, bleeding, and vaginal tearing. By law, confirmed or suspected sexual abuse must be reported to the appropriate authorities.

PATIENTS WITH DISABILITIES

Disabilities may involve cognitive, sensory, and mobility impairments, all of which may create a challenge when performing a pelvic examination. However, the necessity to perform pelvic exams and Pap smears among this population is no different than that of the general female population. In addition to the considerations used when performing breast and pelvic examinations on nondisabled females, the provider must take individual disabilities into account and proceed accordingly. Women with disabilities experience a high prevalence of sexual and/or other forms of abuse, oftentimes from their significant others or caregivers. The following are general considerations to guide examination of women with disabilities:

- When scheduling an appointment for a female with a disability, allow for a realistic span of time to successfully complete the examination. These visits may take a little longer, depending on the nature and degree of the disability.

- Establish a safe, trusting environment by making the patient feel at ease.

- Explain each step of the examination and allow the patient enough time to become comfortable with each step of the process before beginning.

- Cognitive impairment: Careful explanation of the procedure is of utmost importance. In cases of mild dysfunction, the patient may be able to understand the procedure and will likely cooperate. Otherwise, with consent from the legal guardian, sedation may be an option. Do not force the patient to have the procedure when she does not cooperate. You may have to reschedule the exam multiple times before you are successful in getting the patient to cooperate, but it is important not to traumatize the patient.

- Visually impaired patients: Allow the patient to touch any equipment that is nonsterile, especially the speculum. During the pelvic exam, explain what you are doing at each step.

- Hearing-impaired (deaf) patients: For patients who read lips, make sure that the patient can see your mouth or the chaperone's mouth when explaining the procedure. For deaf patients, if the patient does not have a sign language interpreter, it is best to obtain one for the patient if possible. The patient should be able to see the interpreter during the procedure so that the patient may receive any explanations that you provide.

- Mobility-impaired patients: Have someone there to assist with patient transfer onto and off of the exam table, as well as to stand next to the patient during the exam to prevent falls. However, it is important that these patients are allowed privacy during intimate conversations regarding sexual activity, STDs, and IPV or abuse. Women with contractures may require the use of special equipment and/or alternative positioning during the pelvic exam.

VETERAN POPULATION

The provider should ask the patient if they served in the military. If so, the dates and capacity in which they served (e.g., pilot, ground forces, medical services) should be ascertained. Based upon this information, the provider will be aware of what potential hazards or chemicals of warfare the patient may have been exposed to.

Genomics and Genetics

Genomic medicine is an evolving phenomenon in which individual genetic information is integrated with patient care to enhance diagnostic assessment and reasoning, and influence clinical decision-making with the goal of improving health outcomes. Through this process, an increased number of female reproductive disorders have been identified. Aberration from the so-called "normal" assessment of the female reproductive system should consider genetic causes. The physical examination should be driven by the chief complaint, history of present illness, current medical history, past medical history, and family history. Each of these components work in concert to guide the diagnosis and management of the disorder. Some common genetic female reproductive disorders are presented in Table 10.3.

TABLE 10.3
Common Genetic Female Reproductive Disorders

Disorder and Onset	Definition	Clinical Presentation
Hypogonadism: Most often occurs during the expected time of pubertal onset, during the first or second decade of life	Ovarian failure	**Prepubertal:** • Primary amenorrhea • Underdeveloped breasts • Short stature • Eunuchoidism • Infertility **Postpubertal:** • Secondary amenorrhea • Hot flashes • Decreased libido • Mood and energy level changes • Osteoporosis
Endometriosis: Affects women of reproductive age	Implantation and growth of endometrial tissue outside of the uterine cavity	**Pain:** Pelvic, lower abdominal, inguinal, or back pain, dyspareunia, abdominal pain occurring with exercise **Menstrual symptoms:** Dysmenorrhea, menorrhagia, or irregular menstrual bleeding **GI symptoms:** Bloating, nausea, vomiting, and dyschezia **Urinary symptoms:** Pain on micturition and/or urinary frequency
PCOS: Women of reproductive age	A multidimensional disorder characterized by altered metabolism of androgens and estrogens, leading to excess androgen and menstrual irregularities	• Menstrual irregularities • Anovulation • Hyperandrogenism • Hirsutism • Acanthosis nigricans • Infertility • Obesity • Metabolic syndrome • Hypertension • Possibly enlarged ovaries; ovarian cysts • Obstructive sleep apnea

(continued)

TABLE 10.3 Common Genetic Female Reproductive Disorders (*continued*)		
Disorder and Onset	**Definition**	**Clinical Presentation**
Leiomyomata: Occurs in 25% of all women; more common in Black women	Also referred to as uterine fibroids (usually benign); tumors of uterine smooth muscle	• Irregular menses • Pelvic pain • Infertility

GI, gastrointestinal; PCOS, polycystic ovarian syndrome.

Diagnostic Reasoning

Common Differential Diagnoses: Female Genitourinary Complaints	
Diagnosis	**Key History or Physical Examination Differentiators**
Appendicitis	• Abdominal pain/pressure (lower): Caused by inflammation or rupture of the appendix
Bacterial Vaginosis	• Vaginal discharge: Caused by change in vaginal pH and/or irritation to the vaginal mucosa or uterus
Candidiasis	• Vaginal discharge: May be caused by change in vaginal pH, bacteria, and/or irritation to the vaginal mucosa or uterus
Cervical cancer	• Abnormal bleeding: May be caused by disruption of the cervical cells, which leads to friability
Cervicitis	• Abnormal bleeding: May be caused by inflammation and irritation of mucosa • Dyspareunia: May be caused by inflammation and irritation of the vaginal/cervical tissue
Chlamydia	• Vaginal discharge: May be caused by change in vaginal pH, bacteria, and/or irritation to the vaginal mucosa or uterus
Cyst (ovarian)	• Dyspareunia: May be caused by pressure from the enlarged ovary

(continued)

Common Differential Diagnoses: Female Genitourinary Complaints (continued)	
Diagnosis	**Key History or Physical Examination Differentiators**
Cystitis	• Dysuria: May be caused by inflammation and irritation of the tissue near the urethra. • Dyspareunia: May be caused by inflammation of the bladder and urethra
Endometriosis	• Dyspareunia: May be caused by the immobility of the organs related to the scar-tissue formation.
Fibroid	• Abnormal bleeding: May cause heavy bleeding and clot formation • Dyspareunia: Caused by pressure from the fibroid
Gonorrhea	• Vaginal discharge: May be caused by change in vaginal pH, bacteria, and/or irritation to the vaginal mucosa or uterus
Leukorrhea	• Vaginal discharge: May be caused by change in vaginal pH, bacteria, and/or irritation to the vaginal mucosa or uterus
Narrowed vaginal canal	• Dyspareunia: May be caused by a small vaginal opening
Nephrolithiasis	• Dysuria: May be caused by passage of kidney stone fragments and/or inflammation of the urethra
Pelvic inflammatory disease	• Abdominal pain (lower): May be caused by inflammation and scar tissue
Pregnancy	• Abnormal bleeding: Implantation, abnormal implantation
Pregnancy, early	• Abdominal pain (lower): May be caused by uterine enlargement or implantation cramping
Pregnancy, ectopic	• Abdominal pain (lower): May be caused by the conceptus expanding outside the uterus
Prolapse (uterine)	• Dyspareunia: Pressure from relaxed vaginal musculature may lead to pressure sensations.
Rectocele	• Dyspareunia: Pressure from relaxed vaginal musculature may lead to pressure sensations.
Sexually transmitted infection	• Abnormal bleeding: May be caused by inflammation and irritation of mucosa • Dyspareunia: May be caused by inflammation and irritation of the vaginal/cervical tissue • Dysuria: May be caused by inflammation of the tissue near and of the urethra.
Trichomoniasis	• Vaginal discharge: May be caused by change in vaginal pH, bacteria, and/or irritation to the vaginal mucosa or uterus

(continued)

Common Differential Diagnoses: Female Genitourinary Complaints (*continued*)	
Diagnosis	**Key History or Physical Examination Differentiators**
Urinary tract infection	• Abdominal pain (lower): Inflammation and irritation of the of the bladder may lead to discomfort above the pubis symphysis. • Dysuria: May be caused by inflammation and irritation of the tissue near the urethra.
Vaginitis	• Dyspareunia: May be caused by inflammation and irritation of the vaginal/cervical tissue
Vaginitis, atrophic	• Dysuria: Vaginal irritation from the lack of estrogen may cause tissue irritation during micturition. • Dyspareunia: Decreased estrogen leads to increased friction during coitus.

BIBLIOGRAPHY

American College of Obstetricians and Gynecologists. (2019). Practice bulletin No. 213: Female sexual dysfunction. *Obstetrics and Gynecology, 134*, 203–205. doi:10.1097/AOG.0000000000003325

American College of Obstetricians and Gynecologists Committee on Obstetric Practice (Ed.). (2012). *Guidelines for perinatal care (7th ed.)*. Elk Grove Village, IL: American Academy of Pediatrics and Washington, DC: American College of Obstetricians and Gynecologists.

Anh, S. H., Singh, V., & Tayade, C. (2017). Biomarkers in endometriosis: Challenges and opportunities. *Fertility and Sterility, 107*(3), 523–532. doi:10.1016/j.fertnstert.2017.01.009

Atkins, K. A. (2015). *Pathology of uterus smooth muscle tumors*. In R. Masand (Ed.), *Medscape*. Retrieved from https://emedicine.medscape.com/article/1611373-overview#a1

Bates, C. K., Carroll, N., & Potter, J. (2011). The challenging pelvic examination. *Journal of General Internal Medicine, 26*(6), 651–657. doi:10.1007/s11606-010-1610-8

Cleveland Clinic. (n.d.). Female reproductive system. Retrieved from https://my.clevelandclinic.org/health/articles/9118-female-reproductive-system

Cleveland Clinic. (n.d.). Fibrocystic breast changes. Retrieved from https://my.clevelandclinic.org/health/diseases/4185-fibrocystic-breast-changes

Dutton, L., Koenig, K., & Fennie, K. (2008). Gynecologic care of the female-to-male transgender man. *Journal of Midwifery & Women's Health, 53*(4), 331–337. doi:10.1016/j.jmwh.2008.02.003

Dyer, J., Latendresse, G., Cole, E., Coleman, J., & Rothwell, E. (2018). Content of first prenatal visits. *Maternal and Child Health Journal, 22*, 679–684. doi:10.1007/s10995-018-2436-y

El Hayek, S., Bitar, L., Hamdar, L. H., Mirza, F. G., & Daoud, G. (2016). Poly cystic ovarian syndrome: An updated overview. *Frontiers in Physiology, 7*, 124. doi:10.3389/fphys.2016.00124

Gabriel, A. (2018). Breast embryology. In J. N. Long (Ed.), *Medscape*. Retrieved from https://emedicine.medscape.com/article/1275146-overview

Golshan, M. (2018). *Nipple discharge*. In A. B. Chagpar (Ed.), *UpToDate*. Retrieved from https://www.uptodate.com/contents/nipple-discharge

Hooten, T., & Gupta, K. (2019). Acute complicated urinary tract infection (including pyelonephritis) in adults. In S. Calderwood, & A. Bloom (Eds.), *UpToDate*. Retrieved from https://www.uptodate.com/contents/acute-complicated-urinary-tract-infection-including-pyelonephritis-in-adults.

Layman, L. C. (2013). The genetic basis of female reproductive disorders: Etiology and clinical testing. *Molecular and Cellular Endocrinology, 370*(1–2), 138–148. doi:10.1016/j.mce.2013.02.016

Long, W. N. (1990). Pelvic examination. In H. K. Walker, W. D. Hall, & J. W. Hurst (Eds.), *Clinical methods: The history, physical, and laboratory examinations* (3rd ed., pp. 827–829). Boston, MA: Butterworths. Retrieved from https://www.ncbi.nlm.nih.gov/books/NBK286

Lucidi, R. S. (2019). *Polycystic ovarian syndrome*. In F. E. Casey, & R. S. Lucidi (Eds.), *Medscape*. Retrieved from https://emedicine.medscape.com/article/256806-overview

Mayo Clinic Staff. (n.d.). Endometriosis. Retrieved from https://www.mayoclinic.org/diseases-conditions/endometriosis/symptoms-causes/syc-20354656

Mills, B. B. (2017). Vaginitis: Beyond the basics. *Obstetrics and Gynecology Clinics of North America, 44*(2), 159–177. doi:10.1016/j.ogc.2017.02.010

Miranda, A. M. (2018). *Vaginal anatomy*. In T. R. Gest (Ed.), *Medscape*. Retrieved from https://emedicine.medscape.com/article/1949237-overview

National Human Genome Research Institute. (2019). Genomics and medicine. Retrieved from https://www.genome.gov/health/Genomics-and-Medicine

Richard-Eaglin, A. (2018). Male and female hypogonadism. *Nursing Clinics of North America, 53*(3), 395–405. doi:10.1016/j.cnur.2018.04.006

Secretary's Advisory Committee on Health Promotion and Disease Prevention Objectives for 2020. (2010, October 26). *Healthy People 2020: An opportunity to address the societal determinants of health in the United States*. Retrieved from http://www.healthypeople.gov/2010/hp2020/advisory/SocietalDeterminantsHealth.htm

Smeltzer, S. C., Mariani, B., & Meakim, C. (2017). *Assessment of a person with disability*. Retrieved from http://www.nln.org/professional-development-programs/teaching-resources/ace-d/additional-resources/assessment-of-a-person-with-disability

Till, S. R., Schrepf, A. D., & As-Sanie, S. (2018). Characteristics associated with degree of dyspareunia in women with pelvic pain. *Journal of Minimally Invasive Gynecology, 25 (7 Suppl.)*, S89. doi:10.1016/j.jmig.2018.09.181

U.S. Preventive Services Task Force. (2018). Screening for intimate partner violence, elder abuse, and abuse of vulnerable adults: US Preventive Services Task Force final recommendation statement. *Journal of the American Medical Association, 320*(16), 1678–1687. doi:10.1001/jama.2018.14741

U.S. Preventive Services Task Force. (2019). Final recommendation statement: Cervical cancer: Screening. Retrieved from https://www.uspreventiveservicestaskforce.org/Page/Document/RecommendationStatementFinal/cervical-cancer-screening2

Workowski, K. A., & Bolan, G. A. (2015). Sexually transmitted diseases treatment guidelines, 2015. *MMWR Recommendations and Reports, 64(No. RR-3)*, 1–137. Retrieved from https://www.cdc.gov/mmwr/preview/mmwrhtml/rr6403a1.htm

11

ADVANCED HEALTH ASSESSMENT OF THE NEUROLOGICAL SYSTEM

Alexandra Armitage

CHAPTER CONTENTS

(continued)

Overview of Anatomy and Physiology

The nervous system is the master controller of all other systems of the body. It is responsible for communicating with and modulating all systems. Its cells communicate with both electrical and chemical signals. The nervous system is one continuous unit; however, it is divided into the *central nervous system* (CNS) and the *peripheral nervous system* (PNS). The CNS is composed of the brain and spinal cord. It is responsible for interpreting incoming sensory information through the afferent (sensory) nerves and dictating a motor response through the efferent (motor) nerves. The PNS is composed of the nervous system distal to the spinal cord: The nerve roots, plexuses, and distal peripheral nerves. It also includes the cranial nerves.

Motor neurons can be further divided into the *somatic nervous system* and the *autonomic nervous system.*

The somatic nervous system is under voluntary control. Muscles under voluntary control are striated muscles such as the skeletal muscles. The autonomic nervous system consists of visceral motor nerve fibers controlling the heart, smooth muscles, and glands. The autonomic nervous system is further divided into the sympathetic and the parasympathetic divisions. The sympathetic division prepares the body for emergency response, while the parasympathetic division counterbalances the sympathetic system, focusing on activities which take place during rest and relaxation.

HISTOLOGY OF NERVOUS TISSUE

Tissue in the nervous system is made up of neurons, which are excitable and transmit both electric and chemical signals (Figure 11.1). Surrounding and in between the neurons are supporting cells called neuroglia. The neuroglia in the CNS includes astrocytes, microglia, ependymal cells, and oligodendrocytes. In the PNS, the neuroglia are satellite cells and neurolemmocytes (Schwann cells). A bundle of nerve fibers is called a tract in the CNS and a nerve in the PNS.

THE CENTRAL NERVOUS SYSTEM

THE BRAIN

The brain gives meaning to things that happen in the world surrounding us. Through the five senses of sight, smell, hearing, touch, and taste, the brain receives messages, often many at the same time, and is able to respond. Based on the information that it receives, the brain controls thoughts, memory and speech, arm and leg movements, and the function of many organs within the body. The brain is an organized structure, divided into many components that serve specific and important functions.

The brain is made up of two types of cells: *Neurons* and *glial cells*, also known as neuroglia or glia. The neuron is responsible for sending and receiving nerve impulses or signals. Glial cells are nonneuronal cells that provide support and nutrition, maintain homeostasis, form myelin, and facilitate signal transmission in the nervous system. In the human brain, glial cells outnumber neurons by about 50 to one.

The adult brain is divided into the *cerebral hemispheres, diencephalon, brainstem,* and *cerebellum* (Figure 11.2).

The brain is composed of grey matter that surrounds white matter in both the cerebral hemispheres and the cerebellum. The grey matter is called the cortex, and is the consciousness of the mind. The pattern of grey on white matter disappears with the descent through the brainstem where the cortex disappears, but scattered grey matter nuclei are seen within the white matter. The white matter runs in tracts, and its function is not well understood.

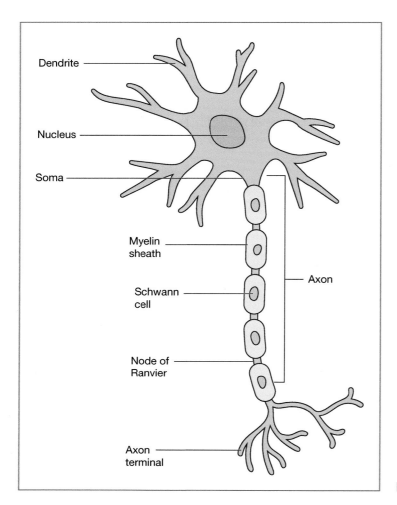

FIGURE 11.1 Anatomy of a motor neuron.

THE VENTRICLES

The brain contains four ventricles filled with cerebrospinal fluid. The lateral ventricles are in the cerebral hemispheres, the third ventricle is in the diencephalon, and the fourth ventricle is in the midbrain and connects with the central canal of the spinal cord. The cerebrospinal fluid is made by the choroid plexus from blood plasma.

THE DIENCEPHALON

The diencephalon consists of the thalamus, hypothalamus, and epithalamus. It encloses the third ventricle.

BRAINSTEM

The brainstem is the lower extension of the brain, located in front of the cerebellum and connected to the spinal cord. It consists of three structures: The midbrain, pons, and medulla oblongata. It serves as a relay station, passing messages back and forth between various parts of the body and the cerebral cortex. Many simple or primitive functions that are essential for survival are located here. Originating in the brainstem are 10 of the 12 cranial nerves that control hearing, eye movement, facial sensations, taste, swallowing, and movements of the face, neck, shoulder, and tongue muscles.

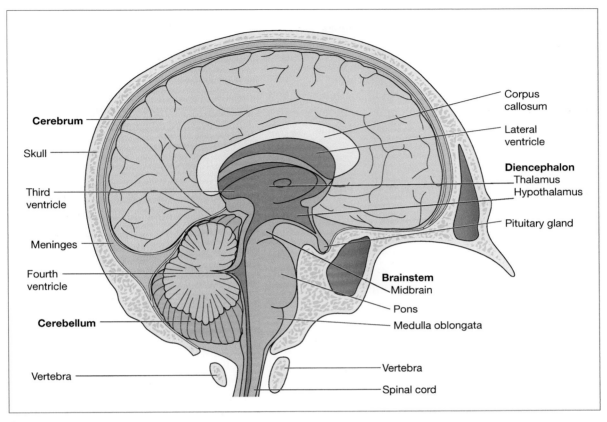

FIGURE 11.2 Anatomy and components of the brain.

CEREBELLUM

The cerebellum is located at the back of the brain beneath the occipital lobes. It consists of two hemispheres, which are separated by the vermis, and is separated from the cerebrum by the tentorium, a fold of dura. The cerebellum is responsible for processing and interpreting impulses from the motor cortex and sensory pathways. It coordinates motor activity into smooth and well-timed movements and helps maintain posture, sense of balance, or equilibrium by controlling the tone of muscles and the position of limbs. The cerebellum is important in one's ability to perform rapid and repetitive action.

CEREBRUM

The cerebrum is made up of the right and left cerebral hemispheres (lobes). The corpus callosum connects the two halves of the brain and delivers messages from one half of the brain to the other.

The cerebral hemispheres have several distinct fissures. By locating these landmarks on the surface of the brain, it can effectively be divided into *lobes*, or regions of the brain. Each hemisphere has a frontal, temporal, parietal, and occipital lobe.

Each cerebral hemisphere receives sensory impulses from, and dispatches motor impulses to, the opposite side of the body. They show lateralization of cortical function. In most people, the left hemisphere is dominant, specializing in language and mathematics. The right hemisphere is more concerned with esoteric functions, such a visual–spatial abilities and creativity.

Frontal Lobes

The frontal lobes are the largest of the four lobes responsible for many different functions. These include motor skills such as voluntary movement, speech, and intellectual and behavioral functions.

Parietal Lobes

These lobes simultaneously interpret signals received from other areas of the brain such as vision, hearing, motor, sensory, and memory. A person's memory, and the new sensory information received, gives meaning to objects.

Temporal Lobes

These lobes are located on each side of the brain at about ear level. An area on the right side is involved in visual memory and helps humans recognize objects and peoples' faces. An area on the left side is involved in verbal memory and helps humans remember and understand language. The rear of the temporal lobe enables humans to interpret other people's emotions and reactions.

Occipital Lobes

These lobes are located at the back of the brain and enable humans to receive and process visual information. They influence how humans process colors and shapes.

HYPOTHALAMUS

The hypothalamus is a small structure that contains nerve connections that send messages to the pituitary gland. The hypothalamus handles information that comes from the autonomic nervous system. It plays a role in controlling functions such as eating, sexual behavior, and sleeping; and regulates body temperature, emotions, secretion of hormones, and movement. The pituitary gland develops from an extension of the hypothalamus downward and from a second component extending upward from the roof of the mouth.

PINEAL GLAND

This gland is an outgrowth from the posterior or back portion of the third ventricle. In humans, it has some role in sexual maturation, although the exact function of the pineal gland in humans is unclear.

PITUITARY GLAND

The pituitary is a small gland attached to the base of the brain in an area called the pituitary fossa or sella turcica. The pituitary is responsible for controlling and coordinating growth and development, as well as the function of various body organs (i.e., kidneys, breasts, and uterus) and glands (i.e., thyroid, gonads, and adrenal glands).

THALAMUS

The thalamus serves as a relay station for almost all information that comes and goes to the cortex. It plays a role in pain sensation, attention, and alertness. The basal ganglia are clusters of nerve cells surrounding the thalamus.

THE SPINAL CORD

The spinal cord is a pathway for both sensory and motor impulses (to and from the brain; Figure 11.3). It is also a reflex center. The spinal cord resides within the vertebral column and is protected by meninges and spinal fluid. The spinal cord starts at the foramen magnum at the base of the skull and terminates at the upper lumbar vertebrae, usually between L1 and L2, where it forms the conus medullaris. In the lumbosacral region, nerve roots from lower cord segments descend within the spinal column in a nearly vertical sheaf, forming the cauda equina.

There are 31 pairs of spinal nerve roots, named for their associated vertebral body. Each pair of nerve roots exits at the corresponding level, innervating distinct dermatomal (Figure 11.4) and myotomal distributions.

THE PERIPHERAL NERVOUS SYSTEM

The PNS includes all neural structures outside of the brain and spinal cord. These include all sensory receptors, peripheral nerves and their ganglia, and efferent motor endings, as well as the cranial nerves.

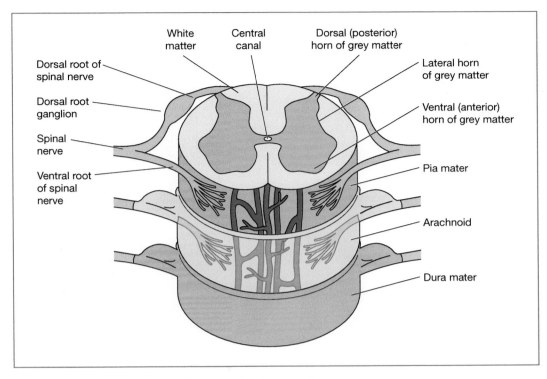

FIGURE 11.3 Spinal cord anatomy.

THE CRANIAL NERVES

There are 12 pairs of cranial nerves which come directly from the brain (Figure 11.5). The first two pairs attach to the forebrain, the other 10 pairs originate from the brainstem. Other than the vagus nerve, which extends into the abdomen, the cranial nerves serve only the head and neck structures. The cranial nerves are numbered, as well as named, from the most rostral to the most caudal.

- CN I, Olfactory: Smell
- CN II, Optic: Visual fields and ability to see
- CN III, Oculomotor: Eye movements; eyelid opening
- CN IV, Trochlear: Eye movements
- CN V, Trigeminal: Facial sensation
- CN VI, Abducens: Eye movements
- CN VII, Facial: Eyelid closing; facial expression; taste sensation
- CN VIII, Auditory/Vestibular: Hearing; sense of balance
- CN IX, Glossopharyngeal: Taste sensation; swallowing
- CN X, Vagus: Swallowing; taste sensation
- CN XI, Accessory: Control of neck and shoulder muscles
- CN XII, Hypoglossal: Tongue movement

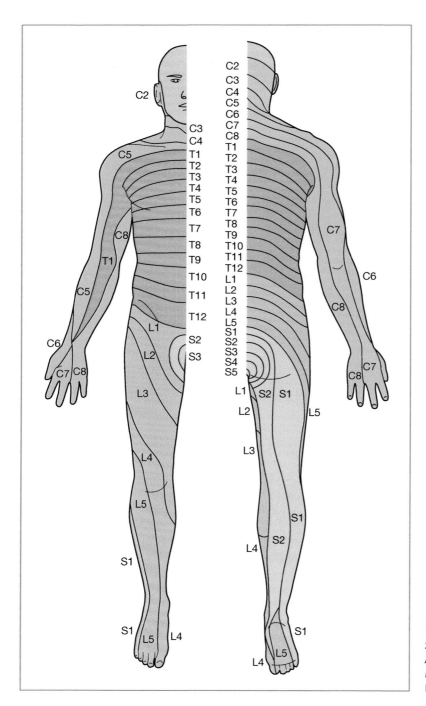

FIGURE 11.4 Dermatome distribution.

Source: Adapted from Armitage, A. (2015). *Advanced practice nursing guide to the neurological exam.* New York, NY: Springer Publishing Company.

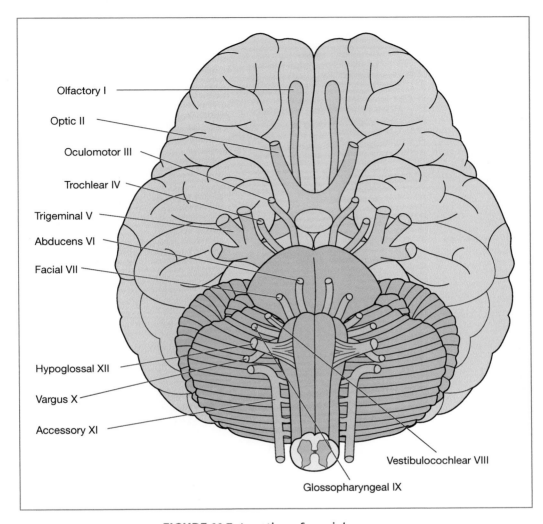

Olfactory I

Optic II

Oculomotor III

Trochlear IV

Trigeminal V

Abducens VI

Facial VII

Hypoglossal XII

Vargus X

Accessory XI

Vestibulocochlear VIII

Glossopharyngeal IX

FIGURE 11.5 Location of cranial nerves.

THE SPINAL NERVES AND PLEXUSES

Thirty-one pairs of spinal nerves, each containing thousands of nerve fibers, arise from the spinal cord supplying all parts of the body. There are eight pairs of cervical spinal nerves, 12 pairs of thoracic nerves, five pairs of lumbar nerves, and five pairs of sacral nerves (Figure 11.6).

The ventral branch (ramus) of each spinal nerve from C1–T1 to L1–S5 interlace, forming complex plexuses. Such plexuses occur in the cervical, brachial, lumbar, and sacral regions and primarily serve the limbs. The interlacing of the ventral rami results in each branch of the plexus containing fibers from several different spinal nerves. This also results in fibers from each ramus traveling to the body periphery via several different routes (branches). Thus, there is redundancy where each muscle in a limb receives its nerve supply from more than one spinal nerve.

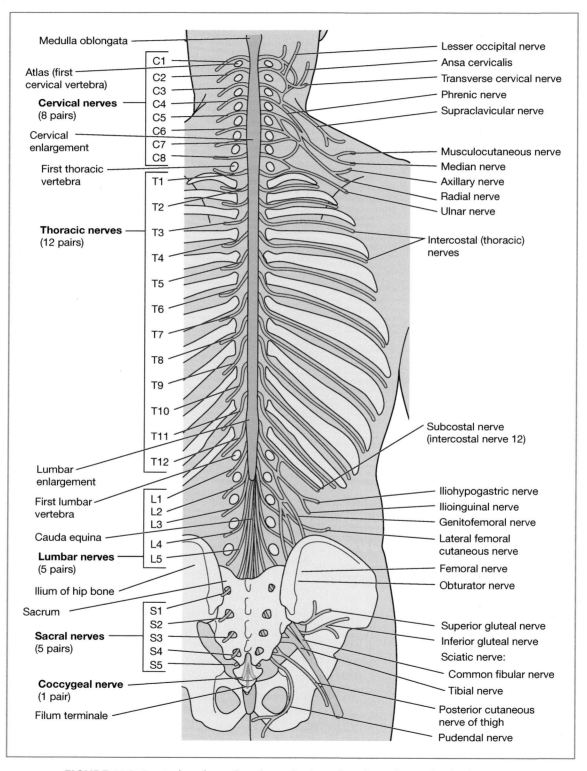

FIGURE 11.6 Posterior view of entire spinal cord and portions of spinal nerves.

THE AUTONOMIC NERVOUS SYSTEM

The autonomic nervous system innervates cardiac and smooth muscle and glands. There are two arms of the autonomic nervous system: The parasympathetic system and the sympathetic system (Figure 11.7). They have antagonistic functions. If one division stimulates the smooth muscle or gland, then the other inhibits it. Through this process of dual innervation, the body is balanced and runs smoothly.

The *parasympathetic system* is most active during nonstressful situations. It is designed to keep the body's energy use low, and it directs vital maintenance activities such as digestion and elimination of feces and urine.

The *sympathetic system* mobilizes the body during times of extreme situations such as fear, exercise, or rage. During these times, energy is focused to quick reactions to a proposed threat. Visceral blood vessels are constricted and blood is shunted to active skeletal muscles and to the vigorous working heart. Lungs dilate, the liver releases more sugar, and pupils dilate.

Screening Health Assessment and Normal Findings

COGNITIVE ASSESSMENT

Mental status evaluation includes the testing of memory, orientation, intelligence, insight, and the general health of the patient's psychic state. Pay special attention to the patient's appearance, communication, and behaviors initially and during the course of the clinical examination. Evaluate conversation for fluency, as well as insightful and goal-directed thinking. Gain an appreciation of the patient's insight into his or her medical condition and ability to express his or her own thoughts.

There are a number of formal tests available for the assessment of cognitive status. Brief screening tests such as the Montreal Cognitive Assessment Test (MoCA; Figure 11.8), Mini-Mental State Examination (MMSE), or the 6-Item Cognitive Impairment Test (6CIT) are concise with standardized scores. One must be aware of the patient's age, education, and primary language as these all influence mental status test scores. The MoCA and 6CIT are the most sensitive to early dementia.

NEUROPSYCHOLOGICAL ASSESSMENT

Neuropsychological assessment is a detailed evaluation of a patient's cognitive, behavioral, and emotional status. These assessments are provided by neuropsychologists. Almost every neuropsychological assessment contains the following components:

- A detailed record review
- A clinical interview
- Neuropsychological testing

A neuropsychological assessment can provide fine-grained information on the patient's cognitive strengths and weaknesses. Results of testing are more sensitive and specific than brief bedside cognitive assessments, but they are also time consuming, taking several hours to complete.

Results may guide a diagnosis and management of dementia, and help counsel a family on what functional activities, such as driving or financial management, might cause the individual difficulties.

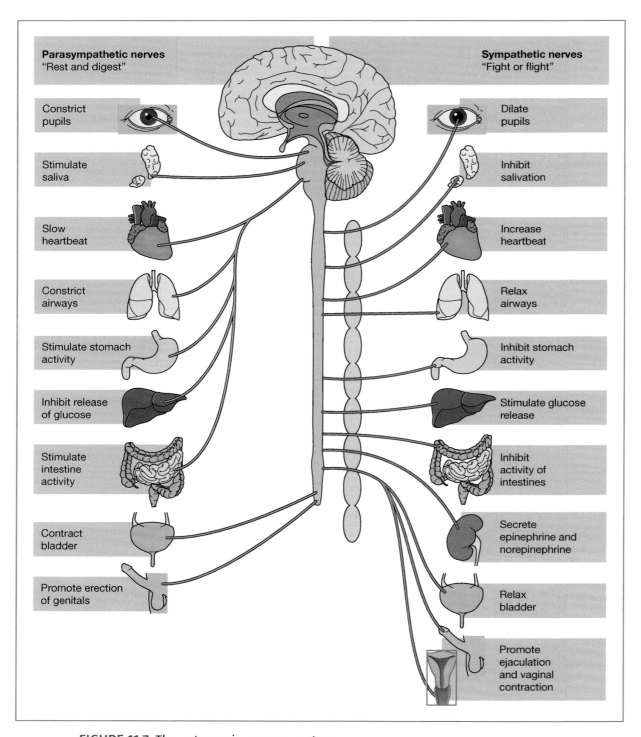

FIGURE 11.7 The autonomic nervous system.

Source: Adapted from Armitage, A. (Ed.). (2018). *A practical guide to Parkinson's disease: Diagnosis and management*. New York, NY: Springer Publishing Company.

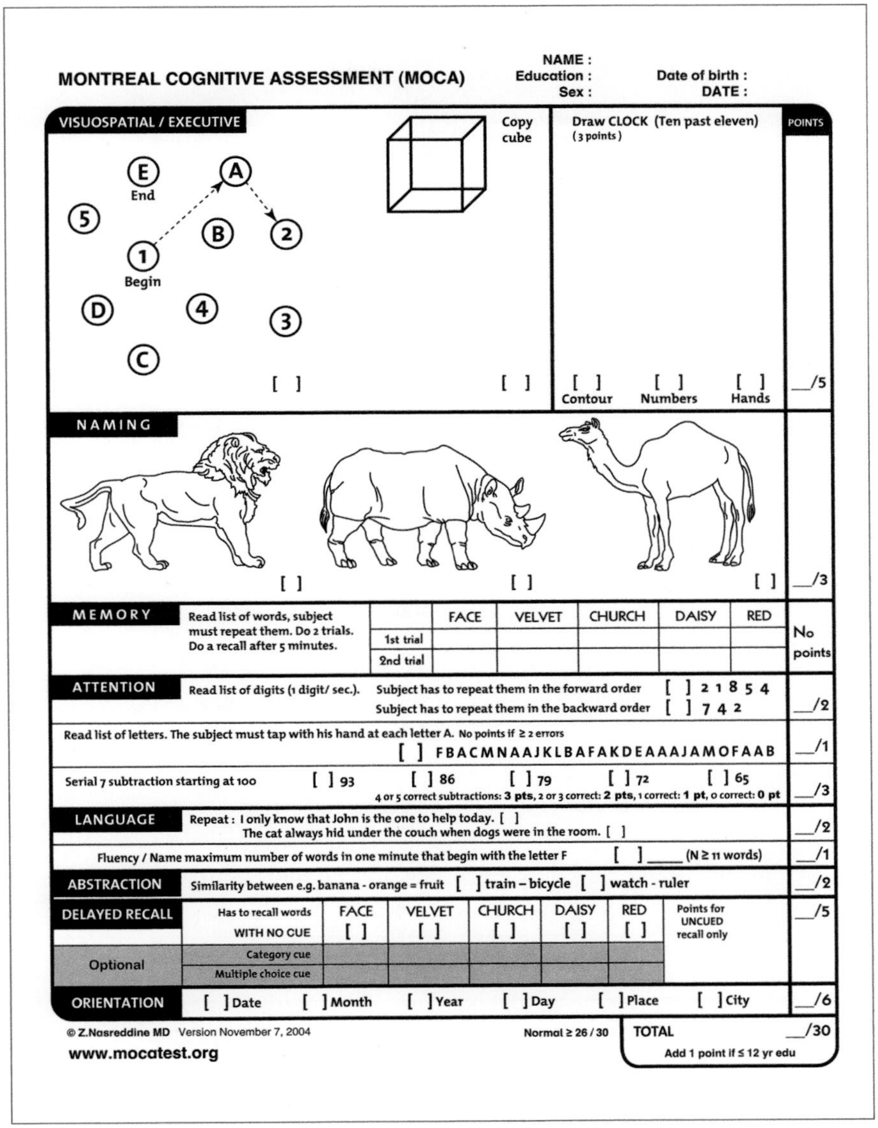

FIGURE 11.8 The Montreal Cognitive Assessment (MoCA) test.

Source: Copyright Z. Nasreddine. Reproduced with permission. Copies are available at https://www.mocatest.org.

CRANIAL NERVE EXAMINATION

Each cranial nerve is to be evaluated independently (Table 11.1).

CN I: The olfactory nerve. The first cranial nerve is a direct extension of the brain. As such, it allows direct access to the brain itself, circumventing the blood–brain barrier. To test cranial nerve I, ask the patient to smell something that he or she should be familiar with, such as coffee, banana, or peppermint. Do not use caustic compounds such as ammonia, as you will not be testing CN I. The pain sensors in the nose are CN V.

CN II: The optic nerve. The pupillary light reflex allows the eye to adjust to various light intensities by changing pupil size with changing light levels. A complete pupillary light reflex requires detection of the light (CN II—afferent nerves) that is relayed to the brainstem. The response is relayed

TABLE 11.1

Special Tests for Cranial Nerves

Cranial Nerve	Clinical Test	Normal Outcomes
CN I Olfactory nerve	Smell (or patient history)	Correct identification of smell
CN II Optic nerve	Pupillary light reflex Visual fields	Pupils constrict on exposure to light Intact as measured by examiner's range of visual field
CN III, IV, and VI Oculomotor nerve Trochlear nerve Abducens nerve	Eye movements to all four quadrants	Full smooth movements in all directions
CN V Trigeminal nerve	Light touch and pinprick	Intact and symmetric
CN VII Facial nerve	Frown or smile	Intact and symmetric facial movement
CN VIII	Fingers rubbed near ear or whisper test	Ability to hear soft sounds
CN IX and X	Gag response and soft-palate elevation	Gag present and soft palate elevates symmetrically
CN XI	Shoulder shrug	Symmetric elevation
CN XII	Tongue protrusion	Symmetric without deviation to either side

back to both eyes with dilation or contraction of the pupils. This is a brainstem-mediated reflex that does not involve the cerebral cortex. The pupillary light reflex is elicited by shining a light into the patient's eye. A normal response is the constriction of the pupils in both eyes.

- **Peripheral vision field testing:** Done at the bedside with confrontation. Have the patient cover one eye and look at your nose. Using the limits of your peripheral vision, ask the patient how many fingers are being displayed.

- **Visual acuity:** Tested with a Snellen chart (Figure 11.9). The patient stands 20 feet from the chart and is asked to read the line with the smallest print that he or she can see. The results are a numeric fraction relative to what a "normal" patient should be able to read at 20 feet. The numerator is always 20, whereas the denominator

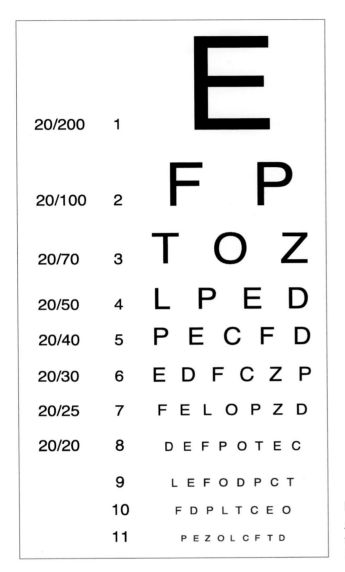

FIGURE 11.9 Snellen chart for visual acuity testing.

Source: Armitage, A. (2015). *Advanced practice nursing guide to the neurological exam* (Figure 3.3). New York, NY: Springer Publishing Company.

is less than 20 for people with high visual acuity and greater than 20 for people with poor vision. Testing is done with corrective lenses, where applicable.

- **Fundoscope exam**: This skill is developed with practice; it looks at the disc, fovea, and retinal surface. CN II is the only cranial nerve that can be seen directly.

CN III, IV, and VI: These are motor (efferent) nerves that, together, control the six muscles of the eye. In addition, CN III innervates the muscles that elevate the upper eyelid and the muscles that control the shape of the lens and size of the pupil. Tested together, ask the patient to look to all four quadrants of the visual field. CN III can further be evaluated by observing the patient's face for eyelid droop and with the pupillary light reflex discussed earlier.

CN V: Best known as the nerve that supplies the brain with sensory input from the face, CN V also has a motor component. This nerve is divided up into three divisions as shown in Figure 11.10. Test by asking the patient to close

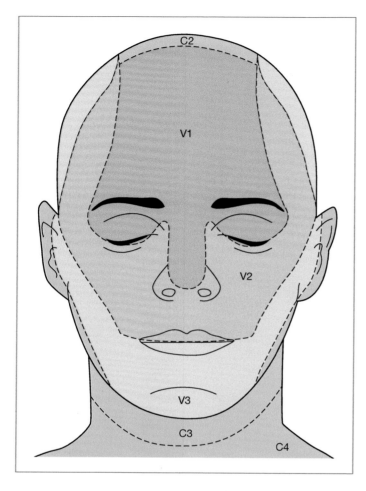

FIGURE 11.10 V1, V2, and V3 dermatomal divisions of CN V.

Source: Adapted from Armitage, A. (2015). *Advanced practice nursing guide to the neurological exam*. New York, NY: Springer Publishing Company.

his or her eyes and then touch the face gently with a tissue or soft paintbrush in each of the three divisions. Touching the left and right side of the face simultaneously allows assessment of symmetry. The motor component of CN V is tested by palpating the temporal and mandibular areas as the patient clenches and grinds his or her teeth. The corneal reflex is elicited using tactile stimulation of the cornea, by touching the eye with a wisp of cotton. The sensory component of the reflex pathway is CN V and the motor component is CN VII.

CN VII: CN VII is involved in almost all movements of the face. In addition, it serves as a source of parasympathetic fibers to the submandibular and sublingual glands, increasing the flow of saliva from these glands. The parasympathetic innervation of the nasal mucosa and lacrimal gland is also supplied by CN VII. It has a sensory component that carries information from the lateral border of the anterior two-thirds of the tongue and the hard and soft palates. It is the moderator of the acoustic reflex and forms the efferent limb of the corneal reflex along with CN V. Testing the muscles of facial expression requires observation of the patient's face at rest, looking for asymmetry; then, looking for symmetry with motion, have the patient smile and then frown.

CN VIII: Sounds are transmitted to the brain through CN VIII. In addition, CN VIII is responsible for a sense of position and movement.

- **Weber and Rinne testing:** This helps to distinguish between conduction problems with the sound waves having trouble getting to the cochlea, and sensorineural deficits, which are problems beyond the cochlea. The Weber test is for unilateral hearing loss. Hold a vibrating tuning fork firmly to the middle of the forehead at the hairline. Ask the patient if one side sounds louder than the other. If the examiner knows ahead of time which side has hearing loss, it may be deduced that if the good side seems louder the damage is sensorineural and if the bad side seems louder the damage is probably conductive. The Rinne test is usually performed in conjunction with the Weber test (Figure 11.11);

it compares the transmission of sound by air conduction versus bone conduction. Strike the tuning fork and hold it firmly to the mastoid so that it is perpendicular to the ear. Ask the patient to tell you when the sound is no longer heard. Quickly reposition the tuning fork parallel to the ear and ask the patient if he or she can hear the tuning fork. If the patient is able to hear the air conduction better than bone conduction, this is a positive response and considered normal. Hearing bone conduction better than ear conduction speaks to a conduction hearing loss, where something is inhibiting the sound waves from reaching the cochlea.

- **Unilateral head impulse test:** This tests the vestibulo-ocular reflex. It is a sensitive and specific test that detects unilateral reduction in functioning of the peripheral vestibular system. Asking the patient to

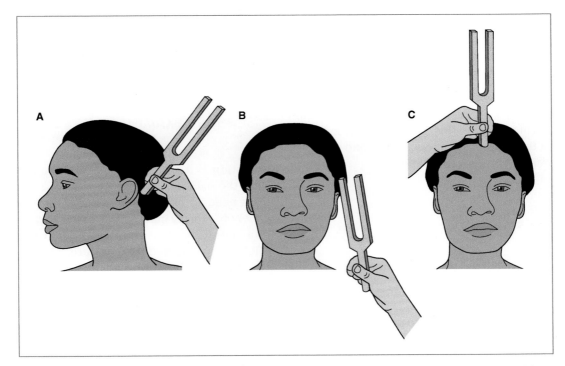

FIGURE 11.11 Positions of the tuning fork during Rinne test (**A** and **B**) and Weber test (**C**).

Source: Adapted from Armitage, A. (2015). *Advanced practice nursing guide to the neurological exam.* New York, NY: Springer Publishing Company.

fixate on a target, turn his or her head very rapidly to one side and observe for corrective eye movements. Repeat with the other side. An intact vestibulo-ocular reflex allows the eyes to remain fixated on their target. When the reflex fails, the patient's eyes move with the head and then correct to fixate on the original target, a saccade. The presence of a saccade indicates vestibular disease as opposed to brainstem disease.

CN IX and X: The glossopharyngeal and vagus nerves travel their course very closely together, so they are generally tested together. Damage to these two nerves is rare, and is best tested by eliciting the gag reflex because the sensory component is mediated by CN IX, and the motor response requires an intact CN X. The gag response is easy to test, yet unpleasant for the patient; consequently, many providers will skip this in preference for symmetrical soft-palate elevation and intact swallow. Intact swallow, however, does not indicate an intact gag.

CN XI: The accessory nerve is a purely motor nerve that innervates the sternocleidomastoid muscle (SCM) and the upper fibers of the trapezius muscles. These muscles are tested against resistance.

CN XII: The hypoglossal nerve controls the tongue, which is key in speech, food manipulation, and swallowing. To test this cranial nerve, ask the patient to stick out his or her tongue and observe for symmetry, without deviation.

MOTOR EXAMINATION

Muscle function is assessed by evaluating three factors: Trophic state (bulk), tone, and strength.

Trophic state: Size, shape, and symmetry of muscles are evaluated by observation.

Tone: Muscle tone is assessed by the passive movement of a limb or an isolated muscle. Ask the

TABLE 11.2 Grading System for Muscle Strength	
5	Movement against full resistance
4 (4−/4/4+)	Movement against some resistance
3	Movement against gravity only
2	Movement with gravity eliminated
1	A trace of voluntary movement
0	No voluntary movement

patient to relax and passively move the limb, noting any resistance, rigidity, or asymmetry between sides.

Strength: Muscle strength is scored according to a standardized grading system from full strength to no voluntary movement at all, as outlined in Table 11.2. The patient pushes and pulls against the provider's resistance, while each muscle group is isolated. The muscle is examined for strength and symmetry.

SENSORY EXAMINATION

Sensation is a subjective test and the results are what the patient says that they are. Leading questions need to be avoided, as they may cause the patient to modify his response. There are four basic skin sensations that are tested: Light touch, pinprick, vibration, and temperature. Proprioception and higher order (cortical) aspects of sensation are also tested.

- Light touch receptors are located superficially under the skin. Touch sensation runs along the posterior tract of the spinal cord. The stimulus required for this test is very light, using a cotton wisp or the lightest touch of the examiner's fingers

- Pinprick tests pain, as the sensory stimulus runs along the spinothalamic tract of the spinal cord. Using a neurotip or an unused safety pin, touch the patient's skin. The patient should be able to make a clear distinction between sharp and dull sensation.

- Temperature sensations also run along the spinothalamic tract to the thalamus. Temperature can be tested with hot (40°–45°C) or cold water (5°–10°C), but in a clinic setting it is easiest to use a cool tuning fork.

Vibration runs along the posterior aspect of the spinal cord. Hold a tuning fork to the bony aspect of the patient's foot and wrist. Ask the patient to tell you when he or she no longer feels vibration, which can then be judged against when the examiner no longer feels the vibration.

Proprioception is the ability to sense body position without having to look. Have the patient close his or her eyes and, holding the patient's big toe on the sides, move the toe up or down. Have the patient identify which direction his or her toe was moved (Figure 11.12). The diseases that typically affect proprioception, such as multiple sclerosis, B12 deficiency, and peripheral neuropathy, tend to affect the lower extremities before the upper extremities so, generally, it is enough to test only the lower extremities.

HIGHER ORDER SENSATION TESTING

Sterognosia is the ability to identify an item by feel. To test stereognosis, ask the patient to close his or her eyes and identify an object that you place in his or her hands.

Graphesthesia is the ability to discern what is written on one's hand without being able to see. Ask the patient to close his or her eyes and identify a number written on the palm of his or her hand with a blunt object. Graphesthesia deficits are indicative of cortical damage.

Extinction is the ability to distinguish two different stimuli simultaneously. Ask the patient to close his or her eyes and, touching the patient once, have him or her point to where the patient was touched. Ask the patient to close his or her eyes again and, touching the patient in two different locations, have him or her identify where he or she was touched.

REFLEX EXAMINATION

Reflexes are a key component of the neurological examination and have the advantage of being an objective test requiring no participation from the patient. When discussing reflex testing in a general clinical examination, one most commonly

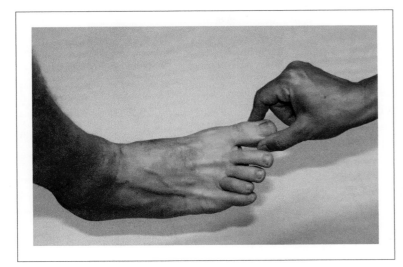

FIGURE 11.12 Testing proprioception by manipulation of the big toe.

Source: Armitage, A. (2015). *Advanced practice nursing guide to the neurological exam.* New York, NY: Springer Publishing Company.

TABLE 11.3
Reflexes Commonly Tested in a Neurological Examination

Reflex	Sensory and Motor Neurons Involved	Type of Reflex
Pupillary	CN II and III	Autonomic reflex
Corneal	CN V and VII	Superficial reflex
Gag	CN IX and X	Superficial reflex
Biceps	C5 and C6	Deep tendon reflex
Triceps	C6 and C7	Deep tendon reflex
Brachioradialis	C6, C7, and C8	Deep tendon reflex
Hoffman's	Spinal cord	Deep tendon reflex
Patellar	L2, L3, and L4	Deep tendon reflex
Achilles	S1 and S2	Deep tendon reflex
Plantar	Corticospinal tract	Superficial reflex
Anal wink	S4 and S5	Superficial reflex

is referring to testing the deep tendon reflexes. Although there are numerous reflexes that can be tested, the most common ones tested in a neurological exam are outlined in Table 11.3.

The pupillary, corneal, and gag reflexes are described in the "Cranial Nerve Examination" section.

Deep tendon reflexes are simple monosynaptic reflexes activated by stretching the tendon or muscle with a sharp tap from a reflex hammer. A reduction in the reflex response indicated a disruption of the reflex arc. Deep tendon reflexes are graded in a semiquantitative manner from 0, no reflex, to 4+ hyperreflexic with clonus. Normal reflexes are 2+ (Table 11.4).

TABLE 11.4
Grading Reflexes

Description	Grade
Mute	0
Hyporeflexic	1+
Normal (standardized patient)	2+
Hyperreflexic	3+
Hyperreflexic with clonus	4+

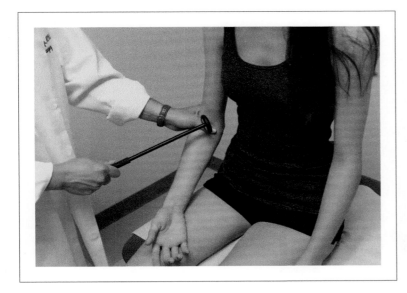

FIGURE 11.13 Testing the biceps reflex.

Source: From Armitage, A. (2015). *Advanced practice nursing guide to the neurological exam*. New York, NY: Springer Publishing Company.

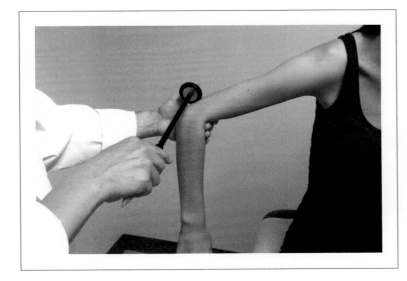

FIGURE 11.14 Testing the triceps reflex.

Source: From Armitage, A. (2015). *Advanced practice nursing guide to the neurological exam*. New York, NY: Springer Publishing Company.

Biceps reflex: Best tested by the examiner placing his or her thumb directly on the biceps brachii tendon and using the reflex hammer to firmly strike the thumb (Figure 11.13). Contraction of the tendon may both be seen and felt.

Triceps reflex: Tested by directly tapping the triceps tendon with the reflex hammer while the arm is relaxed (Figure 11.14).

Brachioradialis reflex: Elicited by striking the brachioradialis tendon (Figure 11.15). The tendon is located on the radial side of the forearm about 4 inches proximal to the base of the thumb.

Patellar reflex: Elicited by striking the patellar tendon, which is located just below the kneecap (Figure 11.16).

Achilles reflex: Elicited by holding the patient's relaxed foot slightly in dorsiflexion with one hand and striking the Achilles tendon with the reflex hammer (Figure 11.17). A normal response is plantar flexion of the foot.

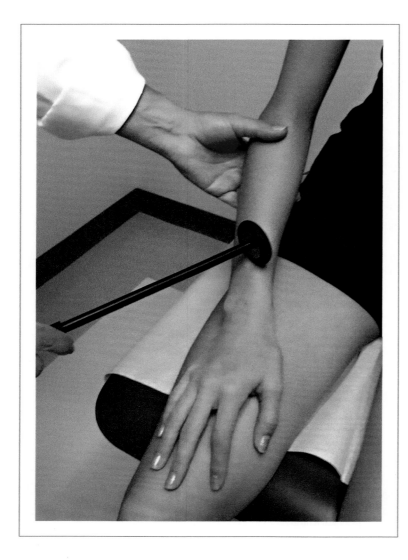

FIGURE 11.15 Testing the brachioradialis reflex.

Source: From Armitage, A. (2015). *Advanced practice nursing guide to the neurological exam*. New York, NY: Springer Publishing Company.

Plantar reflex: Occurs when stimulation of the lateral aspect of the foot and across the ball of the foot and to the base of the great toe causes flexion of the big toe (Figure 11.18).

COORDINATION EXAMINATION

Testing upper extremity coordination can be done simultaneously with testing the patient for a kinetic tremor, with the *finger-nose-finger test*. It is a basic coordination test that is easily executed. Rapid alternating hand movements is a good test of coordination that can elicit some of the subtler changes from baseline. In this test, patients are asked to rapidly slap their hands on their lap, alternating between the dorsal and palmar aspects of their hands (Figure 11.19). This test has the advantage of overcoming possible compensation in a high-functioning patient owing to its speed and its demand to move both hands together.

The *heel-to-shin test* is used to evaluate lower extremity coordination. It requires that the patient trace a path from the top of the kneecap down the

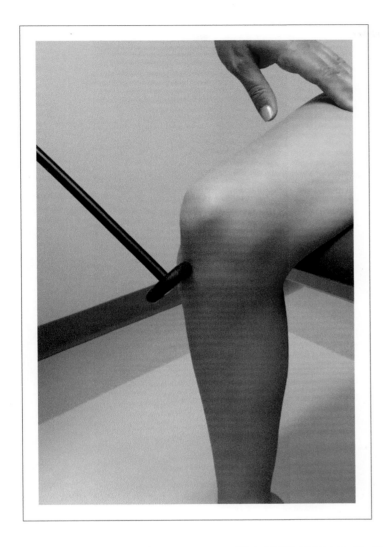

FIGURE 11.16 Testing the patellar reflex.

Source: From Armitage, A. (2015). *Advanced practice nursing guide to the neurological exam*. New York, NY: Springer Publishing Company.

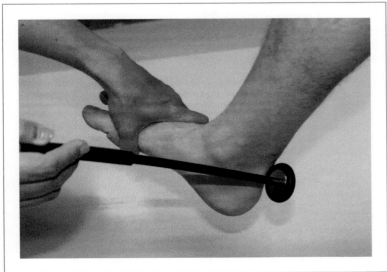

FIGURE 11.17 Testing the Achilles reflex.

Source: From Armitage, A. (2015). *Advanced practice nursing guide to the neurological exam*. New York, NY: Springer Publishing Company.

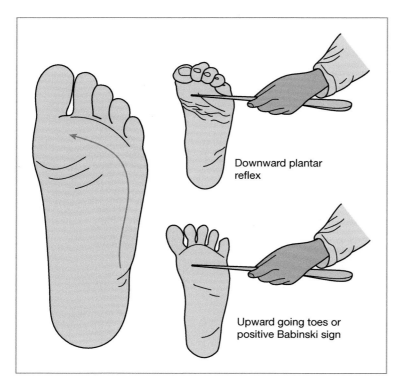

Downward plantar reflex

Upward going toes or positive Babinski sign

FIGURE 11.18 Testing the plantar reflex.

Source: Armitage, A. (2015). *Advanced practice nursing guide to the neurological exam.* New York, NY: Springer Publishing Company.

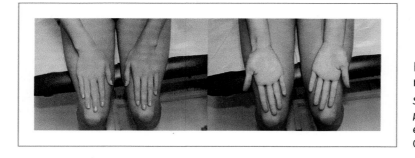

FIGURE 11.19 The hand-slap test (or rapid alternating hand movement test).

Source: From Armitage, A. (2015). *Advanced practice nursing guide to the neurological exam.* New York, NY: Springer Publishing Company.

full length of the shin with his or her heel. It is then repeated on the other side.

GAIT EXAMINATION

Evaluate the patient walking into the clinic. Look for a steady, symmetric gait with regular stride length and good arm swing. Observe the width of the gait; there should be 2″ to 4″ between the patient's heels as the patient walks. Patients widen their gait to improve balance and stability. Wider-based gaits can be indicative of pathology such as vestibular dysfunction, peripheral neuropathy, or a cerebellar lesion.

Length of step, measured from the toe of one foot to the placement of the heel of the other foot, is generally 14″ to 16″. Step length decreases with increased age and conditions such as Parkinson's disease.

Arm swing is a natural part of a walk, and fits the natural rhythm of the walk. While a large part of arm swing is mechanically passive, movements are stabilized by active muscle control. Arm movement is important in overall gait stability. Lack of arm swing is typically seen in diseases that affect movement, such as Parkinson's disease.

Turning problems are common in any gait disorder; generally, turning is more difficult than walking. Make a point of observing how a patient negotiates a 180-degree turn. People without a gait and balance problem can normally turn with one or two steps. Blocked turns (i.e., turns that require more than four steps) are typical of movement disorders such as Parkinson's disease, but can also be seen in frontal gait disorders caused by cerebral or basal ganglia dysfunction. If a patient has less trouble turning than walking forward, a psychogenic disturbance is likely.

Focused Health Assessment and Abnormal Findings

MENTAL STATUS

A score of below 26 on the MoCA evaluation denotes mild cognitive impairment (MCI). When a person scores poorly on either bedside evaluations or a more formal neuropsychological evaluation, coupled with difficulties executing his or her normal activities of daily living, the person can be given a diagnosis of dementia.

DEMENTIA

Dementia is a term that encompasses a number of disease processes; it is not a specific disease. Instead, dementia describes a group of symptoms affecting memory, thinking, and social abilities. A diagnosis of dementia requires that at least two core mental functions be impaired enough to interfere with daily living. They are memory, language skills, ability to focus and pay attention, ability to reason and problem-solve, and visual perception.

Dementia frequently involves memory loss, but not all memory loss is a result of dementia. Memory loss alone does not equate to a diagnosis of dementia. Alzheimer's disease is the most common cause of a progressive dementia in older adults, with vascular dementia and Lewy body dementia following a close second and third. But there are a number of causes of dementia beyond these two diagnoses. Some causes of dementia can be reversed, and, because of this, it is paramount to determine the underlying etiology of the changes in cognitive functioning.

Dementia symptoms vary depending on the cause, but common signs and symptoms include both cognitive and psychological changes (Box 11.1). These changes are frequently noticed by a spouse or close companion, and it is not unusual for the patient to have little to no insight into cognitive difficulties and personality changes.

BOX 11.1 Symptoms Frequently Found in Dementia

Cognitive Changes

- Memory deficits, mostly short term
- Word-finding difficulties
- Visuospatial difficulties
- Problem-solving difficulties
- Challenges completing complex tasks
- Organizational difficulties
- Disorientation, getting lost in familiar places

Psychological Changes

- Depression
- Apathy
- Anxiety
- Executive dysfunction
- Inappropriate behavior
- Hallucinations and delusions

CAUSES OF DEMENTIA

Dementia is a result of damage to the nerve cells in the brain. The symptoms of dementia present differently, depending on the area of the brain affected. Dementias are grouped by the geographic territory that is affected and whether they are progressive or static. Some dementias, such as those caused by a vitamin deficiency or hypothyroidism, might improve with treatment.

PROGRESSIVE NEURODEGENERATIVE DEMENTIAS

Progressive neurodegenerative dementias are not reversible. They are most often a result of protein depositions in the nerve cells that cause irreversible structural damage and ultimately cell death. Especially in older adults, the diagnosis on one type of dementia does not preclude another. Frequently, in the oldest old, a mixed dementia exists with symptoms presenting as a combination of the dementia types.

- **Alzheimer's disease:** Generally this is a geriatric disease in people of age 65 and older, but a young onset variant exists that is much more aggressive in its course and has a strong genetic base.

  Although the cause of Alzheimer's disease is not known, plaques and tangles from beta-amyloid and tau protein, respectively, are often found in the brains of people with Alzheimer's. Vascular factors are also involved which lead to breakdown of the blood-brain barrier.

- **Vascular dementia:** This second most common type of dementia occurs as a result of damage to the vessels that supply blood to the brain.

- **Lewy body dementia:** Lewy bodies are a result of abnormal clumps of α-synuclein protein. The α-synuclein has been found in the brains of people with Lewy body dementia, Alzheimer's disease, and Parkinson's disease. This is one of the more common types of progressive dementia.

- **Frontotemporal dementia:** This is a group of diseases characterized by the degeneration of nerve cells in the frontal and temporal lobes of the brain, the areas generally associated with personality, behavior, and language.

OTHER DISORDERS LINKED TO DEMENTIA

There are a number of other dementias; some are genetic, such as Huntington's disease (untreatable) and Wilson's disease (treatable), while others are structural or metabolic.

- **Huntington's disease:** Caused by a genetic mutation, which results from an abnormally high repeat of cytosine-adenine-guanine (CAG) in the Huntingtin gene. This genetic defect causes an abnormally large production and accumulation of the Huntingtin protein, resulting in certain nerve cells in the brain and spinal cord to waste away. Signs and symptoms, including a severe decline in thinking (cognitive) skills, usually appear around age 30 or 40. This may be preceded by psychiatric symptoms, often confounding the diagnosis.

- **Wilson's disease:** This is a hereditary disease that leads to elevated copper levels in the blood. It presents with multiple symptoms and can lead to cognitive changes and psychiatric symptoms. There are medical treatments, which are lifelong.

- **Traumatic brain injury:** This condition is caused by repetitive head trauma, such as that experienced by boxers, football players, or soldiers. Depending on the part of the brain that's injured, this condition can cause dementia signs and symptoms, including depression, explosiveness, memory loss, uncoordinated movement, impaired speech, and parkinsonism. Symptoms might not appear until years after the trauma.

DEMENTIA-LIKE CONDITIONS THAT CAN BE REVERSED

Some causes of dementia or dementia-like symptoms can be reversed with treatment. These include both metabolic and structural etiologies. As seen in Table 11.5, there are a number of treatable causes of dementia, which drives home the importance of understanding the etiology of a patient's cognitive changes.

TABLE 11.5
Etiologies and Treatable Causes of Dementia

Etiology	Treatable Causes
Infection	Meningitis
Autoimmune	Multiple sclerosis
Metabolic	Low sodium
Endocrine	Hypothyroidism
Nutritional deficiencies	Dehydration B12, B6, or B1
Brain lesion	Tumor Subdural hematoma Normal pressure hydrocephalus
Poisoning	Heavy metals (e.g., lead) Alcohol Recreational drugs
Anoxia	Carbon monoxide poisoning Heart attack

CRANIAL NERVE DYSFUNCTION

CN I: An abnormal response is the inability to smell. This can be seen in a number of neurological conditions such as prodromal Parkinson's disease, Alzheimer's disease, skull-based tumors, and traumatic brain injury.

CN II: The neural pathway that manages the pupillary light reflex runs directly to the midbrain for the sole purpose of light detection to protect the sensitive retina from excess light. The presence of this reflex is one of the most basic tests of brainstem function, and is one of the reflexes tested in determining brain death.

- **Afferent pupillary defect:** Tested by swinging a light from eye to eye. Light shone in the normal eye will cause constriction of both pupils whereas light shone into the defective eye will not, as light detection in the damaged eye is reduced due to damage to the optic nerve. Optic neuritis is overwhelmingly the most common cause of an afferent pupillary defect.

- **Visual field defect:** may result from damage to CN II. The defects will vary depending on the location of the injury (Figure 11.20). Peripheral vision may decrease in migraine with aura events, in patients with cataracts, from lesions at various parts of the optic tract, and patients with eye defects. A patient with a visual acuity of 20/200 or less, with the best corrective lenses, is considered legally blind.

Key abnormal findings in the fundoscopic exam of CN II are summarized in Table 11.6.

CN III, IV, and VI: The primary presenting symptoms when there is damage to CN III, IV, or VI is diplopia. Diplopia is the result of the unyoking of the matching muscles that are innervated by these nerves, leading to a disconjugate gaze. The direction of gaze in which the patient experiences diplopia will depend on which cranial nerve is affected. Damage to the third cranial nerve causes a CN III palsy, which may be partial or complete. A CN III lesion results in ipsilateral ptosis (eyelid droop), a dilated and unresponsive pupil, and the eye looking down and out. A CN III palsy is most commonly due to an ischemic event due to diabetes or hypertension. It is important not to miss an aneurysm pressing on the third nerve presenting as a blown pupil. A blown pupil is considered a medical emergency until proven otherwise.

CN V: Trigeminal neuralgia is a painful spasm of CN V, which may occur in one or more divisions of the trigeminal nerve, most commonly V2 or V3. The pain has a sharp shooting quality lasting a few seconds and may occur repeatedly when severe. The pain may or may not require a trigger.

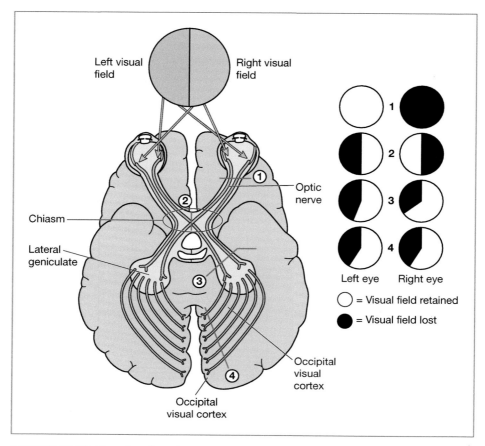

FIGURE 11.20 The visual pathways as seen from above the brain.

Source: From Armitage, A. (2015). *Advanced practice nursing guide to the neurological exam*. New York, NY: Springer Publishing Company.

TABLE 11.6
Key Signs in a Fundoscopic Exam

Change Seen	Interpretation	Possible Etiologies
Papilledema (blurred disc margins with loss of visible venous pulsations)	Increased intracranial pressure	Hydrocephalus, intracranial mass effect from a lesion, idiopathic intracranial hypertension
Disc pallor	Optic atrophy	Multiple sclerosis or neuromyelitis optica
Excessive disc cupping	Increased intraocular pressure	Glaucoma
Microaneurysms	Increased small capillary pressure	Chronic hypertension, diabetic retinopathy
Macular edema	Blood vessels leaking contents into the macular region	Diabetic retinopathy

CN VII: The most well-known abnormality of CN VII is Bell's palsy, an idiopathic paralysis of this nerve. The primary symptoms are a unilateral onset of facial muscle weakness, which involves the forehead as well as the lower parts of the face, plus impairment of taste and hyperacusis. Upper motor neuron lesions may cause a facial palsy, but the clinical presentation differs from Bell's palsy in that there is no forehead involvement. In an upper motor neuron palsy, the lower facial muscles on the contralateral side to the lesion lose voluntary control. The forehead muscles are bilaterally innervated, thereby preserving their function.

CN VIII: Damage to this cranial nerve results in hearing loss or vestibular dysfunction or both.

CN IX and X: A gag reflex tests both CN IX (sensory) and X (motor). When the gag reflex is absent it is generally quite obvious. Patients will find that the cotton swab on their uvula is not bothersome at all, and will remain quite comfortable. The only way to incorrectly assess this test is to poke the patient's throat too hard in an attempt to elicit a response eliciting a pain withdrawal response.

CN XI: Damage to CN XI is rare, but may occur in cases of neck injury, tumor, nerve lesion, or infarction. Shoulder shrug against resistance tests the trapezius component while head rotation against resistance tests the SCM contraction. Lower motor neuron lesions produce weakness of both the trapezius and SCM on the same side. Upper motor neuron lesions produce SCM weakness on the same side as the lesion and contralateral to trapezius weakness.

CN XII: Damage to the hypoglossal nerve causes tongue deviation when the examiner asks the patient to stick out his or her tongue. A lower motor neuron lesion will result in deviation of the tongue toward the side of the lesion, along with fasciculations and atrophy. An upper motor neuron lesion will deviate away from the side of the lesion.

MOTOR ABNORMALITIES

CLINICAL EVALUATION

- **Trophic state:** Atrophy may result from disuse of a muscle or from denervation of the muscle. Hypertrophy is the enlargement of a muscle group that may occur naturally from exercise but may also be pathologic such as in Duchenne's muscular dystrophy.

- **Tone:** Hypertonia is increased muscle tone and manifests as spasticity or rigidity. Muscle tone is assessed by passive movement of the muscle being assessed, or of the limb.

- **Strength:** Lesions in both upper and lower motor neurons can cause weakness. The "Motor Examination" section outlines the testing and gradation of strength; anything less than 5/5 is abnormal. Different presentations result from damage at different levels in the motor system. The motor examination can be a good indication of where the lesion lies as upper and lower motor neuron lesions have distinctive characteristics, as outlined in Table 11.7.

Parkinson's disease is defined by its motor symptoms of increased tone, slowness, and tremor in some patients. Tone is tested by having the patient relax completely and moving his or her elbow and wrist around its own axis. Bradykinesia (slowness) in Parkinson's disease is a progressive slowness of movement in an exercise such as finger tapping. This movement becomes slower or stutters with repetition (known as decrement). This differs from arthritis or stroke that may show slowness, but no decrement is present. To test for resting tremor, have the patient place his or her hands in his or her lap with his or her eyes closed and completely relaxed. Distract the patient by having him or her count backward from 100. With distraction a resting tremor will emerge, seen as a low frequency (4–6 Hz) tremor.

A postural tremor, seen when a patient holds both his or her arms straight out before him or her,

TABLE 11.7
Characteristics of Lower and Upper Motor Neuron Lesions

Clinical Test	Lower Motor Neuron Lesion	Upper Motor Neuron Lesion
Weakness	Yes	Yes
Muscle tone	Decreased/ flaccid	Increased/ spastic
Muscle stretch reflexes	Decreased	Increased
Muscle atrophy	Profound	Minimal
Fasciculations	Present	Absent
Sensory disturbance	Variable	Variable

can be part of the Parkinsonian syndrome and is generally low-to-medium frequency. A physiological tremor is a high-frequency, low-amplitude postural tremor that is not pathologic.

Essential tremor is characterized by a high-frequency kinetic tremor that is tested by having the patient touch from the provider's index finger to his or her nose and back. The tremor is distal and becomes worse when approaching the target.

Observation of the patient during the examination will allow the provider time to see chorea or dyskinesias such as tardive dyskinesia or orobuccolingual dyskinesias. Generally, dyskinesias and chorea are briefly suppressible if the patient makes a conscious effort, but suppression is not sustainable.

SENSORY ABNORMALITIES

CLINICAL EVALUATION

The loss of sensation may be peripheral, such as a peripheral neuropathy, or central in either the spinal cord or the brain. The site of the lesion may be deduced from the physical exam findings (Table 11.8).

Length-dependent peripheral neuropathies, such as those found in diabetes, alcoholism, B12 deficiency, or idiopathic conditions, are predominantly sensory neuropathies, with light touch, pinprick, vibration, and then temperature affected (in that order). These can be profound. Once the nerve damage has advanced up to the calves, the fingertips and then hands and forearms become involved. The lack of electromyography (EMG) findings does not preclude a neuropathy, as the diagnosis is clinical.

Nerve root entrapment causes sensory changes before any motor deficits become apparent. The sensory changes map out in dermatomal distributions (see Figure 11.4) and from this the level of nerve root entrapment may be deduced. Standard light touch and pinprick testing is sufficient.

REFLEX ABNORMALITIES

CLINICAL EVALUATION

Hyperreflexia, an excessive reflex response, may result from a disruption in the CNS damping effect. When this damping is removed, there is nothing to moderate the reflex response. A lesion can affect everything more caudal to it. Typically, hyperreflexia is a result of a central lesion (cord or brain).

Hyporeflexia is the result of peripheral nerve lesion: Nerve root, plexus, or peripheral nerve. Looking for symmetry is important as large muscle-bound patients and heavier patients may appear to have more mute reflexes.

Certain drugs (e.g., stimulants) can influence reflexes. Marijuana can cause marked hyperreflexia, due to disinhibition of the reflex arc. Hyperthyroidism and serotonin syndrome cause hyperreflexia.

SPECIAL TESTS

Hoffman's reflex is an indication of spinal cord irritation; it a pathologic reflex. Hold the patient's hand

TABLE 11.8
Neuropathies Leading to Sensory Changes

Type	Sensory Loss Location	Considerations	Examples
Distal peripheral neuropathy (stocking and glove)	From the toes upward to the feet and calves; hands then become involved	Generally symmetric, presenting as altered sensation	Diabetes, alcohol, or idiopathic; B12 or other metabolic disturbances
Median nerve neuropathy	Thumb, index, and half of the middle finger	EMG is the gold standard diagnostic test. Tinels and phalanges tests used at the bedside have low sensitivity.	Carpal tunnel
Ulnar nerve neuropathy	Fourth and fifth fingers on the affected side	EMG is diagnostic.	Cubital tunnel
Brachial plexus	Entire arm from the point of pressure downward	Can be slow in healing, if at all.	Brachial plexopathy; Saturday night palsy
Trigeminal neuralgia	CN V2 and V3 are the most common.	Challenging to treat medically. Surgical intervention is not a guarantee of symptom remission.	
Impingement of the nerve roots	Pain and loss of sensation; may result in motor weakness	Pain is the most common presenting symptom. Loss of sensation will present in a dermatomal pattern. Loss of strength will present in a myotomal pattern.	Lumber or cervical radiculopathy; cauda equina syndrome
Impingement of the spinal cord	There is no associated pain with cord impingement.	Requires immediate neurosurgical referral. Generally, gait is affected. Concern over a devastating injury if there is further impact on the cord, such as with a fall.	Cervical myelopathy

EMG, electromyography.

completely limp. Flick the tip of the middle finger. Unlike other deep tendon reflexes, this is graded as either present or absent.

Clonus is the rapid, involuntary, rhythmic contraction of a muscle group after a sudden muscle stretch. It is a symptom of spasticity, which occurs as a result of a lesion in the upper motor neurons. Most commonly specific clonus testing is done at the ankles (ankle clonus), but clonus may be elicited with any reflex in both the upper and lower extremities. Ankle clonus is tested by having the patient sit relaxed. With one hand stabilizing the lower leg, the other hand sharply dorsiflexes the foot. Absence of a response is normal. Beating of the foot is documented as 1 beat, 2 beats of sustained clonus (3+ beats).

DISCUSSION

Decreased reflexes occur in Guillain–Barre syndrome as it is the peripheral nerves in GB syndrome that become demyelinated, from distal to proximal. This damage to the peripheral nerves interrupts the reflex arc and a reflex response cannot be elicited.

Heightened reflexes occur in hereditary spastic paraplegia (HSP) and cervical myelopathy. HSP is a group of hereditary, degenerative, neurological disorders that primarily affect the upper motor neurons. The hallmark feature of HSP is progressive weakness and spasticity of the legs. Reflexes are heightened, frequently with spread of the reflex and clonus which can be quite impressive.

Cervical myelopathy is a result of damage to the cervical spinal cord. Part of the myelopathic exam is the presence of symmetric hyperreflexia, due to lack of damping of the normal reflex arc by the central nerve pathways.

COORDINATION ABNORMALITIES

CLINICAL EVALUATION

Speed is an important factor in finger-to-nose and rapid alternating hand tests, as it unmasks ataxic movements. In heel-to-shin testing, speed is not important, but accuracy is.

DISCUSSION

A lesion in the cerebellum is most often associated with loss of coordination (ataxia). However, balance (vestibular system), vision, proprioception, and sequence processing (executive functioning) all contribute to the clinical impression of coordination. The results of coordination testing need to be interpreted contextually, which can challenge integrating them into the final clinical assessment. Known causes of ataxia include stroke, tumor, cerebral palsy, brain degeneration, and multiple sclerosis. Alcohol, drugs, and certain medication also cause ataxia.

GAIT ABNORMALITIES

CLINICAL EVALUATION

Evaluation of a patient starts when the patient first walks into a clinic. It is not always necessary, but special testing can sometimes help distinguish symptoms.

SPECIAL TESTS

Heel and toe walking are tests of provocation. Gastrocnemius muscle testing is best tested by toe walking, and tibialis anterior strength is best tested by heel walking. A patient should be able to bear the full body weight with both.

Tandem walk is a test of balance. This is done by asking the patient to walk a straight line, touching the heel of one foot to the toe of the other foot with each step (Figure 11.21). Patients with balance trouble, reduced sensation in their feet, or lack of proprioception will have particular difficulty with this task since they tend to have wide-based unsteady gaits and become more unsteady when attempting to keep their feet close together.

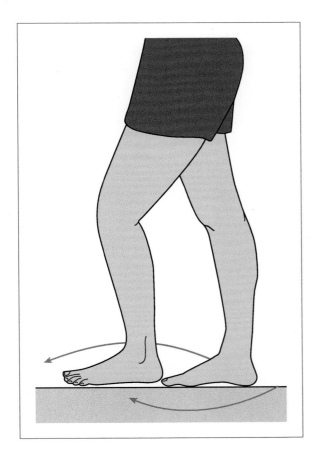

FIGURE 11.21 Tandem walk.

Source: Adapted from Armitage, A. (2015). *Advanced practice nursing guide to the neurological exam*. New York, NY: Springer Publishing Company.

DISCUSSION

Spastic gait is a stiff, foot-dragging quality, caused by long muscle contraction on one side (Figure 11.22). This gait may be seen with many brain and spine lesions, such as brain tumors, multiple sclerosis, and cerebral palsy.

Trendelenburg gait is caused by weakness of hip abductors. This condition makes it difficult to support the body's weight on the affected side. The patient compensates by swinging his or her body over the affected hip to place the center of gravity over the hip, thereby reducing the degree of pelvic drop (Figure 11.23). A Trendelenburg gait is commonly seen in the muscular dystrophies and poliomyelitis.

Hemiplegic gait is a result of weakness to one side of the body. The patient will hold the arm on the affected side adducted and immobile, with circumduction of the affected leg. This is most commonly seen in stroke patients.

A steppage gait is a result of the patient lifting his leg high enough to clear the foot, so that the toe does not catch and the foot does not drag. This is seen in patients with foot drop, as well as those with peroneal nerve injury or L4 nerve root injury. Bilateral causes include amyotrophic lateral sclerosis, the dystrophies, and profound neuropathies.

A hypokinetic gait is one of overall slowness of movement and reduced stride length. This is seen in Parkinson's disease, concomitant with a shuffling gait and en bloc turning.

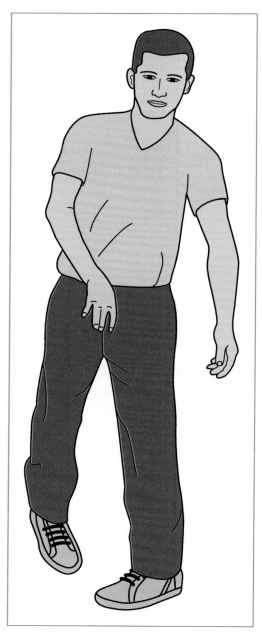

FIGURE 11.22 Spastic gait.

Source: Adapted from Armitage, A. (2015). *Advanced practice nursing guide to the neurological exam*. New York, NY: Springer Publishing Company.

Ataxic gait is characterized by incoordination, resulting in broad-based lurching quality. This gait may be divided into ataxia from a cerebellar lesion or disruption (such as alcohol), or from sensory disruption and severe loss of proprioception. A sensory ataxia may result from a severe peripheral sensory neuropathy and damage to the dorsal columns of the spinal cord.

Antalgic gait is seen in patients who avoid certain movements to avoid acute pain. The compensatory maneuvers are an attempt to achieve reduced weight-bearing time on the painful limb, avoidance of impact loads, reduced joint excursions, and minimization of activity in muscles that span the joint.

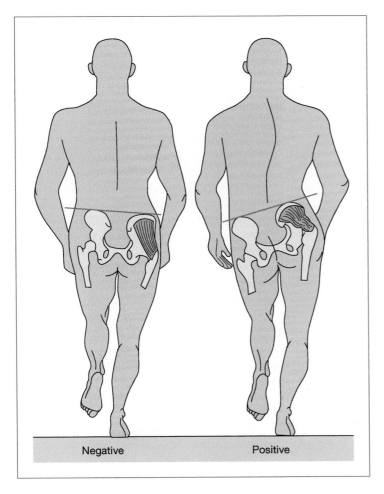

Negative   Positive

FIGURE 11.23 TRENDELENBURG GAIT.

Source: Adapted from Armitage, A. (2015). *Advanced practice nursing guide to the neurological exam.* New York, NY: Springer Publishing Company.

Holistic Assessment

SPECIFIC HEALTH HISTORY

When a patient presents with a neurological complaint, it is imperative to elicit a thorough and accurate chief complaint (CC; in the patient's own words), history of the present illness, and review of systems. When assessing the attributes of the symptom, pay particular attention to the onset and duration for determining if the problem is acute or chronic in nature, for aggravating or alleviating factors for clues into the differential diagnosis, and for associated signs and symptoms, as systems are closely integrated. As with all other body system evaluation, include a detailed and inclusive past medical history (PMH), family history (FH), and social history (SH).

It is important to avoid concluding that someone whose speech is slow or someone with a physical disability that limits mobility is unable to understand and answer questions. Further, it is imperative that the clinician communicates with the person with a disability rather than an accompanying person. Do not assume that all signs and symptoms are due to a preexisting disability or disorder.

SAFETY

The primary safety concern for most neurological patients is risk of fall. In the neurological populations with neurodegenerative disease, such as multiple sclerosis, Parkinson's disease, and Huntington's disease, balance deteriorates as disease progresses due to loss of proprioception, core reflexes, and agility.

Seizure patients are at risk of having an unexpected seizure while doing something that may put their life at risk. Standard seizure precautions are given to all seizure patients, which includes a driving restriction. The ability to enforce this restriction and length of restriction in a seizure-free seizure patient varies by state.

Patients with deteriorating cognition are at risk for poor and impulsive decision-making with limited insight, making them at risk for getting lost or wandering. Many of these patients resist the direction to stop driving, placing themselves and the public at risk. In addition, they may have trouble managing their medications and ultimately need help with their activities of daily living.

MENTAL HEALTH EVALUATIONS FOR THE CHRONICALLY ILL

Neurodegenerative disease comes with significant psychiatric burden, which can be life limiting for the patient and contribute to excessive caregiver burden. Depression and anxiety are commonly seen and should be screened for in all neurological patients. Loss of executive function, depression, anxiety, and emotional lability may be the first presenting symptoms in some disease processes, such as Huntington's disease, which can precede motor symptoms by years.

Impulse control disorders (ICD) and executive dysfunction can make patient management a challenge, bearing in mind some medications, in addition to the neurological illness, can cause ICD. Resolution of the ICD symptoms is slow on discontinuation of these medications. As ICD may be pleasurable, and because many of them are socially undesirable, a patient may be reluctant to disclose impulse disorders to a provider. Patients need to be asked directly with an explanation as to why this is important to discuss.

The hallucinations, on initial presentation in a neurodegenerative disease such as Parkinson's disease or Dementia with Lewy Bodies, are nonthreatening and noninteractive. As the diseases progress, however, this ability to distinguish reality from psychosis is lost and hallucinations can become quite threatening and frightening. Delusions, such as those of infidelity or Capgras syndrome, are difficult to treat medically, and one cannot reason a more moderate perspective with the patient as he or she tends to be firmly rooted in his or her psyche. Although psychosis is part of the disease process itself, a complete medication review is required to ensure that the patient is off all potential offending medications.

Due to the heavy disease burden and caregiver stressors that many neurological diseases bear, community resources such as support groups, seminars, talks, and exercise programs can help a patient learn to care for themselves, and ensure that they and their caregivers do not feel isolated.

The patient's social support system (emotional, driving, daily household management, med management) needs to be considered. As diseases progress, a patient is often able to do less for him- or herself, requiring more assistance. Helping the patient and family recognize these needs is important in ensuring that they are well cared for.

Financial/insurance coverage for new medications, surgeries (e.g., deep brain stimulation), facility placement, or 24-hour caregivers can be complex. Referral to social work for help understanding insurance coverage options and medication assistance, if required, may become necessary as the patient's disease progresses. Social work can also help with understanding the options for advanced care, such as 24-hour in-home coverage versus facility placement.

Medical power of attorney, living will, and release of information to discuss care with relatives should all be in place when a patient is first diagnosed with a neurological illness. Your social worker can help guide the patient and family with this paperwork when a referral is placed.

CASE STUDY

DOCUMENTATION

Chief Complaint: Tremor

History of Present Illness: Mr. Adams presents for the first time to the Movement Disorders Clinic for evaluation of a tremor in his left hand, most especially when he is relaxing in his chair watching television. Recently, he has begun to walk more slowly with a stoop, and his steps are more shuffling. He feels stiff in the mornings when he gets out of bed. He admits that he has not been able to smell for many years, and he has a longstanding issue with constipation and urinary urgency. His wife complains that he moves around in bed at night, acting out his dreams.

Constitutional: No complaints other than those listed in the HPI

PHYSICAL EXAMINATION

General: Pleasant, conversant, and appropriate; well appearing

Cardiovascular: Good perfusion

Pulmonary: Normal excursions

Integumentary: No erythema or ecchymosis is noted.

Mental Status: Fund of knowledge appears intact as grossly tested. No difficulty with repetition or naming. Complex comprehension intact. Affect is normal.

(continued)

(continued)

CRANIAL NERVES

CN I: Deferred

CN II: Pupils equal, round, and reactive. Fundoscopic exam shows intact disc margins.

CN III, IV, and VI: Ocular eye movements intact without nystagmus; no vertical gaze limitation is noted.

CN V: Intact to light touch

CN VII: Face symmetric both with smiling and frowning

CN VIII: Intact to conversational speech and finger rub

CN IX, X, XII: Symmetric elevation of the soft palate, tongue protrusion midline

CN XI: Symmetric elevation of the shoulders

Motor: Adequate bulk. Tone increased on the left upper extremity, with corresponding bradykinesia on the left. Resting tremor noted on the left. No postural tremor of kinetic tremor with finger-nose-finger. Strength 5/5 throughout upper and lower extremities

Sensation: Intact and symmetric to light touch, pinprick, vibration, and temperature in upper and lower extremities

Reflexes: 2+ in upper and lower extremities. Plantar response downward

Coordination: Intact with finger-nose-finger and with heel-to-shin. No dysdiadochokinesia

Gait: Patient is able to rise from a seated position with push off. He has a shortened stride length with a shuffling gait and stooped posture. There is reduced arm swing on the left.

ASSESSMENT

Clinical examination supports his complaints with findings of bradykinesia, rigidity, and resting tremor. These are three of the four cardinal symptoms of Parkinson's disease, and in the absence of any "red flag" signs that would indicate otherwise, you make a diagnosis of idiopathic Parkinson's disease. You spend time with Mr. Adams and his wife reviewing Parkinson's disease and the many effective treatments that exist for symptom control.

Diagnosis: Idiopathic Parkinson's disease

ICD-10-CM Diagnosis Code: G20 Parkinson's Disease

Assessment of Special Populations

ELDERLY POPULATION

Geriatric patients all fall under Medicare, with or without supplemental insurances. This can impact a patient's access to medication as, with specialty drugs, patients quickly fall into the Medicare "donut hole" where they are required to pay for all their medications before catastrophic insurance kicks in. In addition, polypharmacy is common in geriatric patients with many providers reluctant to prescribe medications. Close attention should be paid to the medication prescribed, its side effects in a more sensitive population, and potential interactions with other medications.

PATIENTS WITH DEMENTIA OR COGNITIVE IMPAIRMENT

Patients with dementia or reduced cognitive function require protection. Due to the nature of their disability, the provider is frequently left in a patriarchal role regarding medication decision-making and decision points to change treatments. This comes with increased responsibility.

PATIENTS WITH DISABILITIES

An important point in assessing an individual with a preexisting disability or a diagnosis of a neurological disorder is to avoid attributing all symptoms to the existing disability or neurological disorder. Individuals with preexisting disabilities and neurological disorders are at risk for other disorders that may be unrelated to their existing neurological disorder or disease. Thus, care must be taken to ask the same questions about history and present symptoms that one would ask of other patients. Even if the patient has some degree of cognitive impairment, questions should be directed to the patient rather than to a family member. Family members may be able to fill in information that was not provided by the patient.

Modifications in the examination may be required to accommodate a patient's disability or neurological disorder; safety of the patient during the examination is of top priority to avoid falls and injury.

WOMEN OF CHILDBEARING AGE

Women of childbearing age and the pregnant woman are at much greater risk for medication side effects and the risks of teratogenicity. Antiepileptics are particularly notorious for their birth defect profiles and should be used with caution in women of childbearing age. The necessity of seizure control versus the risk of childbirth defects needs to be carefully weighed.

UNDERSERVED POPULATIONS

Underserved and uninsured populations may have reduced access to care due to transportation issues, difficulty covering medication costs, literacy levels, and language barriers.

VETERAN POPULATION

The provider should ask the patient if they served in the military. If so, the dates and capacity in which they served (e.g., pilot, ground forces, medical services) should be ascertained. Based upon this information, the provider will be aware of what potential hazards or chemicals of warfare the patient may have been exposed to.

Diagnostic Reasoning

Common Differential Diagnoses: Primary Headaches and Facial Pain

Diagnosis	Key History or Physical Examination Differentiators
Cluster headache	Severe orbital or unilateral headaches that occur in clusters for certain periods, lasting from weeks to months, usually followed by long periods of remission. Accompanied by symptoms such as nasal discharge, or red or tearing eyes, sweating, and restlessness
Medication overuse headache	Rebound headache associated with the long-term use of analgesics (>15 d/mo)
Migraine	Commonly lateralizes. Throbbing in nature. Patient is sensitive to light, sound, smells. May or may not have associated aura
New daily persistent headache	Persistent headache for more than 3 days from onset. Bilateral banding pain without associated photophobia and phonophobia. Not aggravated by physical activity
Temporal arteritis	A medical emergency as vision loss can happen rapidly and is irreversible. May cause stroke. Pain over the temporal area with tenderness to palpation, sometimes over the whole scalp. Associated jaw claudication. ERS and CRP are elevated.
Tension headache	Persistent banding or squeezing pain across the forehead or occiput. Associated with psychosocial stressors and inadequate sleep
Trigeminal neuralgia	Episodes of severe shooting pain along the trigeminal nerve lasting seconds to minutes. May have a trigger. Unilateral. Progressive

CRP, C-reactive protein; ERS, erythrocyte sedimentation rate.

Common Differential Diagnoses: Spells

Diagnosis	Key History or Physical Examination Differentiators
Focal seizures	May or may not have impaired awareness. May or may not have motor activity. Focal seizures may progress to generalized seizures.
Generalized seizures	Motor seizures include tonic-clonic seizures. Nonmotor seizures (absence).

(continued)

Common Differential Diagnoses: Spells (*continued*)

Diagnosis	Key History or Physical Examination Differentiators
Pseudoseizures	Psychogenic, nonepileptic seizures are paroxysmal events that may closely resemble a seizure. Clinical symptoms and/or history are incongruent, and the patient is often less responsive to medication. EEG is normal even during an event.
Unknown onset	If the onset of seizure is not known

EEG, electroencephalogram.

Common Differential Diagnoses: Movement Disorders

Diagnosis	Key History or Physical Examination Differentiators
Cortical basal degeneration	Asymmetric parkinsonism with cortical signs, and apraxia
Essential tremor	Tremor (high-frequency and variable amplitude) with action, not present at rest. Strong genetic/familial trends. Exquisitely sensitive to alcohol, which resolves the tremor.
Huntington's disease	Generalized chorea. The severity and age of onset is determined by the repeat number of the aberrant gene. Psychiatric and cognitive symptoms coexist and may predate the diagnosis, leading to misdiagnosis.
Lewy body dementia	Parkinsonism with early cognitive deterioration and hallucinations
Medication-induced "tardive" disorders	Most frequently associated with current or close-past use of a neuroleptic medication. May present as tremor, chorea, orobuccal lingual dyskinesia, or parkinsonism.
Medication-induced tremor	Type of tremor is dependent on the type of medication. Generally, medium-to-high-frequency postural tremor. Presentation may vary. Evaluate patient medication list for offending medications.
Multiple systems atrophy	Parkinsonism with early and profound dysautonomia
Neuropathic gait	Wide-based gait, frequently with imbalance and en bloc turning
Parkinson's disease	Presenting with bradykinesia and tremor and/or rigidity. Falls only occur later in the disease course. Nonmotor symptoms may precede the diagnosis by a decade, but are not diagnostic themselves.

(*continued*)

Common Differential Diagnoses: Movement Disorders (*continued*)

Diagnosis	Key History or Physical Examination Differentiators
Progressive supranuclear palsy	Symmetric parkinsonism and early frequent falls. Coupled with reduced eye movements in the vertical plane and hypometric saccades. MRI demonstrates reduced midbrain size.
Restless leg syndrome	The relentless urge to move one's legs. Occurs at night just before sleep and may wake a patient from sleep. Relieved by walking, returns on lying back down again. As it advances, may occur during the day. Generally symmetric. Rarely may spread to include the upper extremities
Tic disorders	A briefly suppressible urge to move or vocalize. Movements are quick but may be repeated multiple times. Tics change over time. Worse with anxiety. Numerous psychiatric comorbidities, most commonly OCD, ADHD, and GAD
Vascular parkinsonism	Parkinsonism in the lower half of the body. Prominent en bloc turning

ADHD, attention deficit hyperactivity disorder; GAD, generalized anxiety disorder; MRI, magnetic resonance imaging; OCD, obsessive–compulsive disorder.

Common Differential Diagnoses: Dementia

Diagnosis	Key History or Physical Examination Differentiators
Alzheimer's disease	Presenting as a memory problem, patients become deeply amnestic without any related physical disability. Broader cognitive deficits emerge as the disease progresses.
Alcoholism	Severity may vary based on the extremity and duration of alcohol use. Some of the cognitive deficits may be reversible with cessation. Frequently coupled with ataxia due to damage to the cerebellum
B12 deficiency	Coupled with stocking and glove distribution neuropathy and signs of spinal cord myelomalacia
Dementia with Lewy bodies	Cognitive decline before or within 1 year of presenting parkinsonism. Almost all have fully formed hallucinations early in the disease course. Exquisitely sensitive to neuroleptics which may aggravate their mental condition and compound their parkinsonism.
Depression	Not a true dementia, but a very realistic mimic. Treatable with medication, and in extreme cases ECT or TMS

(continued)

Common Differential Diagnoses: Dementia (*continued*)	
Diagnosis	**Key History or Physical Examination Differentiators**
Hypothyroidism	Cognitive slowing and difficulty with comprehension. Coupled with symptoms of hypothyroidism and supporting lab work
Parkinson's disease dementia	Executive dysfunction and word finding prominent. Memory is not as deeply affected and responsive to prompts.
Vascular dementia	Slowed cognitive processing encompassing both memory deficits and executive dysfunction. Coupled with lower body parkinsonism. Patients generally have multiple vascular risk factors.

ECT, electroconvulsive therapy; TMS, transcranial magnetic stimulation.

BIBLIOGRAPHY

Armitage, A (2015). *Advanced practice nursing guide to the neurological exam.* New York, NY: Springer Publishing Company.

Armitage, A. (Ed.). (2018). *A practical guide to Parkinson's disease: Diagnosis and management.* New York, NY: Springer Publishing Company.

Blumenfeld, H. (2002). *Neuroanatomy through clinical cases.* Sunderland, MA: Sinauer Associates.

Fahn, S., Jankovic, J., & Hallett, M. (2011). *Principles and practice of movement disorders* (2nd ed.). New York, NY: Elsevier Saunders.

Gelb, D. J. (2016). *Introduction to clinical neurology* (5th ed.). New York, NY: Oxford University Press.

Goadsby, P. J. (Ed.). (2018). *Headache* (Vol. 24). Hagerstown, MD: American Academy of Neurology.

Goldberg, S. (2004). *The four-minute neurologic exam.* Miami, FL: MedMaster.

Goldberg, S. (2009). *Clinical neuroanatomy made ridiculously simple* (3rd ed.). Miami, FL: MedMaster.

Hoppenfeld, S. (1976). *Physical examination of the spine and extremities.* Upper Saddle River, NJ: Prentice Hall.

Husain, M., & Schott, J. M. (Eds.). (2016). *Oxford textbook of cognitive neurology and dementia.* Oxford, England: Oxford University Press.

Ropper, A. H., & Samuels, M. A. (2009). *Adams and Victor's principles of neurology* (9th ed.). New York, NY: McGraw-Hill.

Siedel, H. M., Ball, J. W., Dains, E., & Benedict, G. W. (2006). *Mosby's guide to the physical examination* (6th ed.). St. Louis, MO: Mosby Elsevier.

12

ADVANCED HEALTH ASSESSMENT OF THE MUSCULOSKELETAL SYSTEM

Karen M. Myrick

(continued)

Wrist and Hand Joints
Spine
Hip Joint
Knee Joint
Foot and Ankle

FOCUSED HEALTH ASSESSMENT AND ABNORMAL FINDINGS
General Musculoskeletal System
Shoulder
Elbow and Forearm
Wrist and Hand
Spine
Hip
Knee
Foot and Ankle

HOLISTIC ASSESSMENT
Specific Health History
Safety
Distress
Nutrition and Exercise
Financial Implications
Spiritual Considerations

CASE STUDY

ASSESSMENT OF SPECIAL POPULATIONS
Transgender Population
Elderly Population
Pediatric Population
Pregnant Population
Patients With Disabilities
Veteran Population
Elite Athlete Population

DIAGNOSTIC REASONING
Common Differential Diagnoses: General Musculoskeletal System
Common Differential Diagnoses: Shoulder
Common Differential Diagnoses: Elbow and Forearm
Common Differential Diagnoses: Wrist and Hand
Common Differential Diagnoses: Spine
Common Differential Diagnoses: Hip
Common Differential Diagnoses: Knee
Common Differential Diagnoses: Foot and Ankle

Overview of Anatomy and Physiology

The musculoskeletal system is composed of the bones, ligaments, muscles and tendons, and supporting soft tissues. The musculoskeletal system functions to provide protection of internal organs, to allow movement, and to generate body heat. A thorough knowledge of the anatomy will guide the clinician in a thorough evaluation of the musculoskeletal system, improving diagnostic accuracy. The history of the present illness (HPI) is of key importance in correctly diagnosing the patient with a musculoskeletal system complaint. The chronicity and mechanism of injury provide pivotal information in arriving at an accurate physical diagnosis.

The joints are the articulation or places where adjacent bones meet. There are three basic classes of joints, based on their function and their structure: Fibrous, synovial, and cartilaginous. Fibrous joints, such as the sutures on the skull, allow minimal movement. Synovial joints, such as the knee joint, allow full movement, and are all contained in a synovial capsule. Cartilaginous joints, such as the joints of the spine, offer some limited movement.

BONES AND LIGAMENTS

The skeleton is made up of 206 bones, which essentially are levers that support the body through movement. The bones of the skull, thorax, and the vertebrae make up the axial skeleton, and the upper and lower extremities make up the appendicular skeleton (Figure 12.1).

The parts of a long bone include the middle or diaphysis, the epiphyseal growth plate in a skeletally immature individual, the end of the bone or the epiphysis, and the area between the epiphysis and diaphysis or metaphysis (Figure 12.2). Bones have a rich blood supply and depend on this blood supply for nutrition.

Ligaments are made up of dense connective tissues that join two bones at an articulation (Figure 12.3). Ligaments have a role in the static stability of a joint, although they also allow motion at a joint.

MUSCLES AND TENDONS

Muscles are attached to and cover the bones. These organs are made up of fibers and bundles called fascicles. The muscles contract through a mechanism involving the filaments of myosin and actin sliding over each other to produce shortening of the muscle fiber.

Tendons are connective tissues that attach skeletal muscles to bone. Tendons that are located in areas with increased motion are generally covered in double-layered tendon sheaths.

OTHER STRUCTURES

Cartilage is avascular tissue of three types: Elastic, fibrocartilage, and hyaline cartilage. Of the three, hyaline cartilage is the most abundant and found on the articulating surfaces of the joints. Elastic cartilage is found in the auricle of the ear and the larynx. Fibrocartilage makes up the intervertebral discs and the symphysis pubis.

Bursae are sacs of synovial fluid that are located in areas of friction, such as the bony prominences of the elbow, greater trochanter of the femur, and knee.

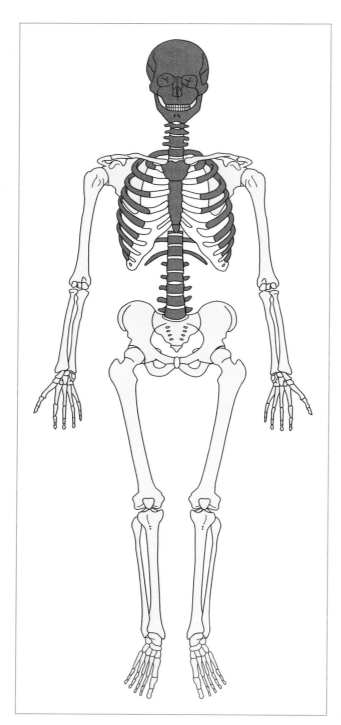

FIGURE 12.1 Axial skeleton and appendicular skeleton. The axial skeleton appears in red.

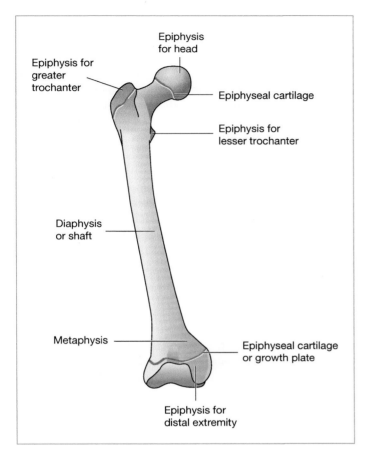

Epiphysis
for head

Epiphysis for
greater
trochanter

Epiphyseal cartilage

Epiphysis for
lesser trochanter

Diaphysis
or shaft

Metaphysis

Epiphyseal cartilage
or growth plate

Epiphysis for
distal extremity

FIGURE 12.2 Anatomy of a long bone.

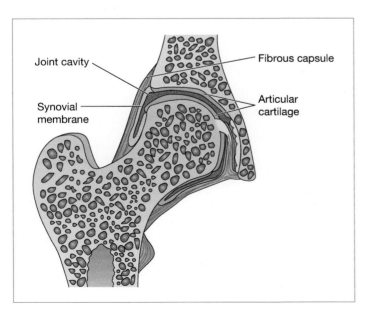

Joint cavity

Fibrous capsule

Synovial
membrane

Articular
cartilage

FIGURE 12.3 Articular cartilage and joint
capsule.

THE SHOULDER

The shoulder is responsible for moving the upper extremity in space, and is pivotal in important functions such as bathing and feeding one's self, as well as sports activities such as throwing.

BONES AND LIGAMENTS OF THE SHOULDER

The shoulder includes the ball and socket glenohumeral joint, the synovial acromioclavicular (AC) joint and the synovial joint, and the synovial sternoclavicular joint. The bones that make up the glenohumeral joint include the glenoid fossa of the scapula and the humerus (Figure 12.4). The shoulder has a large range of motion, and partially this motion is because the humeral head only articulates with approximately one-third of the surface area of the glenoid fossa. The shoulder joint is reliant upon the soft tissues (muscles and ligaments) to provide stability because of this mobility. The AC joint is composed of the acromion of the scapula and the clavicle. The sternoclavicular joint is made up of the clavicle and the sternum.

The ligaments of the shoulder (Figure 12.5) include glenohumeral ligaments (GHL). A joint capsule is a watertight sac that surrounds a joint. In the shoulder, the joint capsule is formed by a group of ligaments that connect the humerus to the glenoid. The ligaments provide the main source of stability for the shoulder joint. The GHL are divided into the superior, middle, and inferior GHL.

The coracoacromial ligament (CAL) connects the coracoid to the acromion. The coracoclavicular ligaments (CCL; trapezoid and conoid ligaments) attach the clavicle coracoid process of the scapula. The transverse humeral ligament (THL) holds the tendon of the long head of the biceps brachii muscle in the groove between the greater and lesser tubercle on the humerus (intertubercular sulcus).

MUSCLES AND TENDONS OF THE SHOULDER

The rotator cuff is made up of four tendons that connect their respective muscles to the humerus. These are listed from the front of the shoulder to the back in the following order: The subscapularis, supraspinatus, infraspinatus, and teres minor (Figure 12.6). Four muscles and their tendons

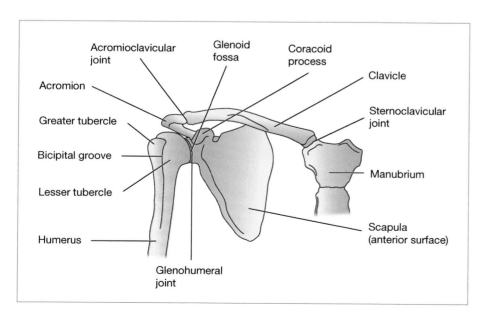

FIGURE 12.4 Bones of the shoulder.

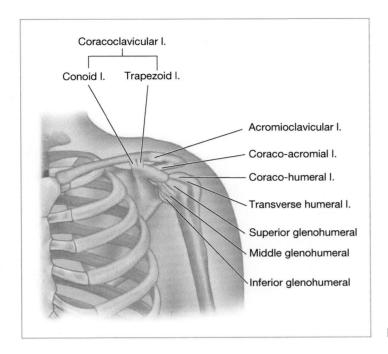

FIGURE 12.5 Ligaments in the shoulder.

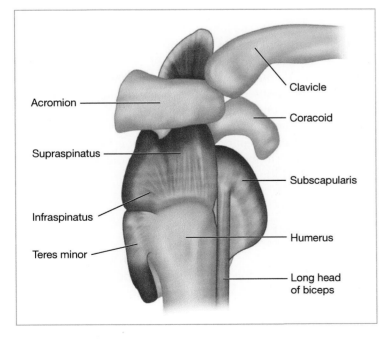

FIGURE 12.6 The rotator cuff.

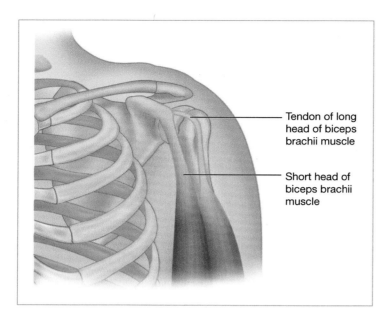

Tendon of long
head of biceps
brachii muscle

Short head of
biceps brachii
muscle

FIGURE 12.7 The long and short head of the biceps.

make up the rotator cuff, which functions to dynamically stabilize the shoulder joint and move the humerus. These muscles are the supraspinatus, the infraspinatus, teres minor, and subscapularis. The supraspinatus inserts on the greater tubercle of the humerus. The infraspinatus and teres minor insert on the greater tubercle. The subscapularis inserts on the lesser tubercle. The tendons of the rotator cuff pass between the moving bones (acromion and humerus).

The biceps tendon attaches the biceps muscle to the shoulder at the coracoid process of the scapula (Figure 12.7).

OTHER STRUCTURES OF THE SHOULDER

The *glenoid labrum* is a fibrocartilaginous rim that attaches around the margin of the glenoid cavity in the shoulder (Figure 12.8). The labrum functions to deepen the socket and provide stability to the shoulder. The labrum is subject to tearing with traumatic injuries to the joint.

The *articular capsule* of the shoulder is fibrous in the outer layer and has an inner synovial layer. The shoulder capsule is lax and subject to allowing the shoulder to dislocate.

The *subacromial bursa* is a synovial fluid–filled sac that separates the acromion from the rotator cuff. The bursa acts to cushion the joint and allow for motion.

THE ELBOW

The elbow functions to position the hand in space and stabilize the lever action of the forearm.

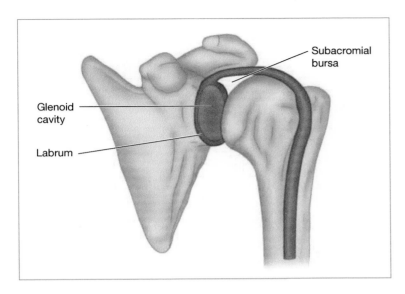

FIGURE 12.8 The glenoid cavity, subacromial bursa, and labrum.

BONES AND LIGAMENTS OF THE ELBOW

The humerus, radius, and ulna bones of the forearm complete the hinge joint articulation of the elbow joint at three articulations (Figure 12.9). These joints are the humeroulnar joint, the radiohumeral joint, and the radioulnar joint.

The ulnar collateral ligament of the elbow connects the distal humerus and proximal ulna on the medial side of the elbow (Figure 12.10). The radial collateral ligament of the elbow connects the lateral epicondyle of the humerus and the annular ligament of the radius. The annular ligament attaches the trochlear notch, encircles the head of the radius, and keeps the radial head in contact with the notch of the ulna (Figure 12.11).

MUSCLES AND TENDONS OF THE ELBOW

The muscles and tendons that comprise and move the elbow are the biceps and brachioradialis, the brachialis, the triceps brachii, the pronator teres, pronator quadratus, anconeus, and the supinator (Figure 12.12). The long head of the biceps brachii originates at the supraglenoid tubercle of the scapula and inserts on the radial tuberosity of the radius. The short head of the biceps brachii

originates on the coracoid process of the scapula and inserts on the radial tuberosity of the radius. The biceps brachii is responsible for flexion of the elbow joint.

The long head of the brachioradialis originates at the lateral supracondylar ridge on the humerus, and inserts on the styloid process of the radius and is responsible for elbow flexion.

The brachialis originates on the anterior surface of the distal half of the humerus and inserts on the coronoid process and ulnar tuberosity of the ulna. The brachialis is responsible for elbow flexion.

The long head of the triceps originates at the infraglenoid tubercle of the scapula and inserts on the olecranon process of the ulna and is responsible for elbow extension. The lateral head of the triceps brachii originates at the posterior surface of the ulna, inserts on the olecranon process of the ulna, and is responsible for elbow extension.

The pronator teres originates at the medial epicondyle of the humerus and coronoid process of the ulna and inserts at the lateral aspect of the radius at its midpoint. The pronator teres is responsible for pronation. The pronator quadratus originates at the distal one-fourth of the ulna and inserts at the distal one-fourth of the radius. It is responsible for forearm pronation. The supinator originates at the lateral epicondyle of the humerus

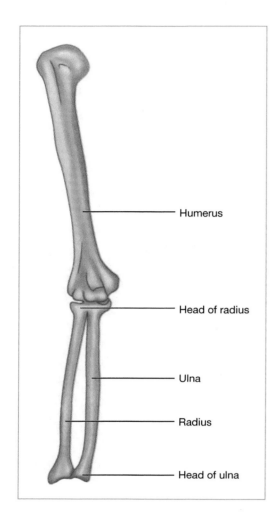

FIGURE 12.9 Bones of the elbow and forearm.

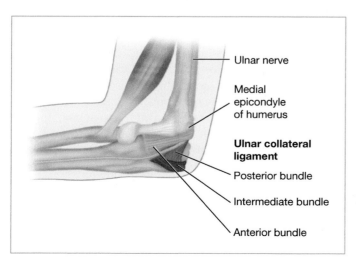

FIGURE 12.10 The ulnar collateral ligament.

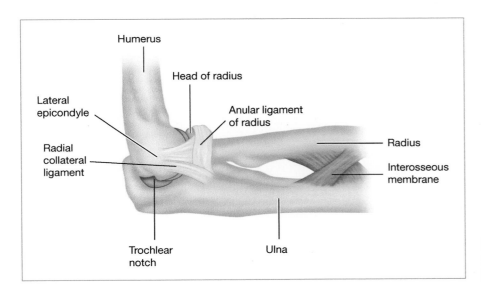

FIGURE 12.11 The annular and radial collateral ligaments.

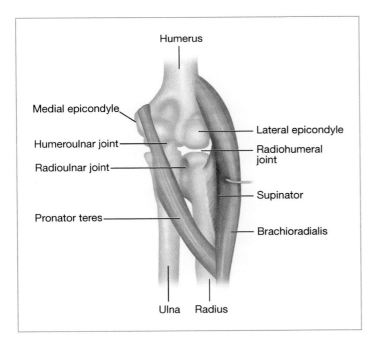

FIGURE 12.12 Muscles and joints of the elbow.

and adjacent ulna and inserts at the anterior surface of the proximal radius. The supinator moves the elbow in supination. The anconeus originates on the lateral epicondyle of the humerus and inserts lateral and inferior to the olecranon process of the ulna.

OTHER STRUCTURES OF THE ELBOW

The olecranon bursa is a thin sac of synovial fluid that cushions the olecranon process, helping the soft tissue structures to glide and move freely (Figure 12.13).

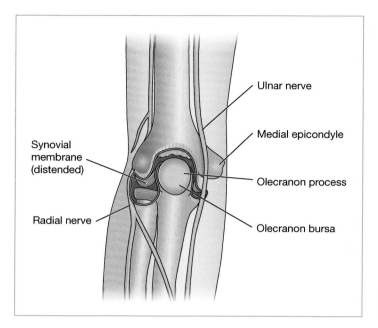

FIGURE 12.13 The olecranon bursa, ulnar, and radial nerves.

HAND AND WRIST

The hand, a highly functioning component of the upper extremity, is responsible for fine motor movement and skills. The wrist joins the hand with the forearm and helps to position the hand in space, allowing for the fine motion that occurs in the human hand.

BONES AND LIGAMENTS

The joints of the hand include the articulation of the metacarpals and phalanges at the metacarpophalangeal joints (MCPs), the proximal articulation of the phalanges at the interphalangeal joints (PIPs), and the distal articulation of the phalanges at the interphalangeal joints (DIPs). The wrist joints include the articulation of the radius and the carpal bones at the radiocarpal joint, the radius and the ulna at the distal radioulnar joint, and the carpal bones at the intercarpal joints (Figure 12.14).

The fingers and thumb joints have collateral ligaments that connect either side of the joints,

preventing sideways movement on the joint (Figure 12.15). The volar plate ligament connects the proximal phalanx to the middle phalanx on the palmar side of the joint (Figure 12.16).

MUSCLES AND TENDONS

The muscles and tendons of the wrist and hand include the two carpal muscles, which are responsible for wrist flexion (Figure 12.17). Two radial and one ulnar muscle are responsible for wrist extension. Supination and pronation result from muscle contraction in the forearm. The thumb moves in flexion, abduction, and opposition by three muscles that form the thenar eminence. Movement in the fingers depends on the action of the flexor and extensor tendons of muscles in the forearm and wrist. The intrinsic muscles of the hand attaching to the metacarpal bones are involved in flexion (lumbricals), abduction (dorsal interossei), and adduction (palmar interossei) of the fingers.

The carpal tunnel is the area in which the forearm muscles and median nerve pass

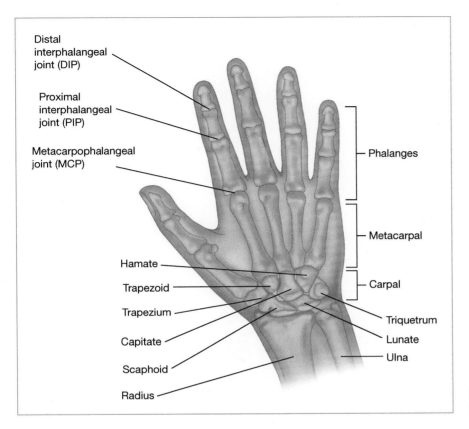

Distal
interphalangeal
joint (DIP)

Proximal
interphalangeal
joint (PIP)

Metacarpophalangeal
joint (MCP)

Phalanges

Metacarpal

Hamate

Trapezoid

Trapezium

Capitate

Scaphoid

Radius

Carpal

Triquetrum

Lunate

Ulna

FIGURE 12.14 Bones of the
hand and wrist.

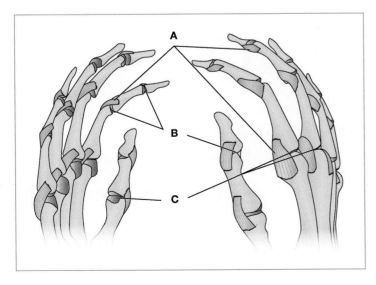

A

B

C

FIGURE 12.15 (**A**) Collateral ligaments of the
finger joints, (**B**) the interphalangeal joints,
and (**C**) metacarpal phalangeal joints.

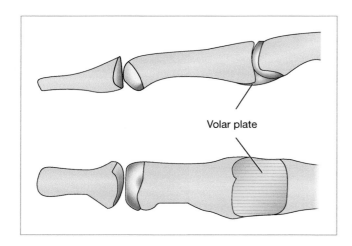

FIGURE 12.16 Volar plate.

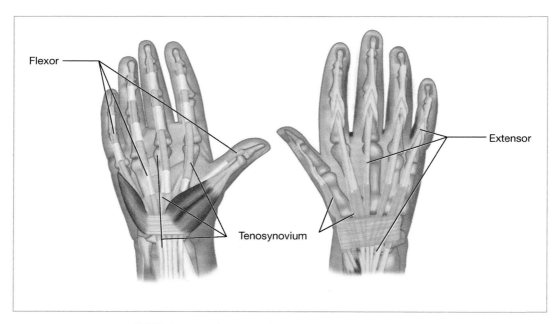

FIGURE 12.17 Flexor and extensor tendons of the wrist.

(Figure 12.18). The transverse carpal ligament holds the flexor tendons and their sheaths in place. The median nerve is below the retinaculum. The median nerve is responsible for innervating the thumb muscles and palmar surface of the thumb (Figure 12.19).

OTHER STRUCTURES OF THE HAND AND WRIST

The triangular fibrocartilage complex (TFCC) is a cartilaginous stabilizer of the ulnar carpal bones and distal radio ulnar joint (Figure 12.20). It absorbs the axial load on the wrist joint.

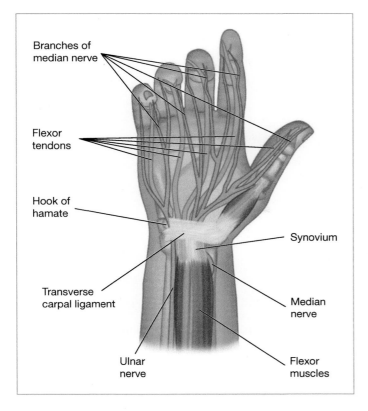

FIGURE 12.18 The carpal tunnel with median nerve.

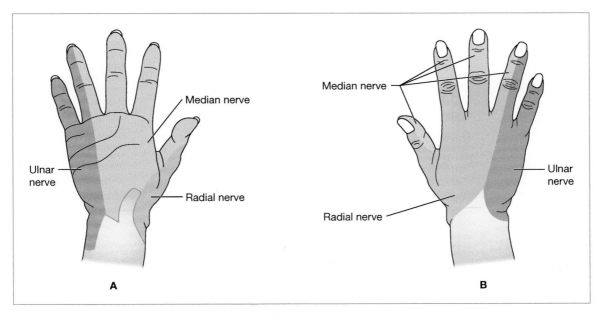

FIGURE 12.19 (A) Volar and **(B)** dorsal innervation of medial nerve.

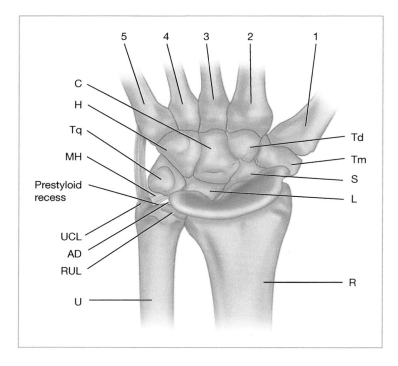

FIGURE 12.20 The triangular fibrocartilage complex of the wrist.

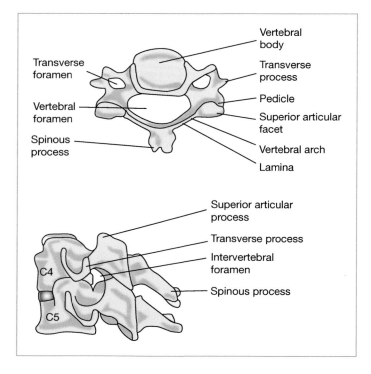

FIGURE 12.21 Vertebral anatomy.

SPINE

The spine is responsible for stability and motion of the trunk and back.

BONES AND LIGAMENTS OF THE SPINE

The 24 bones, the vertebrae, articulate with each other in slightly mobile cartilaginous joints (Figure 12.21). At the junction of the sacrum, the vertebrae are virtually immobile. The vertebrae are connected by ligaments between the spinous processes, between anterior vertebrae and posterior vertebrae, and between the lamina of each adjacent vertebrae (Figure 12.22).

MUSCLES AND TENDONS OF THE SPINE

The muscles that work with the spine include the deep intrinsic or core muscles, the superficial muscles of the back, and the abdominal wall musculature.

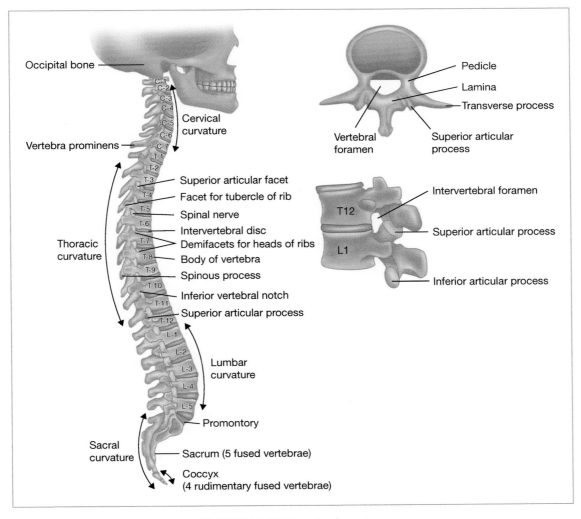

FIGURE 12.22 Vertebral anatomy.

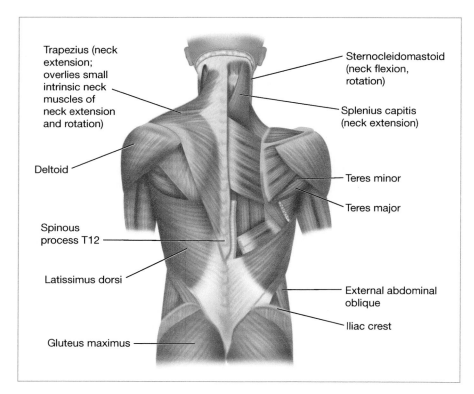

Trapezius (neck
extension;
overlies small
intrinsic neck
muscles of
neck extension
and rotation)

Deltoid

Spinous
process T12

Latissimus dorsi

Gluteus maximus

Sternocleidomastoid
(neck flexion,
rotation)

Splenius capitis
(neck extension)

Teres minor

Teres major

External abdominal
oblique

Iliac crest

FIGURE 12.23 Muscles of
the back.

These include the psoas, erector spinae muscles, latissimus dorsi, levator scapulae, splenius capitis, rhomboid major, quadratus lumborum muscle, splenius cervicis, serratus posterior, rhomboid minor, transversospinales, obliquus capitis, the spinus cervicis, sacrospinalis, and splenius capitis (Figure 12.23).

OTHER STRUCTURES OF THE SPINE

Intervertebral discs separate the vertebrae and provide cushioning. The intervertebral discs are composed of a thick, fibrous tissue—the annular fibrosis—and an inner mucoid softer core, the nucleus pulposus.

The spine encloses the spinal cord, and the nerve roots travel through the vertebral foramen which is an opening between the inferior and superior articulating processes of the adjacent vertebrae.

HIP

The hip is responsible for moving the lower extremities in activities such as walking.

BONES AND LIGAMENTS OF THE HIP

The femoral head articulates with the acetabulum of the hip in a ball and socket joint. The bony landmarks of the anterior surface of the hip include the iliac crest, iliac tubercle, the anterior superior iliac spine, greater trochanter, and pubic symphysis (Figure 12.24). Posterior landmarks include the posterior superior iliac spine, greater trochanter, ischial tuberosity, and the sacroiliac joint (Figure 12.25).

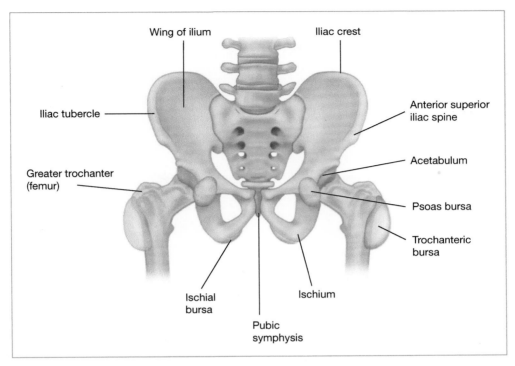

FIGURE 12.24 Bones and ligaments of the anterior hip.

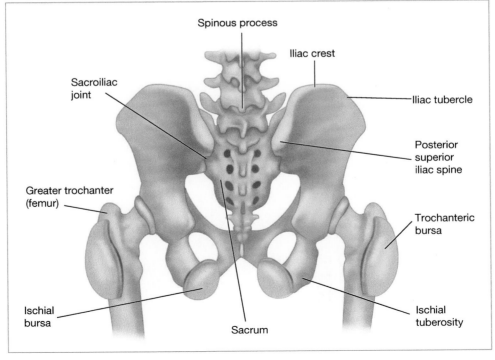

FIGURE 12.25 Bones and ligaments of the posterior hip.

MUSCLES AND TENDONS OF THE HIP

The iliopsoas is a hip flexor; the gluteus maximus functions as a hip extensor (Figure 12.26). The adductor group moves the hip toward the midline of the body. The abductor group (gluteus medius and minimus) moves the hip away from the midline of the body (Figure 12.27).

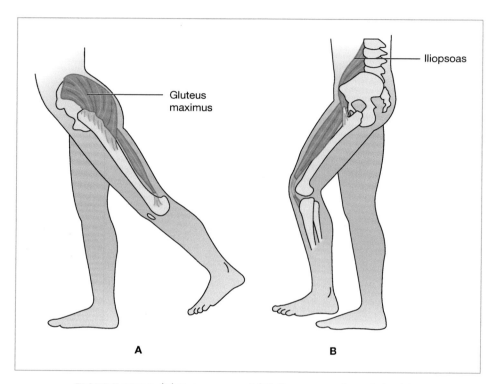

FIGURE 12.26 (**A**) Extensor and (**B**) flexor muscles of the hip.

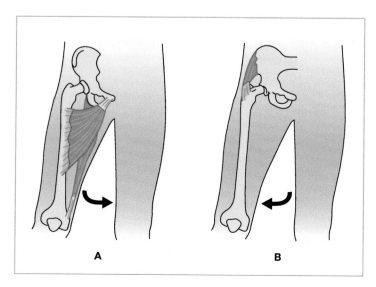

FIGURE 12.27 (**A**) Adductor and (**B**) abductor muscles of the hip.

OTHER STRUCTURES OF THE HIP

The acetabular labrum is a cartilaginous ring that deepens the hip socket. The articular capsule of the shoulder is fibrous in the outer layer and has an inner synovial layer. The trochanteric and ischial bursa is a synovial fluid–filled sac that acts to cushion the joint and allow for motion.

KNEE

The knee is important for flexion and extension of the lower extremity relative to the thigh, and this motion plays a large part in walking.

BONES AND LIGAMENTS OF THE KNEE

The bones of the femur, tibia, and patella articulate to make up the hinge joint of the knee (Figure 12.28). There are essentially three articular surfaces—the medial and lateral femoral and tibial condylar compartments, and the patella femoral joint. The ligaments of the knee play a role in stabilizing the joint in the medial and lateral positions and in the anterior posterior positions. The medial collateral ligament (MCL) and lateral collateral ligament (LCL) provide medial and lateral stability to the knee joint (Figure 12.29). The MCL joins the medial femoral epicondyle to the medial condyle of the tibia. The medial portion of the MCL also attaches to the medial meniscus.

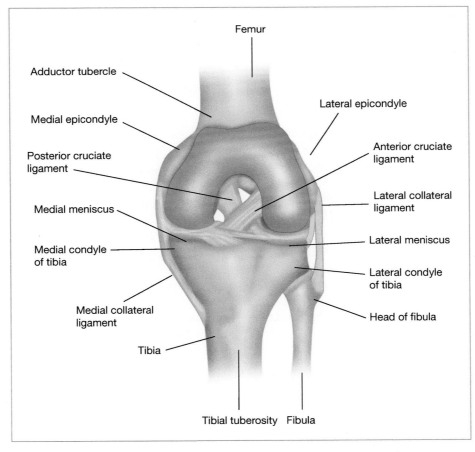

FIGURE 12.28 Anterior view of the bones and ligaments of the knee.

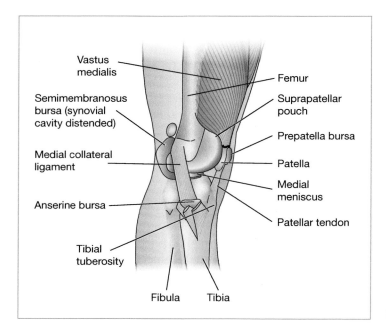

FIGURE 12.29 Medial anatomy of the knee.

The LCL joins the lateral femoral epicondyle and the head of the fibula. The anterior cruciate ligament (ACL) and posterior cruciate ligament (PCL) provide anterior and posterior stability to the knee joint. The ACL crosses at an angle from the anterior medial tibia to the lateral femoral condyle, preventing the tibia from sliding forward on the femur. The PCL crosses from the posterior tibia and lateral meniscus to the medial femoral condyle, preventing the tibia from posterior translation on the femur.

MUSCLES AND TENDONS OF THE KNEE

The quadriceps muscles work to extend the lower extremity at the knee joint, and the hamstring muscles work to flex the lower extremity at the knee joint (Figure 12.30).

FOOT AND ANKLE

BONES AND LIGAMENTS OF THE FOOT AND ANKLE

The tibia and the talus articulate to form the synovial tibiotalar joint, and the talus and calcaneus articulate to form the synovial subtalar (Figure 12.31). The metatarsals articulate with the phalanges, forming the metatarsophalangeal joints, and the phalanges articulate to form the proximal and distal interphalangeal joints, which are synovial joints. The prominent bony lateral malleolus is the distal end of the fibula, and the prominent bony medial malleolus is the distal end of the tibia.

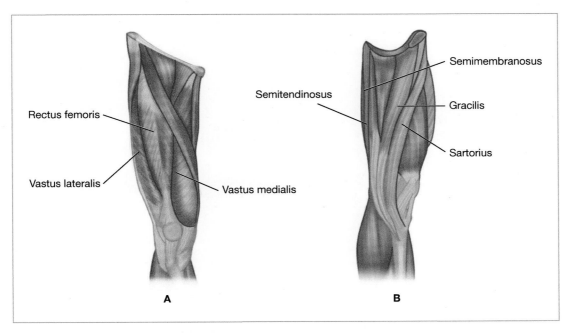

Rectus femoris

Vastus lateralis

Vastus medialis

Semitendinosus

Semimembranosus

Gracilis

Sartorius

A

B

FIGURE 12.30 Flexor and extensor muscles of the knee. (**A**) Anterior view of the quadriceps femorus and (**B**) medial view of the hamstring muscles.

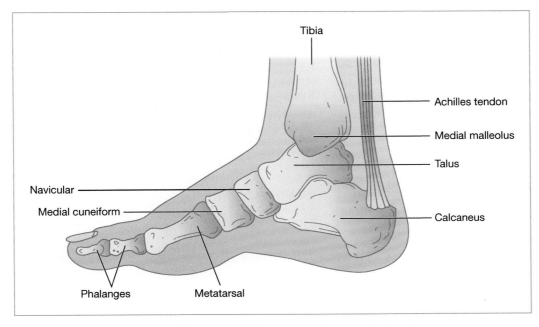

Tibia

Achilles tendon

Medial malleolus

Talus

Navicular

Medial cuneiform

Calcaneus

Phalanges

Metatarsal

FIGURE 12.31 Bones and ligaments of the medial ankle.

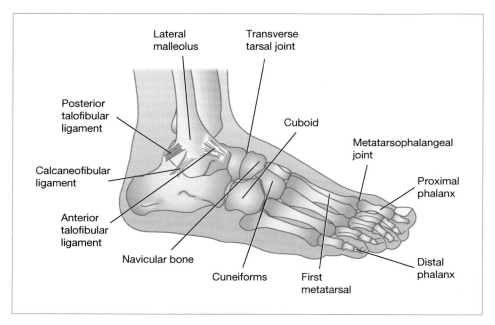

FIGURE 12.32 Bones and ankles of the lateral ankle.

The deltoid ligament connects the medial malleolus to the talus and proximal tarsal bones (Figure 12.32).

The anterior talofibular ligament connects the anterior talus to the lateral malleolus. The calcaneofibular ligament connects the calcaneous and the lateral malleolus. The posterior talofibular ligament connects the talus and the lateral malleolus.

MUSCLES AND TENDONS OF THE FOOT AND ANKLE

Muscles and tendons of the foot an ankle include the gastrocnemius, soleus, plantaris, tibialis posterior, tibialis anterior, extensor digitorium longus, extensor halluces longus, peroneus longus, and peroneus brevis, as well as the dorsiflexors and plantar flexors. The Achilles tendon attaches the gastrocnemius and soleus to the posterior calcaneus.

Screening Health Assessment and Normal Findings

GENERAL MUSCULOSKELETAL SYSTEM

INSPECTION

An assessment of the musculoskeletal system will include an inspection from all sides of the area being assessed, evaluating for deformities, side-to-side differences in symmetrical comparison, limitations in motion, and skin changes including rashes, erythema, edema, and ecchymosis. In a patient with a normally functioning musculoskeletal system, the clinician should expect to find minimal side-to-side differences on inspection, accounting for the patient's dominant side to be slightly more developed. There should be no limitations in motion or skin abnormalities.

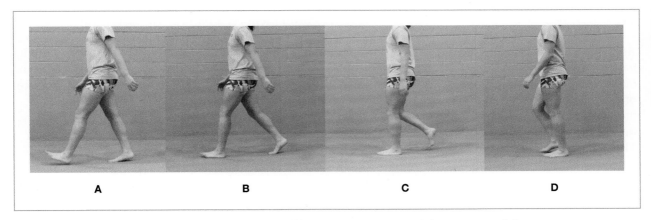

FIGURE 12.33 Stances of gait. (**A**) Heel strike. (**B**) Foot flat. (**C**) Midstance. (**D**) Push off.

EVALUATION OF GAIT

It is important to evaluate the patient's gait, in order to obtain information on the patient's balance, mobility, and to identify any lower extremity abnormalities. The stances of gait include heel-strike, foot flat, mid-stance, and push-off phases (Figure 12.33). The stance phase is noted when the patient has 60% of his or her weight on the foot on the ground, and the swing phase is when the foot moves forward and does not bear weight. In the healthy patient, the gait should be fluid and free of antalgic stances. An antalgic gait is one in which there is shortening of the stance phase relative to the swing phase, and a means for the patient to avoid pain.

PALPATION

Palpate for crepitation, warmth, areas of point tenderness, tone, step off, or nodularity. Pay particular attention to the anatomical landmarks depicting the underlying anatomy. In a healthy patient undergoing a screening examination, the clinician should not be able to identify areas of crepitation or tenderness. Tone should be normal and equal bilaterally, and nodularity is not considered within normal limits.

Palpation should be performed to evaluate for pain, strength, and function. Grading of muscle strength should be performed bilaterally, and documented on a scale of 0 to 5, with 0 being no muscle activity noted with resistance and 5 being normal strength is present (Table 12.1).

TABLE 12.1
Grading of Muscle Strength Testing

Findings on Examination	Grade
No strength or muscle contraction	0
No movement, but muscle contraction noted	1
Movement with gravity	2
Movement against gravity, but not resistance	3
Decreased strength against resistance	4
Normal/full strength	5

RANGE OF MOTION

Active range of motion is measured by asking the patient to move through his or her range of motion on his or her own power. A patient produces active range of motion independently. Passive range of motion is measured by the provider moving the patient's joints through range of motion while the patient is relaxed. The clinician produces passive range of motion. In a healthy patient, the joint range of motion should be within normal limits both actively and passively without discomfort or dysfunction.

SHOULDER JOINT

INSPECTION

Observing the patient from the anterior view, evaluate for abnormal contours and bony prominences. Posteriorly, assess for symmetry and look for atrophy. Healthy patients who present for a screening examination without shoulder pathology should be free of abnormal contours, have symmetrical findings, and not exhibit atrophy.

PALPATION

Begin from a posterior approach and palpate the spine of the scapula from medial to lateral on your patient. Recall the bony landmarks of the anatomy, as the end of the scapula becomes the acromion. Palpate the anterolateral portion of the acromion moving toward the deltoid until you feel the sulcus (Figure 12.34A). The subacromial bursa is in this sulcus. Palpate over the humeral head in the region of the bicipital groove, until your fingers fall into the groove, locating the long head of the biceps tendon (Figure 12.34B).

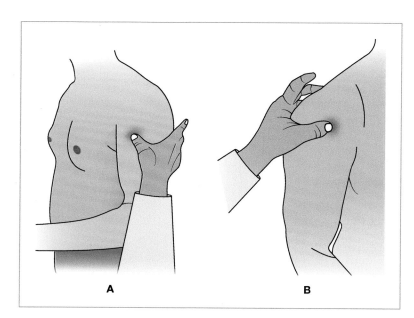

FIGURE 12.34 Palpation of the shoulder joint. (**A**) Sulcus. (**B**) Bicipital groove.

MUSCLE STRENGTH TESTING

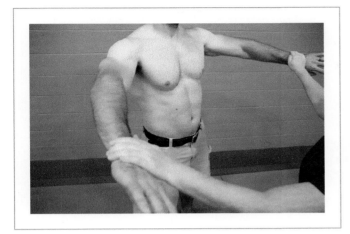

FIGURE 12.35 Supraspinatus muscle strength testing. With the patient in a position of 90 degrees abduction, 30 degrees forward flexion, and internal rotation, elbow extended, and thumb down, ask the patient to resist your downward pressure.

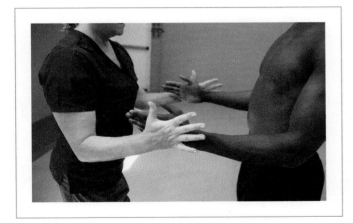

FIGURE 12.36 Infraspinatus and teres minor strength testing. With arm at side and externally rotated to 30 degrees, with a flexed elbow, apply pressure to the forearm and resistance to external rotation.

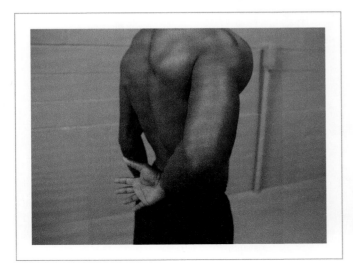

FIGURE 12.37 Subscapularis muscle testing. Lift off test: Place the patient's arm behind back, palm out. Ask the patient to lift away against resistance. A positive test is one in which a patient cannot perform the motion or it is painful.

RANGE OF MOTION: ACTIVE AND PASSIVE

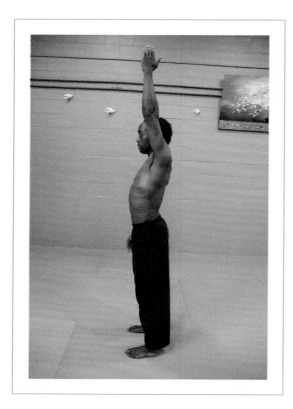

FIGURE 12.38 Range of motion: Forward elevation. Flexion 0 starting position at the patient's side, elevating forward, and raising the arms overhead. Normal is 180 degrees.

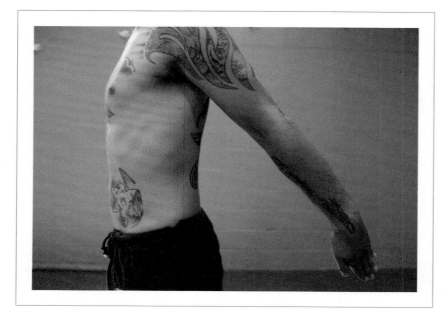

FIGURE 12.39 Range of motion: Extension. Start at 0 and extend straight back. Normal is to 50 degrees.

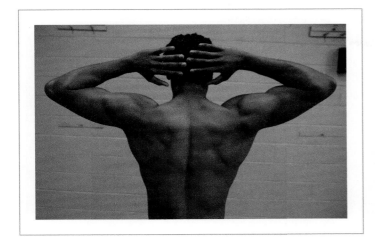

FIGURE 12.40 Range of motion: External rotation. Arm at the side (0 starting position), arm held against thorax, elbow flexed to 90 degrees, and forearm parallel to sagittal plane. Measure by outward rotation of the arm. Ninety degrees is normal.

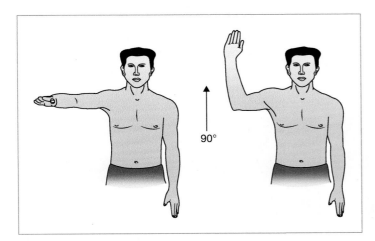

FIGURE 12.41 Range of motion: External rotation. Arm abducted to 90 degrees (0 starting position), arm abducted 90 degrees, aligned with the plane of the scapula, elbow flexed to 90 degrees, and forearm parallel to the floor. Measure by how many degrees the forearm moves away from the floor.

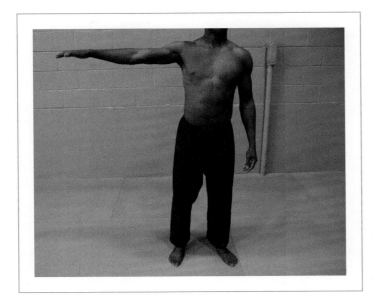

FIGURE 12.42 Abduction of the shoulder. Raising the arms out to the side and overhead. Note that after 90 degrees the scapula is engaged in the motion, and this is no longer pure glenohumeral motion. 180 degrees is normal.

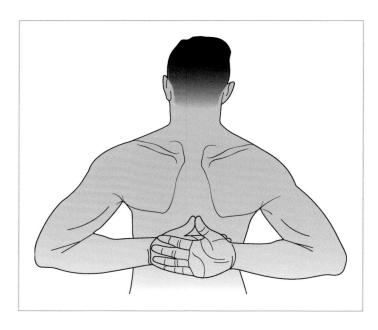

FIGURE 12.43 Internal rotation of the shoulder. Evaluate patient's posterior reach, noting highest midline spinous process that can be reached by hitchhiking the thumb. Ninety degrees is normal.

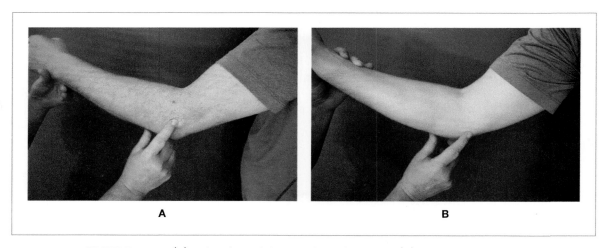

A

B

FIGURE 12.44 **(A)** Palpation of the medial epicondyle. **(B)** Palpation of the lateral epicondyle.

ELBOW JOINT

INSPECTION

Inspect the elbow joint to identify the medial and lateral epicondyles and the olecranon process of the ulna. Inspect for bony deformities, symmetry, and include the flexor and extensor surface of the

ulna and the olecranon process. Note any nodules or skin changes.

PALPATION

Palpate the elbow for any areas of tenderness, noting the bony landmarks of the olecranon process and the medial and lateral epicondyles (Figure 12.44).

MUSCLE STRENGTH TESTING

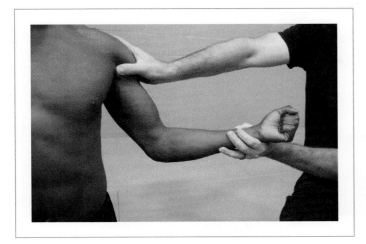

FIGURE 12.45 Testing flexion strength of the elbow: Biceps brachii, brachialis, and brachioradialis. Suggest elbow flexion, having the patient bend his or her elbow.

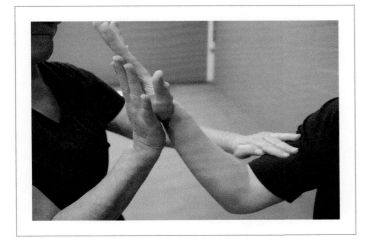

FIGURE 12.46 Testing extension strength of the elbow: Triceps brachii, anconeus. Suggest elbow extension, having the patient straighten his or her elbow.

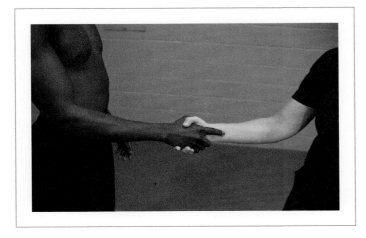

FIGURE 12.47 Testing supination strength of the elbow: Biceps brachii, supinator. Have the patient turn his or her palm up.

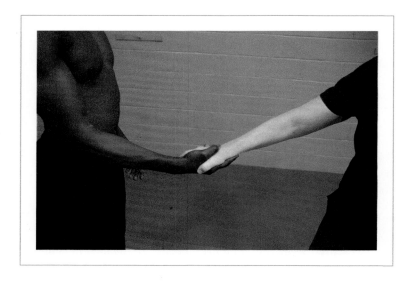

FIGURE 12.48 Testing pronation strength of the elbow: Pronator teres and pronator quadratus. Have the patient turn his or her palm down.

RANGE OF MOTION: ACTIVE AND PASSIVE

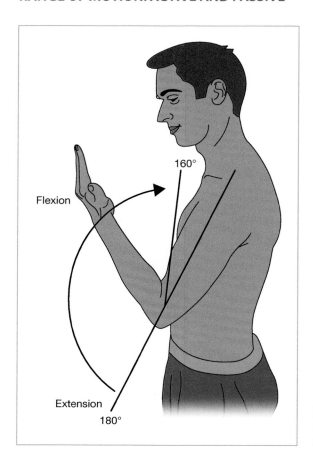

FIGURE 12.49 Flexion and extension of the elbow. One hundred and fifty degrees off flexion is normal, and 0 degrees of extension is normal.

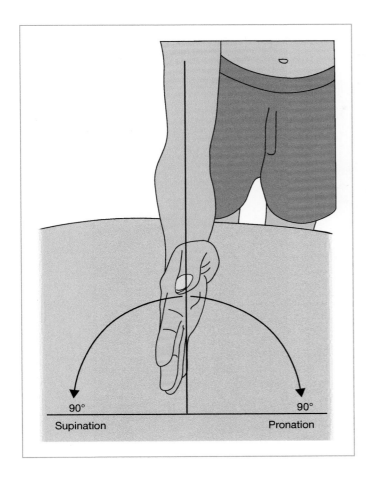

FIGURE 12.50 Supination and pronation of the elbow. Supination and pronation are normal at 90 degrees each.

WRIST AND HAND JOINTS

INSPECTION

In a healthy individual without a condition or injury in this area, inspection should demonstrate symmetry, no findings of atrophy, no swelling, no obvious deformity, and the absence of cords or contractures.

PALPATION

Palpation during a screening examination would assess for areas of soreness with palpation and evaluate the nontender carpal bones, metacarpals, and joints.

MUSCLE STRENGTH TESTING: HAND

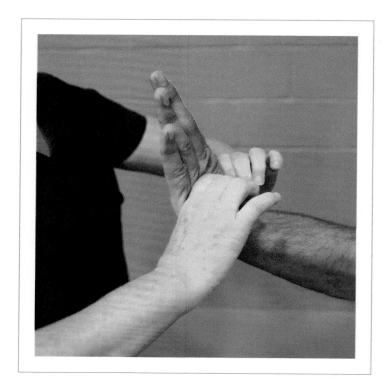

FIGURE 12.51 Testing hand flexion strength: Flexor carpi radialis, flexor carpi ulnaris. Have the patient move the fingers toward the floor with the palm down.

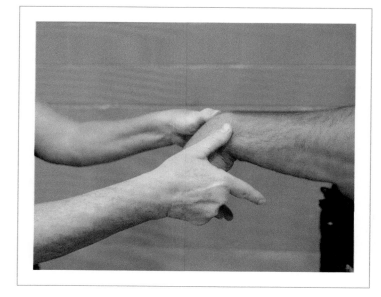

FIGURE 12.52 Testing hand extension strength: Extensor carpi ulnaris, extensor carpi radialis longus, and extensor carpi radialis brevis. Have the patient move the fingers toward the ceiling with the palm down.

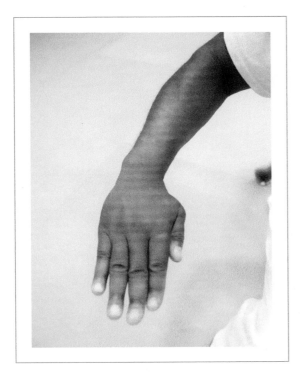

FIGURE 12.53 Testing hand ulnar deviation strength: Flexor carpi ulnaris, adduction, or radial deviation. Have the patient bring the fingers toward the midline with his or her palm down.

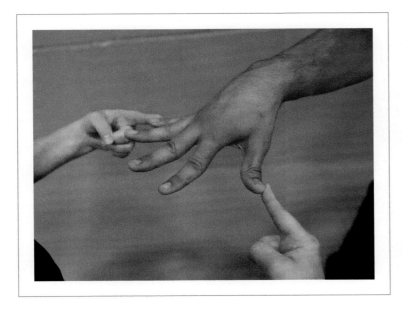

FIGURE 12.54 Testing intrinsic muscle strength: Finger abduction. Ask the patient to hold his or her fingers apart and resist you pushing the fingers in.

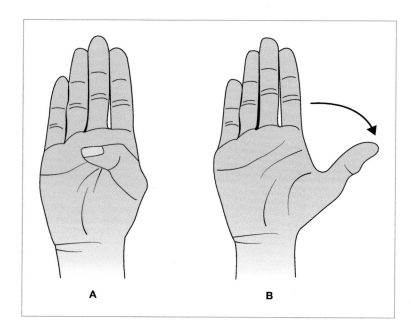

FIGURE 12.55 Testing thumb flexion and extension strength. (**A**) Flexion. (**B**) Extension.

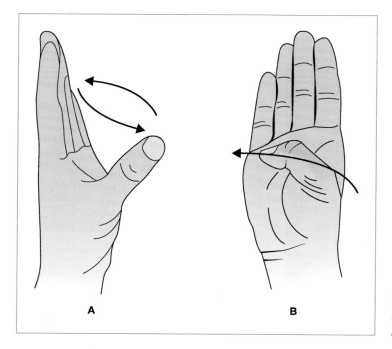

FIGURE 12.56 Testing thumb abduction, adduction, and opposition strength. (**A**) Abduction and adduction. (**B**) Opposition.

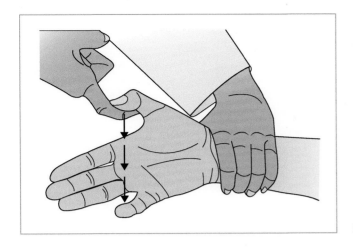

FIGURE 12.57 Testing thumb opposition strength.

MUSCLE STRENGTH TESTING: WRIST

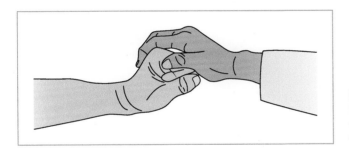

FIGURE 12.58 Testing wrist extension strength: Extensor carpi, radialis longus, and brevis: Have the patient make a fist and resist your pulling toward the floor.

RANGE OF MOTION: ACTIVE AND PASSIVE

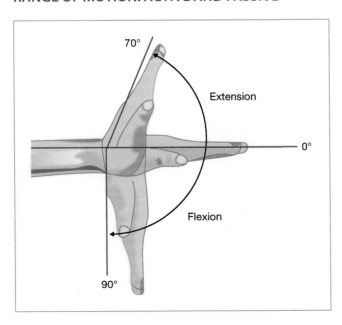

70°

Extension

0°

Flexion

90°

FIGURE 12.59 Wrist range of motion: Flexion and extension.

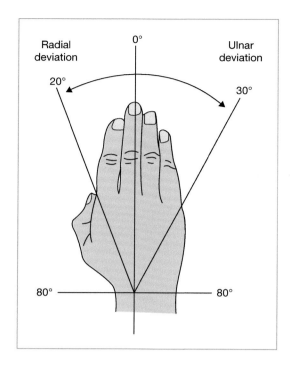

FIGURE 12.60 Wrist ulnar and radial deviation.

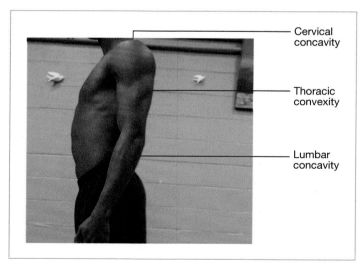

FIGURE 12.61 Normal curvature of the spine.

SPINE

INSPECTION

Inspect for bony deformities, curvature of the spine, and assess the patient's posture and movement (Figure 12.61).

PALPATION

Palpate for areas of tenderness, evaluating soft tissue and bony structures. Palpate each spinous process, as well as over the sacroiliac joints. Evaluate landmarks, including the prominent spinous process of C7 (Figure 12.62), the posterior superior iliac spines and sacroiliac joints (Figure 12.63), and the iliac crests.

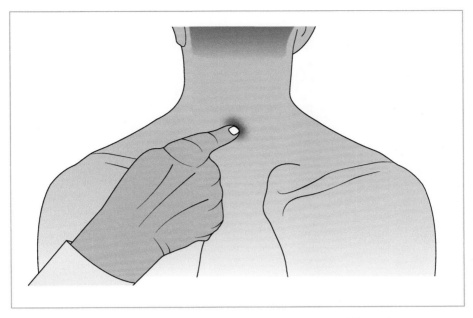

FIGURE 12.62 Palpation of spinous process C7 of the spine.

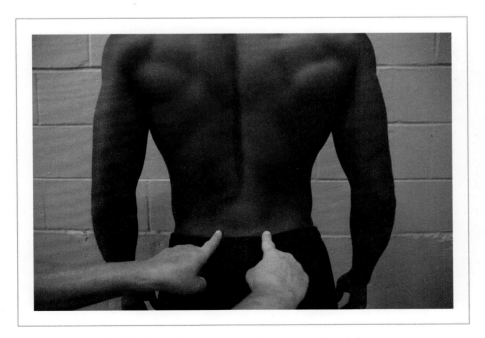

FIGURE 12.63 Palpation of the sacroiliac joints.

MUSCLE STRENGTH TESTING

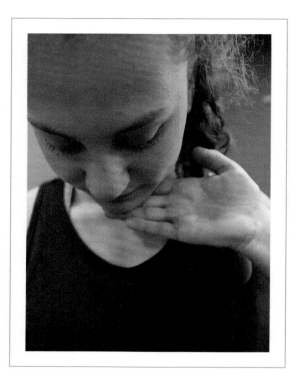

FIGURE 12.64 Muscle strength testing of the neck flexors: Sternocleidomastoid, scalene, and paravertebral muscles. Ask the patient to bring his or her chin to his or her chest.

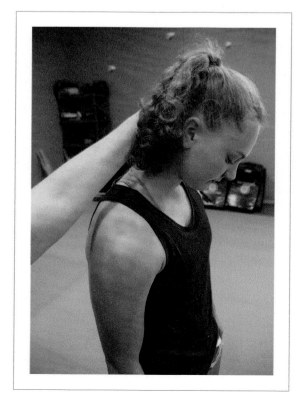

FIGURE 12.65 Muscle strength testing of the neck extensors: Splenius capitis and cervicis. Ask the patient to look up at the ceiling and then look down.

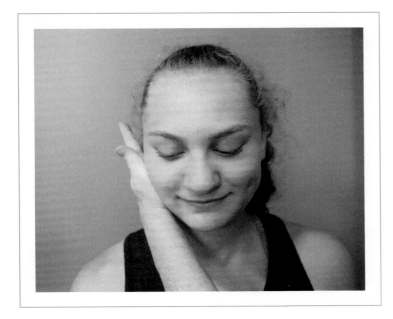

FIGURE 12.66 Muscle strength testing of the neck rotators: Sternocleidomastoid, small intrinsic neck muscles. Ask the patient to look over one shoulder, then the other.

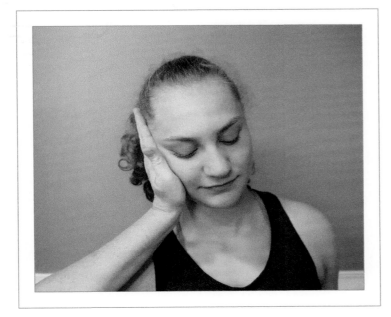

FIGURE 12.67 Muscle strength testing of the neck lateral flexors: Scalenes and intrinsic neck muscles. Ask the patient to bring his or her ear to the shoulder on one side, then the other.

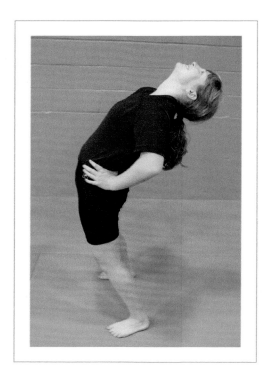

FIGURE 12.68 Muscle strength testing of the spine extensors: Erector spinae and transversospinalis. Ask the patient to bend back.

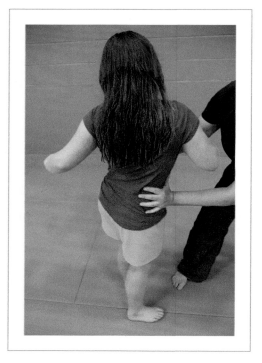

FIGURE 12.69 Muscle strength testing of the spine rotators: Abdominal muscles and intrinsic muscles. Ask the patient to turn to look back over his or her shoulders, one side and then the other.

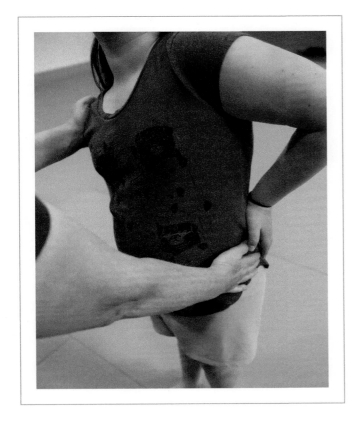

FIGURE 12.70 Muscle strength testing of the spine lateral flexors: Abdominal muscles and intrinsic muscles. Ask the patient to bend to the side, as if to touch the outside of his or her knee with the ipsilateral hand, one side and then the other.

RANGE OF MOTION: ACTIVE AND PASSIVE

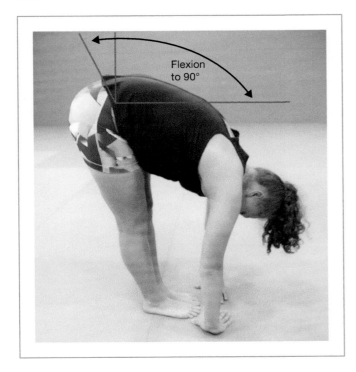

Flexion to 90°

FIGURE 12.71 Spine flexion.

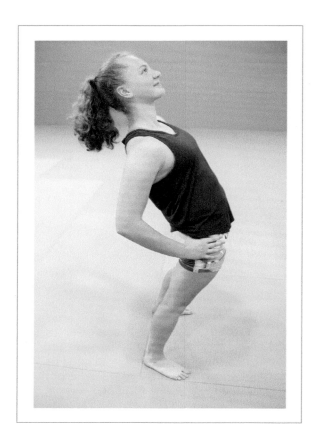

FIGURE 12.72 Spine extension.

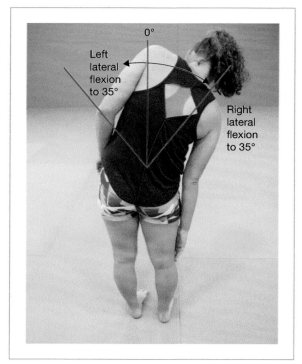

FIGURE 12.73 Spine lateral bending.

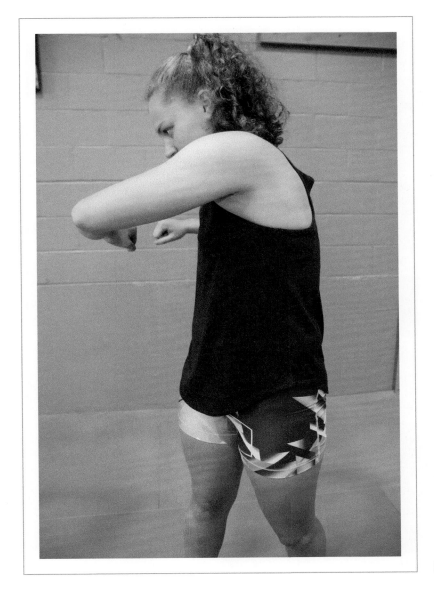

FIGURE 12.74 Spine rotation.

HIP JOINT

INSPECTION

Inspect for bony deformities and symmetry; assess gait.

PALPATION

Assess for areas of tenderness, paying particular attention to bony landmarks.

MUSCLE STRENGTH TESTING

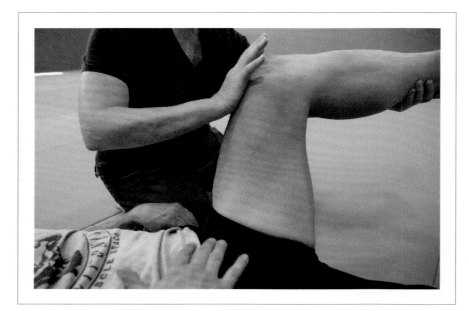

FIGURE 12.75 Testing hip flexor muscles: Iliopsoas. Ask the patient to bend his or her knee toward the chest and hold it against resistance.

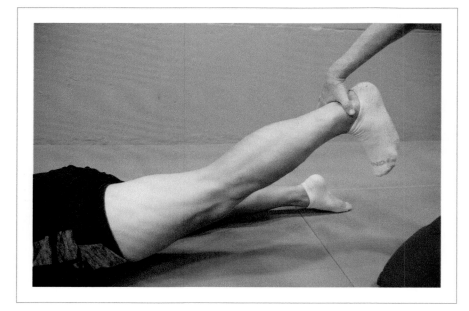

FIGURE 12.76 Testing hip extensor muscles: Gluteus maximus. Ask the patient to lie prone, bend his or her knee, and lift toward the ceiling.

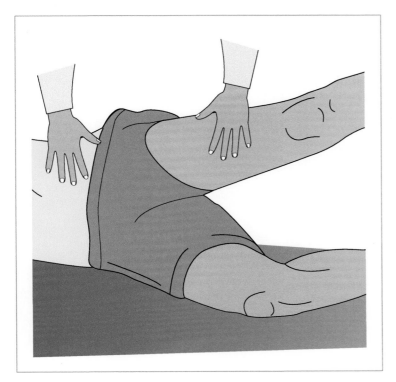

FIGURE 12.77 Testing hip abductor muscles: Gluteus medius and minimus. Ask the patient to lie supine, and to move his or her leg away from the midline of the body.

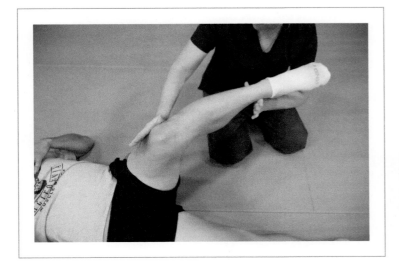

FIGURE 12.78 Testing hip internal rotator muscles: Internal and external obturators, quadratus femoris, superior and inferior gemelli. Ask the patient to lie supine, bend the knee, and to turn the leg out at the hip joint away from the midline of the body.

RANGE OF MOTION: ACTIVE AND PASSIVE

Normal is 120 degrees of flexion and 10 to 20 degrees of extension.

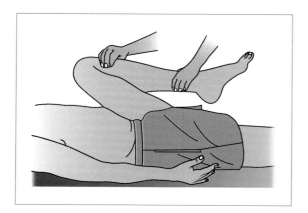

FIGURE 12.79 Hip flexion.

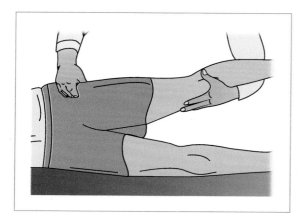

FIGURE 12.80 Hip extension.

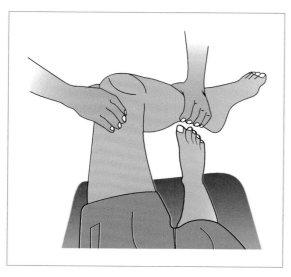

FIGURE 12.81 Internal and external rotation. Normal is 40 degrees of internal rotation and 45 degrees of external rotation.

KNEE JOINT

INSPECTION

Inspect for bony deformities, alignment, and symmetry. Observe the gait.

PALPATION

Assess for areas of tenderness, paying particular attention to bony landmarks.

MUSCLE STRENGTH TESTING

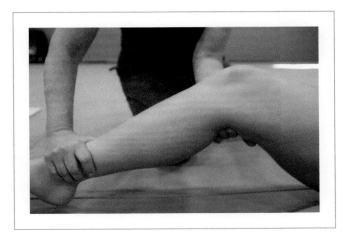

FIGURE 12.82 Testing knee extensors: Quadriceps, rectus femoris, and vastus medialis. Ask the patient to be in a seated position and to extend the knee over side of table against resistance.

RANGE OF MOTION: ACTIVE AND PASSIVE

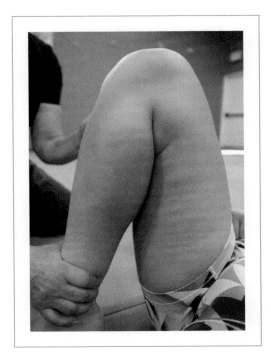

FIGURE 12.83 Knee flexion. Normal flexion to 135 degrees.

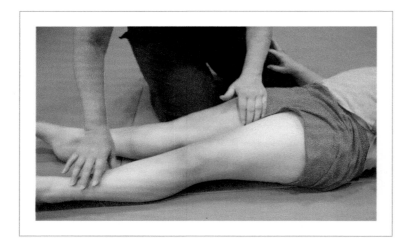

FIGURE 12.84 Knee extension. Normal extension to 0 degrees.

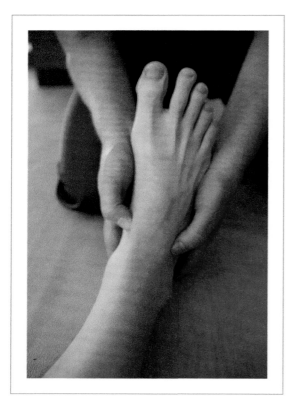

FIGURE 12.85 Ankle palpation.

FOOT AND ANKLE

INSPECTION

Look for bony deformities, symmetry, or swelling.

PALPATION

Palpate for areas of tenderness (Figure 12.85). Note landmarks and correlate the clinical findings with the underlying anatomy.

MUSCLE STRENGTH TESTING

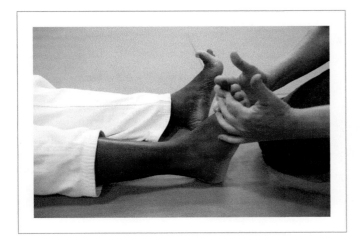

FIGURE 12.86 Testing ankle dorsiflexion: Tibialis anterior, extensor digitorum longus, and extensor hallucis longus. Ask the patient to point his or her foot toward the ceiling.

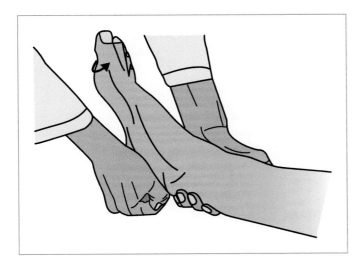

FIGURE 12.87 Testing ankle inversion: Tibialis posterior and anterior. Ask the patient to bend his or her heel inward.

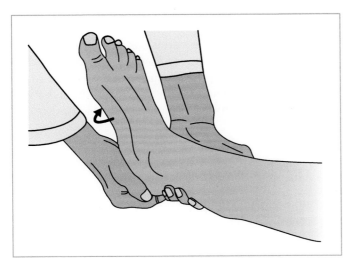

FIGURE 12.88 Testing ankle eversion: Peroneus longus and brevis. Ask the patient to bend his or her heel outward.

Focused Health Assessment and Abnormal Findings

GENERAL MUSCULOSKELETAL SYSTEM

When a patient presents to the provider with a focused chief complaint (CC) in the musculoskeletal system, the following health assessment techniques with their rationales would be performed.

INSPECTION

Look for any erythema or ecchymosis over the area of complaint. Evaluate for deformity or asymmetry. Identify scars from previous injury or trauma. Assess for any change in movement patterns or gait. A biomechanical analysis of the patient's gait may lead you to see that the gait is antalgic, with a shortened stance phase, or limitations of movement in one joint, affecting the others. Without normal range of motion in the ankle, limited ankle rocker, or dorsiflexion may lead to lifting a knee higher during the swing phase of gait, or a loss of knee flexion may cause the patient to rotate their hip to compensate, for example.

PALPATION

When there is an abnormal condition of an injury of part of the musculoskeletal system, the clinician will palpate areas of tenderness that clinically correlate with the patient's CC, and with the anatomical structure that is involved in the patient's condition or injury. With inflammation, areas of warmth are palpable, and the clinician can identify and compare the temperature of structures both proximal and distal to the area being evaluated, and areas on the uninvolved limb to the area of involvement. Areas of step off, palpated as a loss in continuity in palpation, may be felt by the clinician's hands on assessment, which may be indicative of a joint separation, a tendinous or ligamentous disruption, or muscle tear.

Muscle strength testing: Using the grading scale in Table 12.1, a patient with a CC involving the musculoskeletal system will likely also display loss of muscle strength associated with his or her injury or condition. It is important to grade the muscle strength of the muscles that move the joint involved, and to compare this strength to the contralateral, or uninvolved, side.

SPECIAL TESTS

The specific joints of the musculoskeletal system have a variety of advanced or special tests that help clinicians to identify the underlying condition or injury. These special tests will be described for each joint.

Assess the patient for ligamentous tears. Ligaments tear rather than stretch when exposed to stresses beyond their degrees of freedom. Ligament tears are graded 1 to 4, with 3 being a complete tear, and 4 being a bony avulsion (Figure 12.89).

RANGE OF MOTION

When a patient presents to the clinician with a complaint that involves the musculoskeletal system, a limitation in his or her active and/or passive range of motion is central in the clinician's differential diagnostic process. The variations in range of motion from normal are closely associated with the actual injury or disease process that is causative. For example, an equal loss of both active and passive range of motion is found in adhesive capsulitis (frozen shoulder).

FRACTURES

When describing a fracture, the first thing to mention is what type of fracture it is. Generally,

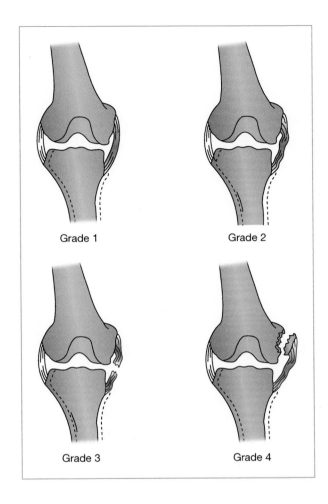

Grade 1

Grade 2

Grade 3

Grade 4

FIGURE 12.89 Grades of ligament tears 1 to 4.

these can be split into the categories of complete, incomplete, and Salter–Harris. A complete fracture is one in which the fracture goes all the way through the bone. These can be oriented in several ways: Transverse, oblique, spiral, or comminuted. Figure 12.90 illustrates the types of fractures: A transverse fracture goes straight across the bone, an oblique fracture produces a fracture in a line across the bone, and a spiral fracture produces a corkscrew type of fracture. A comminuted fracture is one that consists of more than two parts to the fracture. There can be segmental or butterfly types of comminuted fractures, and a fracture can be impacted. Incomplete fractures occur when the whole cortex is not disrupted and

generally consist of buckle (Torus) or greenstick fractures. A buckle fracture is of the concave surface, which involves bony compression of the cortex on one side with the opposite cortex remaining intact.

Fractures are described by the bone that is involved and what part of the bone is affected, the diaphysis, the metaphysis, or the epiphysis (see Figure 12.2). The diaphysis is the shaft of the bone, the metaphysis the portion of the bone that widens next to the growth plate, and the epiphysis is the end of the bone adjacent to the joint.

It is also important to describe what has happened to the bone during the fracture, identifying displacement. In general, when describing a

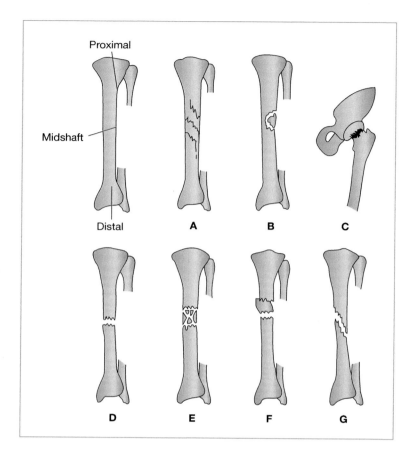

Proximal

Midshaft

Distal   **A**   **B**   **C**

D   **E**   **F**   **G**

FIGURE 12.90 Types of fractures: (**A**) Spiral, (**B**) butterfly, (**C**) impacted, (**D**) transverse, (**E**) comminuted, (**F**) segmental, and (**G**) oblique.

fracture, the body is assumed to be in the anatomic position and the injury is then described in terms of the distal component displacement in relation to the proximal component. Displacement can include any angle, translation, or rotation to the distal component.

Note if the joint surface is involved by the fracture or not. If the fracture does extend to the joint, early referral to a specialist is recommended as the patient will likely have a different treatment than if the fracture is extra-articular.

Salter–Harris fractures are fractures that involve the growth plate in the skeletally immature patient and are classified into five types (Figure 12.91). Torus and buckle fractures are incomplete fractures that are most likely to occur in the skeletally immature patient (Figure 12.92).

SHOULDER

INSPECTION

In the anterior view, inspect for AC separation—a prominent distal clavicle, and evaluate for step off at the AC joint.

PALPATION

The deformity of an anterior shoulder dislocation—this is a prominent acromion and anterior fullness of the deltoid swelling in the glenohumeral joint which may indicate infection or synovitis.

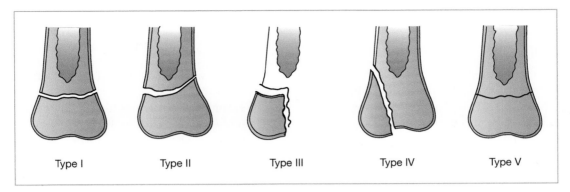

FIGURE 12.91 Salter–Harris classification.

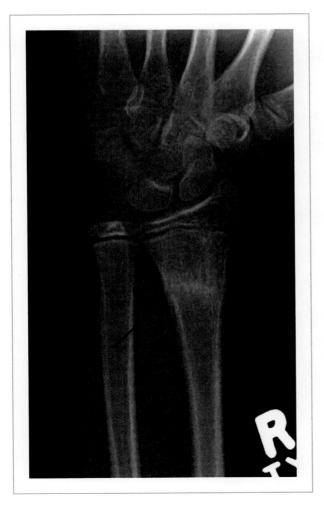

FIGURE 12.92 Buckle (Torus) fracture. Note that the opposite cortex is intact.

SPECIAL TESTS

IMPINGEMENT TESTS

Hawkins impingement test (Figure 12.93): Elevate shoulder to 90 degrees, flex the elbow to 90 degrees, and place the forearm in a neutral position. Support the arm, and then internally rotate the humerus. The test is considered positive if the patient's pain is reproduced with maximal internal rotation. Sensitivity: 79%; specificity: 59%.

Neer impingement test (Figure 12.94): Elevate the arm in forward elevation, then depress the scapula. A positive test is noted when the patient has pain with full forward elevation. Sensitivity: 79%; specificity: 53%.

O'Brien's test for labral tears: Elevate the arm to 90 degrees, adduct arm to 30 degrees, and keep the thumb up—resist downward force (Figure 12.95A). Turn thumb down and resist downward force (Figure 12.95B). A positive test is identified when patients describe pain with the thumb in the down position more than the thumb up. Sensitivity: 75%; specificity: 90%.

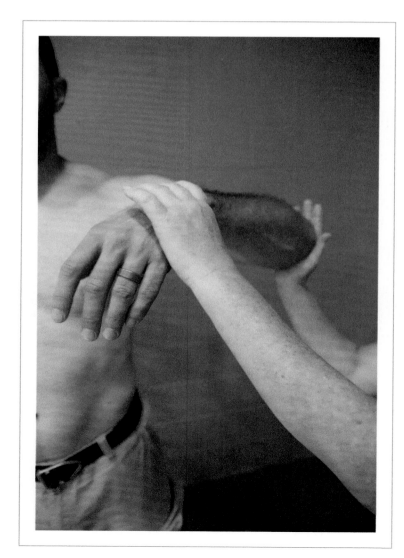

FIGURE 12.93 Hawkins impingement test.

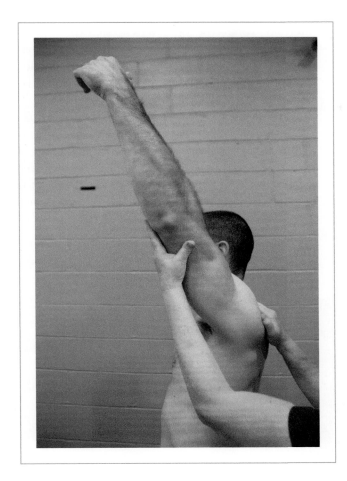

FIGURE 12.94 Neer impingement test.

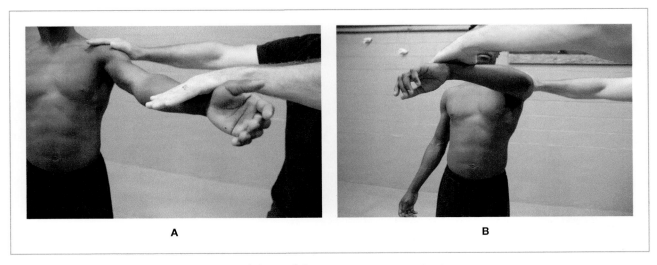

A   B

FIGURE 12.95 (**A**) and (**B**) O'Brien's test for labral tears.

ROTATOR CUFF INTEGRITY TESTS

Lift-off test (subscapularis; Figure 12.96): Ask the patient to stand and place his or her hand behind the back, with the back (dorsum) of his or her hand resting in the mid-lumbar spine region. Have the patient lift his or her hand straight off the back. A positive test is noted when the patient cannot perform the motion, or it is painful. Sensitivity: 60%; specificity: 92%.

Jobe test (supraspinatous test; Figure 12.97): Ask your patient to stand, place arms in 90 degrees of abduction and 30 degrees of forward flexion, and internally rotate the shoulders so that the thumbs are pointing down. Ask the patient to resist your downward pressure. A positive test is noted when the patient cannot resist the downward pressure. Sensitivity: 86%; specificity: 66%.

Lag sign test (external rotation; infraspinatus; Figure 12.98): Ask the patient to stand with the arms externally rotated to 20 degrees, with the elbow at the sides and elbows flexed to 90 degrees. Have the patient resist your inward force. A positive test is noted when a patient cannot resist the inward force. Sensitivity: 70%; specificity: 100%.

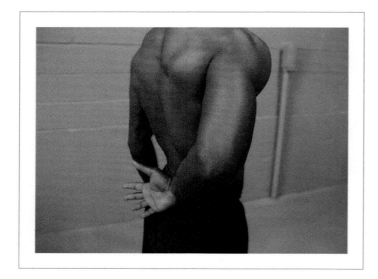

FIGURE 12.96 Lift-off test.

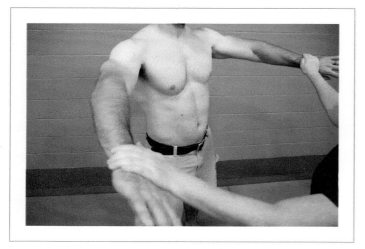

FIGURE 12.97 Jobe test.

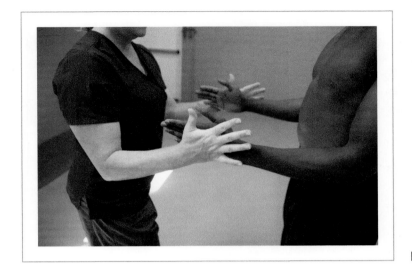

FIGURE 12.98 Lag test.

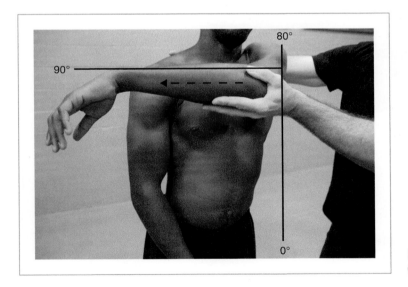

FIGURE 12.99 Cross-body adduction test (scarf sign).

AC JOINT PROBLEM TEST

Cross-body adduction test (scarf sign; Figure 12.99): Ask the patient to place his or her arm across the body and assist him or her with maximal crossing of the arm. A positive test is when pain is demonstrated in the ipsilateral AC joint. Sensitivity: 77%; specificity: 79%.

SHOULDER STABILITY TEST

Apprehension sign (Figure 12.100): Place the arm in 90 degrees of abduction and maximum external rotation. A positive test is when the patient demonstrates apprehension or guarding when the shoulder is in this position. Sensitivity: 88%; specificity: 50%.

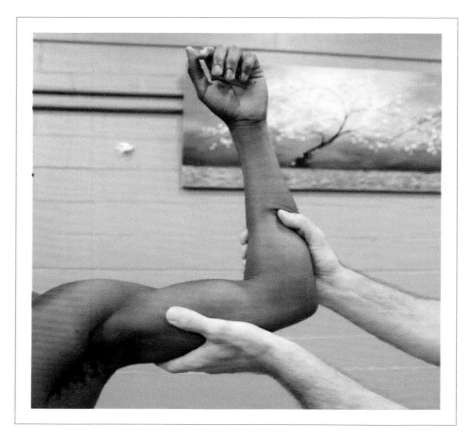

FIGURE 12.100 Apprehension sign.

BICEPS TENDON PATHOLOGY TESTS

Yergason test (Figure 12.101): Ask the patient to hold the arm in a neutral position with the elbow flexed to 90 degrees. Have the patient externally rotate and supinate the arm against resistance. Pain in the bicipital groove is positive for biceps tendon pathology. Sensitivity: 43%; specificity: 79%.

Speed test (Figure 12.102): Have the arm in 60 degrees of flexion, and the patient's elbow flexed to 20 to 30 degrees with the forearm in supination. Resist forward flexion of the arm while palpating the patient's biceps tendon over the anterior aspect of the shoulder. A positive test is when the patient has pain with palpation. Sensitivity: 50%; specificity: 67%.

ELBOW AND FOREARM

INSPECTION

Localized swelling over the olecranon—olecranon bursitis, nodules over the extensor surface of the ulna—gouty tophi, or rheumatoid nodules.

PALPATION

Evaluate for tenderness at the medial or lateral epicondyle with epicondylitis.

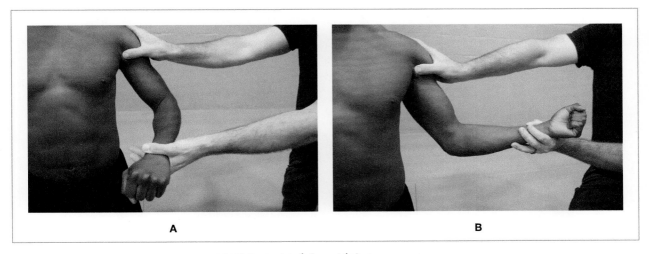

FIGURE 12.101 (**A**) and (**B**) Yergason test.

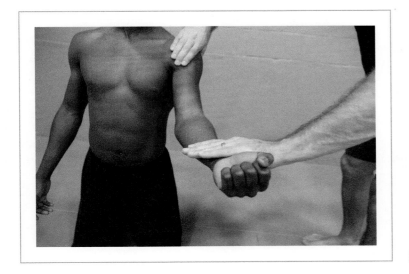

FIGURE 12.102 Speed test.

SPECIAL TESTS

Milking maneuver (Figure 12.103): Ask the patient to elevate the arms to 90 degrees of shoulder flexion, elbows bent, and cross the affected arm over the unaffected arm. Have the patient grasp the thumb of the affected arm and slowly extend the arm at the elbow. Pain or gapping at the ulnar side of the joint is consistent with an ulnar collateral ligament injury. Sensitivity: 100%; specificity: 75%.

WRIST AND HAND

INSPECTION

Inspect for any swelling over the wrist joint on the dorsal or volar surface looking for ganglion or synovial cysts. Evaluate for flexion deformities of the metacarpal phalangeal joints.

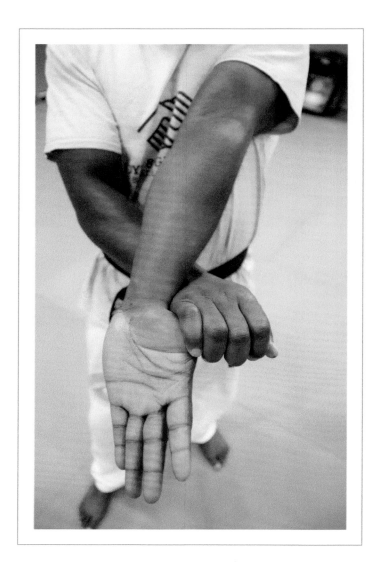

FIGURE 12.103 Milking maneuver.

PALPATION

Palpate for cords on the palmar aspect of the hand for Dupuytren's contractures (typically in the third or fourth fingers).

SPECIAL TESTS

Evaluate the rotational alignment of the hand and wrist, looking for the fingers to be in a slightly flexed position at rest, and pointing toward the scaphoid (Figure 12.104). Evaluate for the ulnar deviated posture in rheumatoid arthritis.

With trauma, palpate the anatomic snuffbox for tenderness (Figure 12.105). Tenderness in this area is indicative of a scaphoid fracture. Palpate for catching and locking at the A1 pulley with trigger fingers (Figure 12.106). Palpation of a nodule at the area of the pulley is indicative of a trigger finger.

Finkelstein test (Figure 12.107): Ask the patient to make a fist and ulnarly deviate the wrist. There will be pain with De Quervain's tenosynovitis.

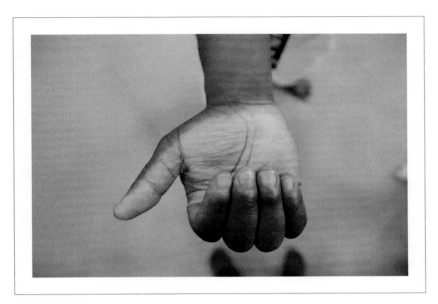

FIGURE 12.104 Rotational alignment assessment.

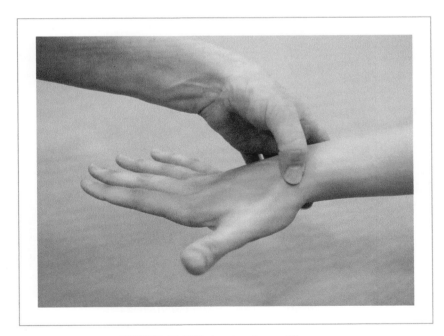

FIGURE 12.105 Anatomic snuffbox.

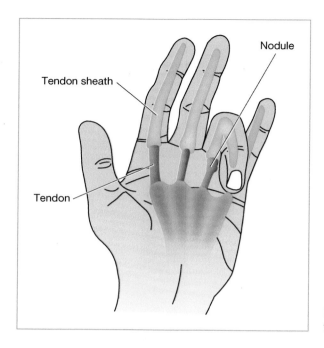

FIGURE 12.106 Palpation at the A1 pulley to assess for a trigger finger nodule.

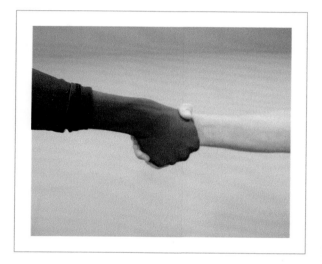

FIGURE 12.107 Finkelstein test.

Tinel's sign test (Figure 12.108): Percuss the carpal tunnel for paresthesias into the hand in carpal tunnel syndrome, for Tinel's sign. A positive test is indicated by the reproduction of paresthesias in the median nerve distribution with percussion.

Phalen's test (Figure 12.109): Should be performed for suspected carpal tunnel; ask the patient to hold his or her flexed wrists pressed together for at least 60 seconds, or until any symptoms arise. A positive test is indicated by reproduction of the patient's symptoms at or before the 60-second time mark.

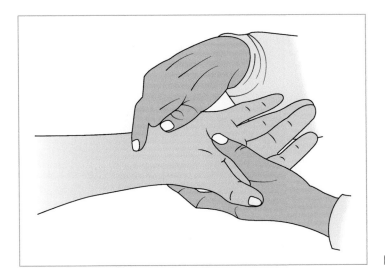

FIGURE 12.108 Tinel's sign test.

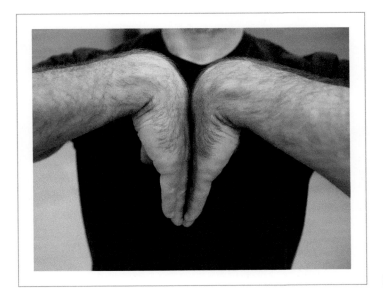

FIGURE 12.109 Phalen's test.

SPINE

INSPECTION

Inspect for loss of lumbar mobility, or pain with movement. The immobility of the lumbosacral junction increases the mechanical stress at L5 and S1, increasing the likelihood of disc herniation or spondylolisthesis of L5 on S1. Evaluate for curvature of the spine, laterally in scoliosis and anterior-posterior in kyphosis. Look for hairy patches, lipomas, and birthmarks that may overlie a spina bifida or bony defect.

PALPATION

Palpate for any bony tenderness; this may be indicative of a compression or burst fracture.

SPECIAL TESTS

Straight leg raise test (Figure 12.110): Ask the patient to lie supine. The motion is passive; the clinician should be moving the patient's leg. Elevate the leg from 0 degrees to 80. A positive test is when the patient describes pain that radiates down the leg when the leg is elevated between 30 and 70 degrees. Pain felt in the opposite leg may be indicative of a large disc herniation. Sensitivity: 52%; specificity: 89%.

Spurling test (Figure 12.111): Ask the patient to rotate and extend his or her neck to one side. Apply a gentle axial load to the neck. A positive test is noted when the patient has reproduction of his or her radiating symptoms. Sensitivity: 30%; specificity: 93%.

HIP

INSPECTION

With trauma or pain, evaluate for external rotation as in femoral neck fracture or anterior dislocation. Internal rotation with posterior hip dislocation may be present.

PALPATION

Palpate for pain over the greater trochanter, which may be consistent with greater trochanteric bursitis.

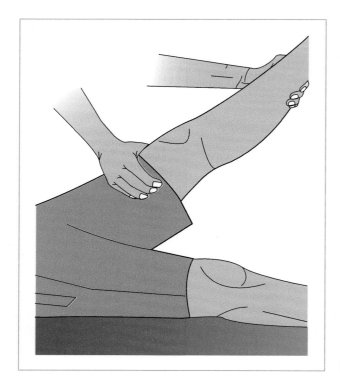

FIGURE 12.110 Straight leg raise test.

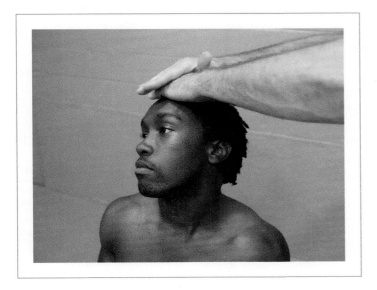

FIGURE 12.111 Spurling's test.

SPECIAL TESTS

The Hip Internal Rotation with Distraction (THIRD) test (Figure 12.112): A positive test is noted when the patient has pain with internal rotation of the hip that is then relieved with distraction of the hip and internal rotation.

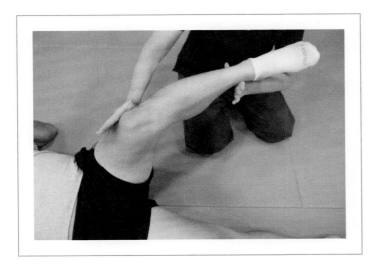

FIGURE 12.112 THIRD test. THIRD, The Hip Internal Rotation with Distraction.

KNEE

INSPECTION

On the patient's anterior aspect of his or her knees, look for effusion, varus or valgus deformity, or muscle atrophy. On the patient's posterior aspect of the knee, evaluate for varus or valgus deformity, atrophy, or hypertrophy.

PALPATION

Fullness in the popliteal fossa—Baker's cyst; pain with palpation over the anserine bursa—bursitis; pain with palpation over the patellar tendon—tendinitis.

SPECIAL TESTS

Apprehension sign (Figure 12.113): Once seated, have the patient extend his or her knee, attempt to displace patella laterally, and flex knee to 30 degrees. A positive test is indicated by the patient exhibiting apprehension with this maneuver.

Flexion pinch test (Figure 12.114): Accurate test, with increased accuracy with posterior horn tears (which are most common). A flexion pinch test is performed by fully flexing the patient's knee (135 degrees). A positive test is indicated by the patient experiencing pain when the knee is flexed.

Valgus stress test (Figure 12.115): Evaluates the patient for MCL laxity.

At 0 and 30 degrees of knee extension, exert a valgus stress to the knee joint. Opening of the joint is considered a positive test, and opening at 0 degrees indicates that more than the MCL is damaged; usually, the ACL is injured as well.

Varus stress test (Figure 12.116): Evaluates the patient for an LCL injury. At 0 and 30 degrees of knee extension, exert a varus stress to the knee joint. Opening of the joint is considered an abnormal test.

Lachman's test (Figure 12.117): Performed with the patient's knee in 30 degrees of flexion. The femur is stabilized with one hand, and the other

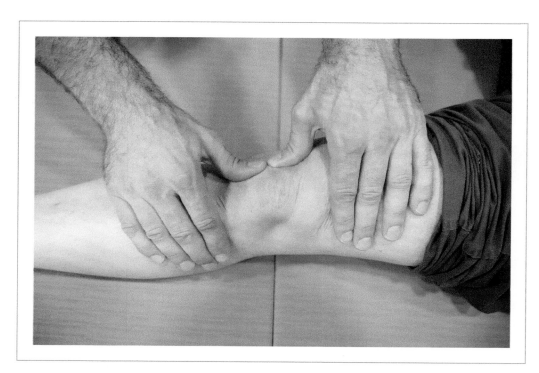

FIGURE 12.113 Apprehension sign.

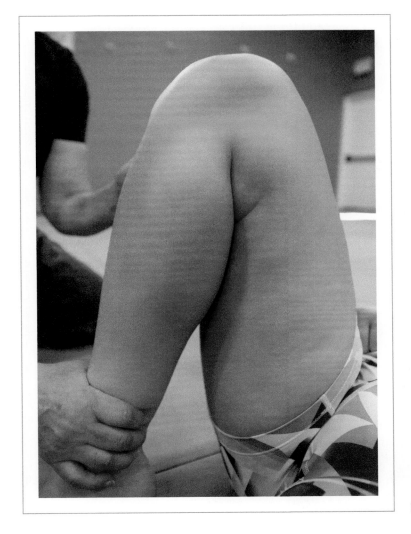

FIGURE 12.114 Flexion pinch test.

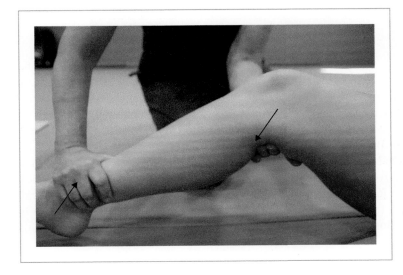

FIGURE 12.115 Valgus stress test.

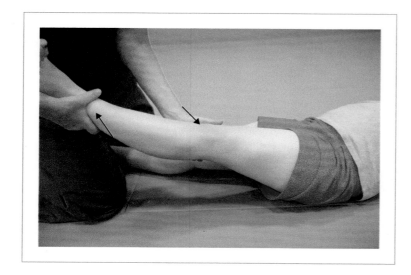

FIGURE 12.116 Varus stress test.

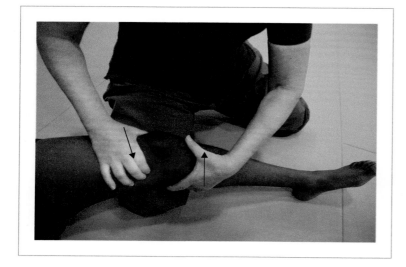

FIGURE 12.117 Lachman's test.

hand is used to apply force to the tibia, in an attempt to displace the tibia forward on the femur. A positive test is one in which there is a soft end point, and/or increased translation of the tibia on the femur. Sensitivity: 84% to 87%; specificity: 93%.

Anterior drawer test: May also be used for ACL injury. The test is less sensitive than the Lachman's test. With the knee bent to 90 degrees, pull forward on the tibia and attempt to displace the tibia forward on the femur. A positive test is one in which there is displacement of the tibia in an anterior direction, and/ or a soft end point. Sensitivity: 48%; specificity: 87%.

Posterior drawer test for PCL injury (Figure 12.118): With the knee bent to 90 degrees, push backward on the tibia and attempt to displace the tibia backward on the femur. A positive test is one in which there is displacement of the tibia in a posterior direction, and/ or a soft end point.

Pivot shift test (Figure 12.119): Performed when the knee is flexed; an axial load in the direction of the knee is exerted by the examiner, and a val-gus force is also applied. A positive test is one in which there is instability of the joint noted with this motion.

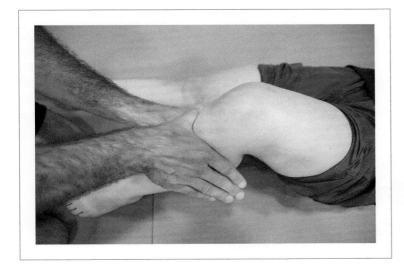

FIGURE 12.118 Posterior drawer test.

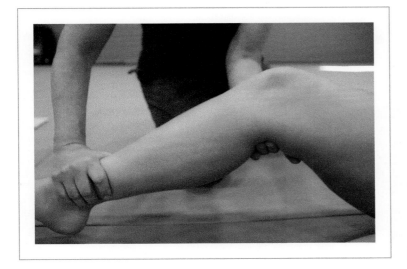

FIGURE 12.119 Pivot shift test.

FOOT AND ANKLE

DIRECTED QUESTIONS

Foot pain increases, first thing in the morning; plantar fasciitis.

INSPECTION

Toe raise that does not result in recreation of the longitudinal arch—pes planus.

PALPATION

Bony tenderness associated with a fracture, or tenderness localized to the lateral or medial ligaments, which are associated with a sprain.

SPECIAL TESTS

Thompson's test (Figure 12.120): Performed with the patient in a kneeling position. The calf is squeezed, and the foot is noted to passive plantar flex in a negative test. A positive test is one in which the foot does not move when the calf is squeezed.

Anterior drawer test (Figure 12.121): Apply an anterior force to the foot with the tibia stabilized. A positive test is one in which there is displacement of the tibia in an anterior direction, and/or a soft end point.

Morton's squeeze test (Figure 12.122): Performed by compressing the metatarsal heads. A positive test is indicated by pain between the metatarsal heads, or a click is felt.

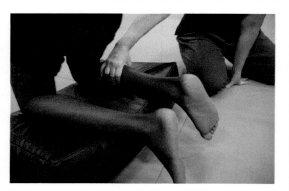

FIGURE 12.120 Thompson's test.

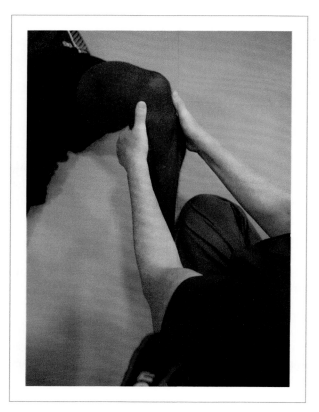

FIGURE 12.121 Anterior drawer test.

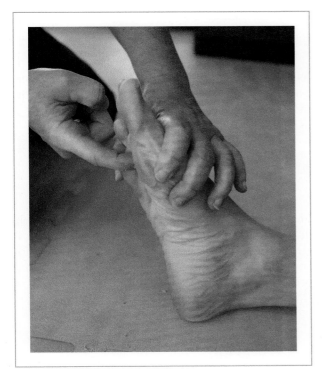

FIGURE 12.122 Squeeze test (Morton's neuroma).

Holistic Assessment

SPECIFIC HEALTH HISTORY

When a patient presents with a musculoskeletal complaint, it is imperative to elicit a thorough and accurate CC (in the patient's own words), HPI, and review of systems (ROS). When assessing the attributes of the symptom, pay particular attention to the onset and duration for determining if the problem is acute or chronic in nature, for aggravating or alleviating factors for clues into the differential diagnosis, and for associated signs and symptoms, as systems are closely integrated. As with all other body system evaluation, include a detailed and inclusive past medical history (PMH), family history (FH), and social history.

SAFETY

Identifying patients who are at risk for a fall is one musculoskeletal system–specific safety concern. This identification also needs to take into consideration conditions such as osteoporosis, and to identify individual goals such as athletic return to play conditions.

DISTRESS

It is important to identify and understand the effect that the condition or injury is having on the patient's life. Is this an elite athlete who will risk losing a scholarship or championship due to his or her condition? Identify any functional limitations.

NUTRITION AND EXERCISE

Regarding the musculoskeletal system, particular attention needs to surround the diet and exercise habits of the patient. Inquire as to whether or not your patient has a diet that is adequate in meeting his or her daily requirements for calcium, which is integral to bone health and remodeling. Ask about exercise habits, paying particular attention to weight-bearing exercise for the reduction in the risk of osteoporosis, and important for long-term bone health. Assess exercise habits for trends of overuse injuries.

FINANCIAL IMPLICATIONS

Ask the patient if there are any financial implications because of his or her injury or condition. Inquire about the patient's ability to work.

SPIRITUAL CONSIDERATIONS

Identify areas where the patient has turned for help in the past, including his or her faith and support circles. Ask the patient about his or her habits for coping with difficult times, and if the patient has provisions for self-care.

CASE STUDY

DOCUMENTATION

Chief Complaint: Joint stiffness, bilateral knees, and right shoulder

History of Present Illness: Onset was slow and atraumatic. Location is both knees and the right shoulder. Duration over the last 6 months, stiffness is aggravated by sitting for long periods of time, or keeping the arm in one position for an extended period. Also notes that stiffness is the worst first thing in the morning. Discomfort is alleviated with some steady, nonimpact activity, such as walking or swimming. There are no other associated symptoms.

REVIEW OF SYSTEMS

Constitutional: No complaints of fever, chills, or malaise

Integumentary: Denies rashes or lesions

Neurological: Denies numbness, tingling, paresthesia, or weakness

(continued)

(continued)

PHYSICAL EXAMINATION

General: Well appearing, no acute distress

Integumentary: No erythema or ecchymosis is noted

Neurological: Triceps reflexes are 2+ and equal bilaterally, whereas patellar reflexes are 1+ and equal bilaterally. Sensation is intact to light touch proximally and distally, and equal bilaterally.

Musculoskeletal: Inspection reveals no atrophy or abnormality. With palpation, the patient has some sensitivity over the medial and lateral joint line, for both the anterior and posterior aspect of the knee. Mild tenderness is felt with palpation of the shoulder over the subacromial bursa. Mild crepitation is noted with bilateral knee and right shoulder palpation. Range of motion is full in the knees and shoulders with mild discomfort at the extremes of motion in bilateral knees and right shoulder. Muscle strength testing demonstrates 5/5 strength in knees and shoulders.

Diagnosis: Knee osteoarthritis bilaterally and right shoulder osteoarthritis

ICD-10-CM Diagnosis Code: M17.0 Bilateral Primary Osteoarthritis of Knee

ICD-10-CM Diagnosis Code: M19.011 Primary Osteoarthritis, Right Shoulder

Assessment of Special Populations

 ## TRANSGENDER POPULATION

When caring for the transgender population, the clinician will need to consider the effects of hormone replacement/supplementation such as testosterone on the musculoskeletal system, and the bulking of muscle or change in body mass or weight.

Transgender individuals may also be practicing techniques to express their gender such as postural changes, tucking or binding, or using prostheses. Be aware of specific patient practices, in order to understand the risks that are unique to them.

The implications on the musculoskeletal system are important to consider, including the effect of hormone treatment on osteoporosis risks. Osteoporosis is a concern more for premenopausal female to male transgender individuals. For men, osteoporosis becomes more of a concern later in life. Pay particular attention to your male to female transgender patients for the potential of osteoporosis.

ELDERLY POPULATION

When examining the elderly population, be aware of age-related changes including a Dowager hump, osteoporosis, osteoarthritis, and atrophy (Figure 12.123). Assess the patient for fall risk. Aging places the patient at an increased risk for osteoarthritis and degenerative tendonitis and tears.

PEDIATRIC POPULATION

The pediatric patient has unique findings in the musculoskeletal system. Note the normal progression of lower extremity alignment progression in Figure 12.124.

Additional physical examination techniques that are specific to the pediatric population include the

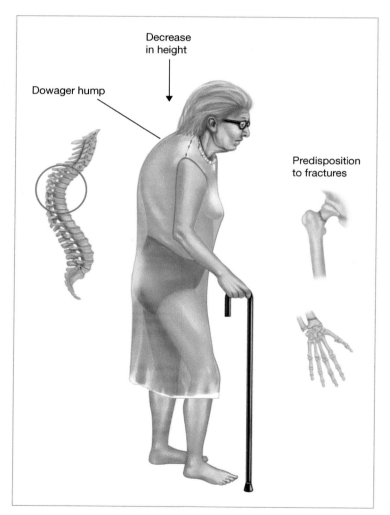

FIGURE 12.123 Common physical examination findings with the elderly.

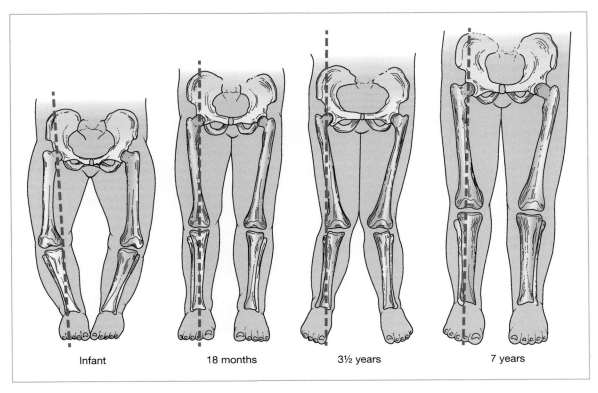

FIGURE 12.124 Normal progression of lower extremity alignment.

Ortolani and Barlow tests for hip dysplasia. The Ortolani test is used in an attempt to identify a dislocated hip that can be reduced in the acetabulum. The Barlow test is used to identify a loose or lax hip joint that can be pushed out of the acetabulum with gentle pressure. Pediatric patients have open growth plates, or epiphyses. The pediatric patient is at increased risk for injury in these vulnerable areas.

PREGNANT POPULATION

The pregnant patient will have unique physical assessment findings and CCs in the musculoskeletal system. In addition to the demands of her changing body structure, the hormone relaxin is released from the beginning of the pregnancy which helps enable the pelvis to expand during the birth by increasing the laxity in the ligaments around the pelvis. The hormone also has an effect on all other joints, presenting the increased possibility for injury. Often, pregnant patients will experience musculoskeletal pain that is associated with the laxity that occurs in the joints. Commonly, sacroiliac joint laxity is experienced, or round ligament pain. A careful history and physical examination will assist you in developing differential diagnoses to include this discomfort.

PATIENTS WITH DISABILITIES

It is important to conduct a thorough history to understand the abilities of your patient, as well as his or her baseline functioning and current somatosensory experience. Ask the patient's perception of his or her functional limitations.

With this information taken into consideration, you will have the ability to appropriately assess the musculoskeletal system of the patient.

Assess the potential for risk of falls, balance issues, muscle weakness, secondary conditions such as sequelae from poorly fitting prosthetic devices, decreased ability to exercise, and pressure ulcers. Understand what accommodations the patient has in place in the home and in his or her work or active life.

VETERAN POPULATION

A detailed history of your patient's military experience, including deployments and service, should be obtained. Pay particular attention to locations that have exposure to known toxic chemicals or hazardous materials, and any vibratory or traumatic injuries that may have been sustained. Depending upon the job title and experience, assess the likelihood of risk and risk level of exposure to certain repetitive activities or chemical agents. For example, do you have a veteran whose job was repetitive jumping (out of helicopters), or were other repetitive activities part of his or her job? The physical assessment of the veteran should include evaluating for diseases and conditions related to the potential exposure of conditions or agents that may cause cancer, arthritis, or long-term disability. Ask the veteran about his or her perceived health and needs. Be particularly aware of inquiring about injuries and chronic pain, as well as substance abuse and mental health.

ELITE ATHLETE POPULATION

The elite athlete is considered to be one who has competed at a varsity, professional, international, or national level. This level of athlete would be at risk for overuse injuries and would also have unique return to play criteria.

Diagnostic Reasoning

Common Differential Diagnoses: General Musculoskeletal System	
Diagnosis	**Key History or Physical Examination Differentiators**
Dislocation	A dislocation is a complete loss of joint articulation
Osteoarthritis	Crepitation, decreased range of motion, and progressive symptoms that are worse after being sedentary or immobile; somewhat better with movement
Recurvatum deformity	Increased hyperextension of a joint, typically seen in the knee or elbow
Subluxation	Slippage of a joint within its articulation
Valgus deformity	The distal part of the limb is directed away from the body midline
Varus deformity	The distal part of the limb is directed toward the midline of the body

Common Differential Diagnoses: Shoulder	
Diagnosis	**Key History or Physical Examination Differentiators**
AC separation	Palpable step off at the acromioclavicular joint History of trauma is common
Adhesive capsulitis	Decreased range of motion both active and passive Passive external rotation <50% compared with unaffected side
Biceps tenosynovitis	History of overuse and pain with palpation of the tendon in the groove
Cervical radiculopathy	Positive Spurling's maneuver, radiating pain
Clavicle fracture	History of trauma and bony tenderness
Impingement syndrome	Pain when sleeping on affected side; pain with overhead activity
Instability	History of at least one episode of dislocation, positive sulcus sign
Osteoarthritis	Decreased range of motion, insidious onset Generalized shoulder pain with restriction in all activities Common in the 55–75 year age group
Rotator cuff tear	Pain located in outer arm and weakness with muscle strength testing. Decreased active range of motion
Rotator cuff tendinitis	Pain located on the outer arm and limited range of motion Common in the age group 35–55

AC, acromioclavicular.

Common Differential Diagnoses: Elbow and Forearm	
Diagnosis	**Key History or Physical Examination Differentiators**
Medial and lateral epicondylitis	Pain with palpation over either the medial or lateral epicondyles
Olecranon bursitis	Localized cystic swelling over olecranon
Ulnar collateral ligament tear	History of trauma, throwing sport, complaint of instability

Common Differential Diagnoses: Wrist and Hand

Diagnosis	Key History or Physical Examination Differentiators
Carpal tunnel syndrome	Symptoms of numbness and tingling, history of overuse, nighttime awakening
De Quervain's tendonitis/ tenosynovitis	Pain with movement of the thumb and over the radial side of the wrist. History of overuse
Dupuytren contracture	Progressive palpable cord on the volar aspect of the hand with flexion deformities of 1–3 of the fingers
Ganglion cyst	Complaints of swelling over the dorsal or volar aspect of the wrist
Osteoarthritis	Insidious onset of stiffness. Heberden's nodules
Scaphoid fracture	Pain at the anatomic snuffbox is indicative of scaphoid fracture
Trigger finger	Triggering or catching of the fingers or thumb when moving through ROM, palpable nodule on the A1 pulley that moves with the patient's finger in ROM

ROM, range of motion.

Common Differential Diagnoses: Spine

Diagnosis	Key History or Physical Examination Differentiators
Ankylosing spondylitis	History of progressive stiffness in the back and straightening of the spine
Cauda equina syndrome	Rare condition that occurs with approximately 2% of all herniated discs. The condition is considered a medical emergency, and is evidenced by bowel and/or bladder dysfunction, reduced sensation in the saddle area, or sexual dysfunction
Degenerative disc disease	Older at age of onset, progressive worsening of back pain and symptoms
Lumbar disc syndrome radiculopathy/sciatica	Radiating pain traveling within a dermatome
Lumbar fracture	History of trauma and bony point tenderness
Lumbar sprain and pain	Low back pain without radiculopathy

(continued)

Common Differential Diagnoses: Spine (*continued*)

Diagnosis	Key History or Physical Examination Differentiators
Sacroiliac joint syndrome	Pain over the sacroiliac joint in the low back
Scoliosis	Curvature of the spine
Spondylolysis	History of overuse and pain
Spondylolisthesis	Pain that is intermittently worse with movement
Syringomyelia	Findings on MRI of pockets of fluid within the spinal canal

Common Differential Diagnoses: Hip

Diagnosis	Key History or Physical Examination Differentiators
Greater trochanteric bursitis	Pain directly over the greater trochanteric bursa with palpation, history of overuse of trauma
Labral tear	Catching pain in a younger patient
Osteoarthritis	Progressive stiffness and pain in the older patient
Slipped capital epiphysis	Skeletally immature patient with hip pain, typically active and overweight

Common Differential Diagnoses: Knee

Diagnosis	Key History or Physical Examination Differentiators
ACL tear	History of an injury with a planted foot and hyperextension or valgus load. Immediate joint effusion after injury
Baker's cyst	Fullness in the popliteal fossa
Bursitis (prepatellar, pes anserine)	History of overuse or trauma is typical, and tenderness is observed with palpation directly over the bursa.

(continued)

Common Differential Diagnoses: Knee (*continued*)	
Diagnosis	**Key History or Physical Examination Differentiators**
Collateral ligament tear	History of valgus or varus injury with a blow to either side of the knee, laxity
Meniscal tear	History of twisting injury with swelling the day after injury, clicking and popping with possible catching
Osgood–Schlatter	Pain over the tibial tubercle in a skeletally immature patient
Osteoarthritis	Progressive stiffness and pain in the older patient
Patellar tendinitis	Tenderness over the patellar tendon with a history of jumping sports such as basketball
PCL tear	Fall onto a flexed knee, joint effusion, laxity

ACL, anterior cruciate ligament; PCL, posterior cruciate ligament.

Common Differential Diagnoses: Foot and Ankle	
Diagnosis	**Key History or Physical Examination Differentiators**
Achilles tendinitis	Pain over the Achilles tendon with a history of overuse
Ankle fractures	Bony tenderness with a history of trauma and inability to weight bear
Ankle sprain	History of twisting injury with pain and swelling
Gout	Exquisite pain over the first MTP (most common)
Hallux valgus/bunion	Deformity at the first MTP with valgus positioning of the great toe
Medial tibial stress syndrome	Pain over the medial lower extremity with a history of overuse and pes planus deformity
Osteoarthritis	Progressive stiffness and pain in the older patient
Plantar fasciitis	Pain over the bottom of the foot or feet that is worse first thing in the morning and after sitting for a period of time

MTP, metatarsophalangeal.

BIBLIOGRAPHY

Armstrong, A., & Hubbard, M. (2016). *AAOS essentials of musculoskeletal care*. Burlington, MA: Jones & Bartlett.

Bickley, L. S. (2013). *Bates' guide to physical examination and history taking* (11th ed.). Philadelphia, PA: Lippincott Williams & Wilkins.

Buchanan, B., & Hughes, J. (2019). Tennis elbow (lateral epicondylitis). In: *StatPearls* [Internet]. Treasure Island, FL: StatPearls Publishing.

Chaudhari, A., Jamison, S., McNally, M., Pan, X., & Schmitt, L. (2014). Hip adductor activations during run-to-cut maneuvers. *Journal of Sport Sciences, 32*(14), 1333–1340. doi:10 .1080/02640414.2014.889849

Cohn, R., Lerebours, F., & Strauss, E. (2015). Sports hernia and extra-articular causes of groin pain in the athlete. *Bulletin of the Hospital for Joint Diseases, 73*(2), 90–99. Retrieved from http://hjdbulletin.org/files/archive/pdfs/BHJD%2073(2)2015%20pp%20 90-99%20Cohn%20Lerebours%20Strauss.pdf

Daniels, J. M. (Ed.). (2015). *Common musculoskeletal problems: A handbook* (2nd ed.). Cham, Switzerland: Springer International Publishing.

Dunn, J., Kusnezov, N., Orr, J., Pallis, M., & Mitchell, J. (2016). The boxer's fracture: Splint immobilization is not necessary. *Orthopedics, 39*(3), 188–192. doi:10.3928/01477447-20160315-05

Goolsby, M. J., & Grubbs, L. (Eds.). (2019). *Advanced health assessment: Interpreting findings and formulating differential diagnoses* (4th ed.). Philadelphia, PA: F. A. Davis.

Joyce, C., Kelly, J., Chan, J., Colgan, G., O'Briain, D., Mc Cabe, J., & Curtin, W. (2013). Second to fourth digit ratio confirms aggressive tendencies in patients with boxers fractures. *Injury, 44*(11), 1636–1639. doi:10.1016/j.injury.2013.07.018

Kohyama, S., Kanamori, A., Tanaka, T., Hara, Y., & Yamazaki, M. (2016). Stress fracture of the scaphoid in an elite junior tennis player: A case report and review of the literature. *Journal of Medical Case Reports, 10*. doi:10.1186/s13256-015-0785-3

Kruse, A., Stafilidis, S., & Tilp, M. (2017). Ultrasound and magnetic resonance imaging are not interchangeable to assess the Achilles tendon cross-sectional-area. *European Journal of Applied Physiology, 117*(1), 73–82. doi:10.1007/s00421-016-3500-1

Mosler, A., Weir, A., Eiral, C., Farooq, A., Thorborg, K., Whiteley, R., . . . Crossley, K. (2018). Epidemiology of time loss groin injuries in a men's professional football league: A 2-year prospetive study of 17 clubs and 606 players. *British Journal of Sports Medicine, 52*(5), 292–297. doi:10.1136/bjsports-2016-097277

Myrick, K. (2014). Clinical assessment of ankle sprains. *Journal of Orthopaedic Nursing, 33*(5), 249–250. doi:10.1097/NOR.0000000000000086

Myrick, K. (Ed.). (2017). *Orthopedic and sports medicine case studies for nurse practitioners*. New York, NY: Springer Publishing Company.

Park, Y., Jeong, S., Choi, G., & Kim, H. (2017). How early must an acute Achilles tendon rupture be repaired? *Injury, 48*(3), 776–780. doi:10.1016/j.injury.2017.01.020

Rambau, G., & Rhee, P. (2017). Evaluation and management of nondisplaced scaphoid waist fractures in the athlete. *Operative Techniques in Sports Medicine, 24*, 87–93. doi:10.1053/j.otsm.2016.01.005

Rhodes, J., & Peterson, S. (2017). *Advanced health assessment and diagnostic reasoning* (3rd ed.). Burlington, MA: Jones & Bartlett.

Roberson, T., & Tokish, J. (2016). Acromioclavicular joint injuries in the contact athlete. *Operative Techniques in Sports Medicine, 24*(4), 254–262. doi:10.1053/j.otsm.2016.09.004

Rockwood, C. (1984). Injuries to the acromioclavicular joint. In C. A. Rockwood & D. P. Green (Eds.), *Fractures in adults* (2nd ed., pp. 860–910). Philadelphia, PA: J.B. Lippincott.

Santilli, O., Nardelli, N., Santilli, H., Tripoloni, D., Santilli, O. L., Santilli, H. A., & Tripoloni, D. E. (2016). Sports hernias: Experience in a sports medicine center. *Hernia, 20*(1), 77–84. doi:10.1007/s10029-015-1367-4

Tosti, R., Rossy, W., Sanchez, A., & Lee, S. (2016). Burners, stingers, and other brachial plexus injuries in the contact athlete. *Operative Techniques in Sports Medicine, 24*(4), 273–278. doi:10.1053/j.otsm.2016.09.006

Weinberg, D., Williamson, D., Gebhart, J., Knapik, D., & Voss, J. (2017). Differences in medial and lateral posterior tibial slope: An osteological review of 1090 tibia comparing age, sex, and race. *American Journal of Sports Medicine, 45*(1), 106–112. doi:10.1177/0363546516662449

Zellers, J., Cortes, D., & Silbernagel, K. (2016). From acute Achilles tendon rupture to return to play- a case report evaluating recovery of tendon structure mechanical properties, clinical and functional outcomes. *International Journal of Sports Physical Therapy, 11*(7), 1150–1159. Retrieved from https://www.ncbi.nlm.nih.gov/pmc/articles/PMC5159638

INDEX

Pages containing figures and tables are indicated by an *f* or *t*, respectively.